PALLIATIVE CARE

Palliative Care:

The Management of Far-Advanced Illness

Edited by Derek Doyle

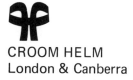

CROOM HELM
London & Canberra

THE CHARLES PRESS, PUBLISHERS
Philadelphia

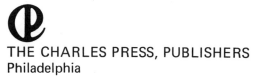

© 1984 Derek Doyle
Croom Helm Ltd, Provident House, Burrell Row,
Beckenham, Kent BR3 1AT

Croom Helm Australia Pty Ltd,
28 Kembla Street, Fyshwick,
ACT 2609, Australia

and
The Charles Press, Publishers, Suite 14K,
1420 Locust Street, Philadelphia,
Pennsylvania 19102

British Library Cataloguing in Publication Data

Palliative Care.
   1. Terminal care
   I. Doyle, Derek
   362.1'75   R726.8

ISBN 0-7099-0836-9

Library of Congress Catalog Card Number
83-073015

ISBN 0-914783-02-5

Printed and bound in Great Britain

CONTENTS

CONTRIBUTORS

Norman C. Allan, MB, ChB, FRCPEdin, FRC Path, Consultant Haematologist, Western General Hospital, Edinburgh

Michael Bond, PhD, FRCS, FRCPsych. DPM, Professor of Psychological Medicine, University of Glasgow

Audrey Boyle, MA, DipSocSt, AIMSW, Senior Social Worker, Northern General Hospital, Edinburgh

Marion Buchanan, RGN, NA(H) Cert, Principal Nursing Officer, Royal Hospital for Sick Children, Edinburgh

Ian Campbell, BSc, MB, ChB, FRCPEdin, Consultant Physician, Victoria Hospital, Kirkcaldy, Scotland

Fiona Cathcart, MA, MSc, ABPsS, Senior Clinical Psychologist, Rehabilitation Unit, Astley Ainslie Hospital, Edinburgh

Elizabeth L. Cay, MD, FRCPsych, DPM, Consultant in Rehabilitation Medicine, Lothian Health Board, Scotland

Derek Doyle, MB, ChB, MRCPEdin, FRCGP, Medical Director, St Columba's Hospice, Challenger Lodge, Boswall Road, Edinburgh, Clinical Teacher, University of Edinburgh Medical School

Elizabeth A. Edwards, BSc, SRN, SCM, HVCert, Chief Area Nursing Officer, Dumfries and Galloway, Scotland

James Farquhar, MD, FRCPEdin, Professor of Child Life and Health, University of Edinburgh

Niall D.C. Finlayson, MB, ChB, PhD, FRCP, FRCPEdin, Consultant Physician, Royal Infirmary, Edinburgh, and Honorary Senior Lecturer, Department of Therapeutics and Clinical Pharmacology, University of Edinburgh Medical School

David C. Flenley, PhD, FRCP, FRCPEdin, Professor of Medicine, Respiratory Diseases, University of Edinburgh

Jennifer M. Henderson, SRN, RGN, SCM, DN (Lond), Nursing Sister, Dumfries Royal Infirmary, Dumfries, Scotland

Ernest Jellinek, DM, FRCP, FRCPEdin, Consultant Neurologist, Edinburgh Northern Hospital Group, and Senior Lecturer, University of Edinburgh Medical School

Ivan Lichter, FRCS, FRACS, Associate Professor, Department of Surgery, University of Otago Medical School, Dunedin, New Zealand

David Lyall, BSc, BD, PhD, STM, Chaplain, North Lothian Hospitals, Edinburgh

Michael Matthews, MA, MD, FRCP, FRCPEdin, Consultant Cardiologist, Western General Hospital, Edinburgh

Balfour M. Mount, MD, FRCS (C), Professor of Surgery and Director of Palliative Care Services, McGill University and Royal Victoria Hospital, Montreal, Quebec, Canada

Derek Murray, MA, BD, PhD, Senior Chaplain, St Columba's Hospice, Edinburgh

Mary Parker, SRN, SCM, BTA, Cert., Nursing Officer, Dumfries and Galloway Health Board, Dumfries

John Smyth, MA, MD, MSc, FRCPEdin, Professor of Medical Oncology, University of Edinburgh

Peter J. Swarbrick, MB, ChB, MRCGP, Fellow in Rehabilitation Studies, University of Edinburgh, General Practitioner, Livingston

Ian Thompson, BA, PhD, Senior Educationalist, Scottish Health Education Group, Woodburn House, Canaan Lane, Edinburgh

Eric Wilkes, OBE, FRCP, FRCGP, FRCPsych, Professor of Community Health, University of Sheffield, and General Practitioner, Sheffield

Robin Winney, BSc, MB, ChB, FRCPEdin, Consultant Physician, Medical Renal Unit, Royal Infirmary, Edinburgh

FOREWORD

Balfour M. Mount

I was heading home for dinner. It was 6.30 and the end of a long day. As I passed his room, I glanced through the open door. Max looked restless, even agitated. Conscience and the urge to continue on my way jousted fleetingly for supremacy. Conscience, or rather, something about the anguished look in Max's eye, won. At 56, although he was aphasic and largely hemiplegic, due to brain metastases from his carcinoma of the lung, there was still something commanding about his bearing. A 'presence', you might say. He was a big man. He had always been dynamic. Husband, father, businessman, amateur boxer, philanthropist, racing enthusiast, teacher of young Jewish Montrealers regarding traditions Jewish, Max had a streak of proud independence that prompted our Palliative Care Service team to hold back rather than offer a helping hand as he laboured the few feet from bed to toilet. Better for him to do it himself!

As I settled beside him on the bed, we embarked on an exercise in frustrated communication that left me half an hour later none the wiser regarding the cause of his evident turmoil. He could manage a single monosyllabic protest that sounded like 'have'. Finally we turned again to a pencil and paper and he wrote 'Max'. A second line was unintelligible, while a third appeared to be 'horse'. When I was still unable to comprehend he finally laboured into print the words 'I horse'.

It suddenly hit me! I understood. With an overwhelming rush of feeling I responded, 'Max, I understand! Your saying, "I horse". If I were a horse you would shoot me. Why do you let it go on?'

From somewhere at the core of his being came a welling affirmative groan that was punctuated by a sweep of his one good arm. I shall never forget that gesture. With one motion his outstretched hand swept the quadrants of his small universe, expressing more eloquently than pages of prose or a symphony of sound, 'I used to be able to work, play, relate to my friends, make love with my wife, now all I have are these four damned walls! Why do you let it go on?'

My response was unintentional. Struck by the enormity of his dilemma, my eyes filled with tears. A momentary impulse to hide my feelings passed as Max, that paragon of truncated independence,

1

responded to *me* by putting *his* arm around me.

What is palliative care? It is attention to detail. Active listening. It involves assessment of psycho-social and spiritual, as well as physical, needs. Good palliative care as it applied to Max included the development of a comprehensive treatment plan and the setting of daily achievable treatment goals; the monitoring of medications for confusion, increased intracranial pressure, bowel activity and bed-time sedation; liaison with family members and close friends as they integrated the reality, with all its complex implications, of a life that would be Max-less. But as is frequently the case, the patient was to teach me that good palliative care is more than these things. Without intent, as it turned out, I had done the one thing for my patient that could have made a difference at that moment in his life. In unwittingly revealing my feelings for him, he was given the opportunity to give to me: to have his own personhood reinforced by being able to give to someone else: to have his integrity as a moral agent validated — still able to give to others; not simply able to receive! We both grew a little in that moment.

How do we palliate our patients' lives? There are only three admissible therapeutic goals: to cure, to prolong life and, when these ends are out of reach, because of the limitations of our current therapeutic armamentarium, to focus on the quality of remaining life.

But how do we foster quality in our patients' lives? Our understanding of the issues involved has been assisted by a variety of writings. Two that I have found particularly helpful are by the Viennese psychiatrist Viktor Frankl and the American physician Eric Cassel. First, Viktor Frankl's landmark contribution *Man's Search for Meaning* (1963) was written in eight days of creative outpouring after Frankl was freed from Auschwitz. It tells us something of the essence of the motivational drive that lies at the germinal centre of our being. To understand the significance of man's search for meaning is to become motivated to help our patients experience an enhanced context of meaning in their lives and thus an improved quality of life.

Second, I wish to recommend Eric Cassel's insightful article 'The nature of suffering and the goals of medicine' (1982). It reminds us of the varied dimensions of the 'whole persons' we are privileged to treat — for to palliate effectively we must tend the whole person, and only in understanding the concept of personhood can that be fully accomplished.

Derek Doyle has now added to the above resources in a most helpful way. *Palliative Care, the Management of Far-Advanced Illness*, fills an important need in the medical literature. The word 'palliate' comes from the Latin *pallium* meaning cloak. As a verb, it originally implied 'to cloak' or 'to hide', but later took on the meaning 'to improve the quality of'. For the more than 70 per cent of us who die in institutions and for many others who will die at home this work will provide our physicians with an indispensable guide to our needs. Here is a book that pulls together in one accessible, readable and practical volume strands of medical knowledge that relate to those problems that lie outside the traditional curative and life-prolonging concerns of modern medical practice. John Hinton (1972) observed: 'we emerge deserving of little credit; we who are capable of ignoring the conditions which make muted people suffer. The dissatisfied dead cannot noise abroad the negligence they have experienced.' This volume will be a major aid towards erasing that negligence.

References

Cassel, E.J. (1982), 'The nature of suffering and the goals of medicine', *New England Journal of Medicine* (18 March), pp. 306, 639–45

Frankl, V.E. (1963), *Man's Search for Meaning*, Pocket Books, New York

Hinton, J. (1972), *Dying*, 2nd edn, Harmondsworth, England, Penguin, p. 159

INTRODUCTION

It is interesting to reflect on the changing book titles and subject matter of medical books in the last century. These changes reflect the birth of new specialties, the development of new care regimes, the introduction of hundreds of new drugs and techniques and, to some extent, the changed objectives of both doctors and nurses.

Who would have thought, a hundred years ago, that we would have such new and exciting specialties as immunology, medical oncology, transplantation surgery and radiotherapy, each with a fast-growing bibliography of its own? It is no wonder, in our age of antibiotics and antimitotics, that we devote so much of our energy and time to the curing of our patients. The changing pattern of so many diseases, some halted and others brought under control or into remission, has every right to cheer us, as it has done our patients. Many of the killers of last century are now tamed.

Such progress, however, should not blind us to the fact that there remains only a handful of diseases which we truly *cure*; for the majority of patients we must aim for long-term control of the disease, hopefully to give them many years of happy and useful life. There will always be those who need our skills and our love as the end of life comes in sight, for whatever we have achieved in recent years, we have not found, nor ever shall find, the secret of immortality for our patients. We shall always be challenged to care for those we cannot cure. Such is the meaning of 'palliative care'.

This surely is one of the titles which, for a different reason, would not have been given to a book last century. Palliation was, after all, the only objective of our forefathers, who had so few of our diagnostic, pharmacological and surgical tools. To them fell the honour of relieving suffering and restoring peace to patients whose life was often all too short. That anyone should have prepared a book on what was, in effect, the basic ethos of all they did, would have amazed or amused them. Today, in the view of my colleagues and myself, such a book is essential. We deceive ourselves if we believe we are only here to cure. We diminish our caring role if we are skilful only with those who will live as the result of our attention.

What do we mean by 'palliative care'? We have chosen to focus on those last years and months of life when death is foreseeable rather than merely a possibility, looking at the pattern of physical, emotional, social and spiritual suffering which may be present, and which should and can be relieved. Deliberately we speak of 'care' rather than just 'palliation' as a reminder that such patients need more than skilfully applied pharmacology or psychotherapy – they need that warmth and depth of human contact and concern which is described as 'care'.

Why, it might be asked, is the book not entitled 'Terminal Care', that phrase now so widely used and popularised by the hospice movement, another of the great medical events of this century? Our reasons are threefold. First and quite simply, because we hope our book will be of help to colleagues in North America, where 'palliative care' is a term more commonly used and understood. The second and more important reason is that we want to get away from the focusing of attention principally on the final *weeks* of life, which too many colleagues have come to regard as the domain of modern terminal care. It is our feeling that much remains to be learnt about how to enhance and maintain the quality of life for our patients long before they retire to their deathbeds. Our third reason is that through popular use 'terminal care' has come to be associated with cancer care. We believe most fervently that those suffering from advanced disease, whatever its underlying pathology, deserve the same care and devotion as those with malignant disease.

Inevitably we make reference in many sections of this book to the teaching and principles of hospices. We are particularly concerned with their timely reminder to us all that *total care means team care*, with due and equal attention to each facet of human experience – physical, emotional, social and spiritual. We have learnt from them that attention to fine detail bears dividends, that a patient and his family may suffer in ways we do not always recognise, that most would probably elect to be cared for at home longer than we choose to believe, and that emotional involvement in the care of our patients, far from being unprofessional or dangerous, may be positively therapeutic for our patients and exciting for the professionals. As the editor, one of my hopes is that, through this book, 'hospice-type care' will be seen as practicable wherever we serve these patients and that many colleagues, even in hospices, will be reminded – as I have been – that hospices have not taught us a new principle but rather rediscovered and highlighted an age-old one. Though we must strive for cure, we must not strive any the less to care and give of ourselves, our skills and our love, when cure is impossible and life is short. Hospices have no monopoly of compassion as will be seen by the sensitive, but truly scientific, contributions from many of my colleagues working in general hospitals, who have so willingly contributed to this book.

Such a subject as *palliative care* throws up phrases and expressions which, though commonly used, themselves demand definition. Thus we have sought to explore in some depth the concept 'Quality of Life' with a chapter by a Professor of General Practice, himself a hospice physician. We have looked at the ethics of palliative care through the eyes of a moral philosopher whose professional work and research has been in medical circles; we have focused on bereavement, an issue which cannot be avoided, and communications as understood by a thoracic surgeon in New Zealand. In addition, we have sought to explore the realities and the potential of team care with chapters by distinguished nurses, hospital chaplains and a senior social worker.

As editor, I have not sought to impose my ideas upon my colleagues (nor would they have permitted it), nor insisted on any uniformity of style. There are even divergent opinions but, in such a difficult field, this is as it should be. To be dogmatic would be to oversimplify or miniaturise a subject which is, and always must remain, complex, complicated and demanding of all we cherish as members of the caring professions.

I acknowledge my indebtedness to authors and publishers who have consented to the inclusion of their work and findings; to my colleagues who have put so much thought and time into writing their chapters; to our publishers Croom Helm for their unfailing courtesy and patience; and most of all to our many patients who have taught us out of all proportion to what we have tried to do for them or indeed what we deserve.

Derek Doyle

1 THE 'QUALITY OF LIFE'

Eric Wilkes

Introduction

Our health-care delivery system was designed to deal at first with an age of infection and trauma, and it is adjusting slowly but surely to the succeeding era of chronic disease. Polio and diphtheria have almost vanished with smallpox. Infections like tuberculosis and whooping cough still wait for their chance, but it is now the chronic diseases that form the main burden to doctor, patient and society at large.

There are two things therefore that dominate the modern medical scene. One is the need to adjust to the apparently inexorable progress of the degenerative diseases, but to give battle against them. This means that all appropriate therapeutic advances must be tested and used, and involves the education of doctors and of patients into what is, for the time being, susceptible to palliation and what is not. Secondly, it requires a courageous adjustment and resignation to the imperfections of mortality, for which we receive little in the way of either encouragement or preparation.

But while we encounter now a very different spectrum of need, the basic design of the health-care system still remains geared to the acute short-term hospital admission. The day hospitals and the community services have to manage with resources that are, by comparison, inadequate and deprived.

There are, however, some helpful aspects intrinsic in such a system. It is not profitable to over-diagnose or over-treat, as can — arguably — be claimed to be the case in the USA. The British family doctor may be just as greedy as his American counterpart, but he has rather less opportunity. If the British general practitioner is at times uncaring and out of date, this is to some degree a protective reaction to intolerable pressures. But it is also, through the design of the system, an economy.

Nor is it all the doctors' fault. When orthopaedic out-patient departments had six-month waiting lists, patients in one district were asked after a few months if they still wanted their appointment now due in another six weeks' time. A considerable proportion did not take up their deferred consultation. This may have been an unjustifiable delay for some patients, some may have transferred to private care, but many exacerbations of chronic disease surely had settled without treatment in a manner beneficial to the nation's economy and possibly to the patient.

In fact, medicine is not always worth having. Only the inactive drugs are safe and every medical intervention carries a risk that needs to be weighed against possible benefits rather more thoughtfully than is often done. The present education of doctors is only now beginning to include an increased interest in evaluation: but poorly substantiated enthusiasm from doctors is more often encountered than cautious humility, and is usually a great deal more popular with patients and relatives. Everyone likes to feel there is an answer, especially if they can be involved in taking some of the credit for it. So younger doctors tend to refer, admit or investigate more cases than the older doctors. There is no good evidence that the outcome for their patients is any better, but there is evidence that − coincident with, if not consequent on, vocational training schemes − younger doctors have a more sensitive approach than some of their more elderly colleagues.

This area of relationships and communication is where some of the greatest changes need to be made in the next decade. One can review the present scene perhaps most clearly by restricting the discussion to the doctor's approach to malignant disease.

Survey of Doctors

A series of questions was put by postal questionnaire to the consultants and general practitioners of two cities in the north Midlands of England, one of which was a teaching centre. Over a third of the doctors replied, and clearly the questions were largely inapplicable to the work of many (anaesthetists, radiologists, pathologists) who did not respond.

Of the 258 replies, 167 were from general practitioners and 118 were from hospital consultants. The sample was reasonably representative of the British medical establishment in that it was neither young nor female. Of the respondents 11 per cent were women, 10 per cent were overseas graduates and only 14 per cent had been medically qualified for less than ten years.

When we asked if these colleagues normally told cancer patients their real diagnosis, 44 per cent of the consultants and 25 per cent of GPs said they did. Some 24 per cent of consultants and 30 per cent of

GPs did not normally tell, although 30 per cent of consultants and 41 per cent of GPs would tell if the patient pressed them to do so. A third found it difficult to generalise about their policy and when all were asked about their last case, half had been told and half had not — a finding that agrees closely with the patients' preferences described by Spencer Jones (1981). Two-thirds of the doctors would listen to the relatives' advice about telling or not telling, but would not consider the advice binding. Some 53 per cent of consultants did not take advice from the family doctor about what they should tell — the practical difficulties of doing so are daunting enough to require no description — and 56 per cent of the family doctors found the communication from the consultants concerning what and who had been told was inadequate and unsatisfactory, and this was even worse in the teaching centre.

The main factors influencing the behaviour of the doctors were their personal and clinical experience (69 per cent), rather than their medical-school teaching (6 per cent). The only cases of unanimity were in acknowledging the right of patients not to be told if they so indicated, and in the doctors' denial that any change in their policy was likely in the near future.

When the doctors were asked how much the poor-prognosis cases worried them, 53 per cent said slightly, 22 per cent agreed that they worried a great deal, and another fifth (including a fifth of the GPs) considered such a reaction was not applicable to them.

A third of the consultants often encouraged their capable junior doctors to hold discussion with such patients, but 39 per cent did so rarely or never. When asked if they encouraged capable and experienced nursing colleagues to hold discussions with such patients, a third of the consultants and a fifth of the GPs did so often, but 40 per cent of consultants and 34 per cent of GPs did so rarely or never.

Inevitably, such a miniscule excursion into medical attitudes can give a wrong impression. The basic reaction seems to be one of a characteristically sturdy pragmatism, but there are some interesting points that merit further comment. In an age when patients often require to know more about their own problems, that 25 per cent of consultants and 30 per cent of GPs do not tell them may be more justifiable in special and selected cases rather than as a rule of thumb. We must be anxious that what could be a timid conservatism is depriving the patient not only of information but also of solace and support. Not telling the patient can tell a very great deal.

Furthermore, there are indications that the senior doctors tend to delegate such difficult interviews to their juniors and that although they may hesitate about getting personally involved, they are not always prepared to delegate such duties to capable senior nursing colleagues. This is a potent cause of resentment both on the wards and in the community. Just because the reaction of a bull in a china shop may not be appropriate, the behaviour pattern of the ostrich will not solve any problems either.

Involvement

When a general practitioner lives in his community, it is much easier for him to see his patients as people. When he lives away and conducts sessional medicine with minimal visiting, especially as part of a group, then a subtle change in the relationship may ensue, and the use of an out-of-hours deputising service may help to compound that change. It has been said that such practice is now as impersonal as the out-patient department, lacking only the latter's clinical reliability.

In a recent (as yet unpublished) series of interviews with newly bereaved relatives, only a quarter of the relatives expressed gratitude to their family doctor for the care given. Ann Cartwright reports a further diminution in the general practitioner's readiness to be involved in social or pastoral problems (Cartwright and Anderson, 1979). It is surely in this context that a fifth of the general practitioners in the survey could feel that any emotional involvement with cancer sufferers was inapplicable to them. Such a withdrawal may not save them from long hours of work, an inhibited family life, and a high alcoholism rate. This may be inevitable in a free-access system operating in an area of high-density population and all the social disruption that that implies. But it does bring the future pattern of general practice somewhat into question.

It may be eccentric to say this when we have never had so many highly qualified and well-trained doctors in family medicine as we have now. After a decade of vocational training major improvements have been effected and one can, in more optimistic moments, see many more as a consequence of a snowball effect.

Yet two out of three consultations still end with a prescription, the six-minute consultation is a damaging imperative, and one could say that the main result of the first years of vocational training has been to make the good practice rather better. We have not touched the more deprived practices and the updating of isolated practitioners remains an unsolved problem. This is not all, of course, the doctor's fault. We may be more scapegoats than sinners.

A major complicating factor in modern general practice is that we are contractually obligated to look after the patient who knocks at our door, even if there are others less demanding yet in greater need. We have not yet adjusted to supplying the administrative structure necessary for the anticipatory care of the population for whom we are responsible. Although the hospital diabetic clinics are overwhelmed by the increasing number of cases, the community care of diabetes is even more unreliable. Our follow-up of cases with a recent acute myocardial infarction hovers between being over-cautious or indifferent in rehabilitation, we connive at unnecessary delays in getting back to work, and we ignore the spouse as routinely as we ignore the husband of a patient with a mastectomy. Hypertensive cases are undiagnosed, untreated or uncontrolled. Psychiatric cases and their families remain fairly unsupported. It may well be the best primary-care system in the world, but its triumphs are often in spite of the system rather than because of it. We have such a burden of transient illness that the major chronic problems are displaced and neglected.

Such a situation gives the hospitals — which have their own enormous unsolved problems of relationships and teamwork and vast but shrinking budgets — an opportunity to extend their activities further into the community. First, this is of political importance in the battle for resources, and secondly, it is genuinely enough the only way in which the required expertise can be brought to the bed-side of patients in need, but still in their own homes. Therefore we have seen a proliferation of stoma nurses, psychiatric nurses, diabetes nurses, and even, in Britain, health visitors who attend oncology out-patients in an attempt to provide that continuity of support which the doctors have so conspicuously failed to deliver.

So long as the family doctor visits the really sick minority so rarely, either on the ward or in the home, and remains overwhelmed by the workload of the cough bottle and the sick note, so long as the hospital consultant remains more concerned — as with his pressures he must be — with diagnosis and treatment and rapid discharge, then the patient is likely to fall into the holes in the network of care. It will be difficult for nursing colleagues to fill the gap, when they are so often excluded from sharing in the most important areas of patient management. The fact that so many acute hospital admissions are really acute exacerbations of chronic pathology makes teamwork between doctor and nurse, and between community and hospital services, more important than ever before.

Co-operation

There is anecdotal evidence that in the hospitals the professional relationships between doctor and nurse are not so good as they were a quarter of a century ago. It is traditional to blame the Salmon re-organisation for this, but that was more a symptom than a cause.

Of course it is always difficult, at a time of changing expectations, to be sure. Certainly, there is more blatant discontent from the nurses about inadequate pain control, but that may be due to their greater contact with the realities at the bed-side: and the nurses cannot themselves be blameless. The commonest cause for dissatisfaction among recently bereaved relatives (in 22 per cent of cases) was with the generally uncaring attitude of the hospitals.

Some admission procedures may be administratively sound and yet sociologically disastrous. Some of the routines for collecting the effects or the death certificate are equally unjustifiable. In an attempt to rationalise the use of scarce, expensive professional labour, the use of ward clerks, ward orderlies and the exclusion of nurses from non-nursing duties have further distanced the personal elements of care. And nurses who lack confidence can evade patients as well as the doctors.

In the community the more rapid discharge from hospital has not always been matched by an increase in the community nursing establishment and the nurse has therefore to operate under pressures that impose a concentration on the purely physical aspects of care.

The relationships in the primary health-care teams may not be as satisfactory as the general practitioners believe, and the concept of the nurses as the doctor's handmaiden still lingers. The diffuse geographical spread of the practice population leads to a waste of nursing time and often there is no forum where such difficulties and irritations can be shared or clinical problems brought towards a common management policy. One must be grateful and surprised that so much team-work has been brought to reality with so little training or preparation among so many practices.

Yet the doctor–nurse relationship at times limps along as lamely as the community–hospital relationship. Here, it is still common to wait for weeks to hear about the death of one's hospitalised patient, so the obituary columns of the local paper are essential and required reading.

The Doctor-Patient Relationship

If we are conscious of the difficulties involved in such professional partnerships, we need at the same time to pay far more attention to the most crucial partnership of all — that between the doctor and his patient. So many problems require a mutual respect, and this may be difficult to sustain if all the two parties see of each other is the contact needed for intermittent crises intervention.

In a British city sustaining some 250 general practitioners, over 2 million consultations in general practice will take place each year. Arising from this, there will be some 50 complaints arriving at the Family Practitioner Committee yearly and only three or four of these will go on to the formal complaints procedures. This is an enviable situation and says much for the effective work of the doctors and the tolerant understanding of the patient. None of this makes headlines, for it is there all the time.

What gives real cause for concern, however, is that among these 50 complaints are examples of a rudeness and a lack of understanding that must give the doctors in their turn sleepless nights. So besieged with trivia do the doctors feel that they sometimes request patients to attend their surgery headquarters when they are becoming paraplegic or have only hours to live: and although it may be their contractual obligation to deliver medical care, it is not part of that obligation to do so kindly or with tact. It would clearly be comically unhelpful to have surgeons weeping in sympathy before their patients come to theatre: yet we need to remark that some of us are liable to an emotional atrophy that can diminish our own lives as well as our patients' care.

It is often not realised in our exceptionally lonely society how families, in their turn, need to be shown how to respond. We need to cherish and nurture family relationships that one may once have taken for granted. When, for example, one is asked by patients to tell their child that they are about to die soon, this must be done simply and without hurry, a genuine opportunity offered for further questions, and the relative asked to repeat back the salient points about the case. But if one is briefing a child — from age 7 to 70 — about a dying parent, this is not enough. The child needs to discuss whether they should not go in and kiss their parent, and hug them, and tell me they will help cherish them and be with them, for this is their privilege and their right: and this can add enormously to the quality of the last few days or weeks. Yet this is rarely taught or practised.

Quality of Life

It is perhaps because of this stunted emotional environment in which our chronically ill patients so often have to live that discussions have surfaced so much of late arguing that the quality of life is more important than its mere duration. The quality, like beauty, must be very much in the eye of the beholder, and what seems a sad and restricted day of bedfast dependence can still be rich. If most patients can enjoy a cup of tea and a chat, and perhaps even a short walk around the living room or garden, life still is sweet, at any rate so long as symptom control is reasonable.

Pain control is not difficult for the vast majority of patients — nausea and vomiting, weakness, dysphagia and tenesmus can be far more intractable than pain — and the home-based nebuliser, the potent diuretics and the adroit use of opiates can do as much for the breathlessness as we have achieved in the field of analgesia.

Yet symptom control is by no means the only dominating factor. The combination of paralysis with pride, the impossibility of independence or cleanliness with malignant fistulae, the progressive course of motor neuron disease, the long time-scale of the years of encroachment by the disseminating breast cancer, or the sheer frailty of age — these can be intolerable at times and lead patient and relative, rightly and calmly, to accept death as the only possible answer.

Such acceptance may be genuine and yet intermittent. The grandchild's christening or the daughter's visit can temporarily transform the world. It therefore can be equally difficult to assess with any accuracy the quality of life for someone we know well or for a stranger. This has not deterred nursing colleagues from making such an attempt (Wilkes, 1981). In a Sheffield hospice's assessment of 500 consecutive admissions, in views based largely on the observed quality of relationships and adequacy of pain control, 29 per cent of patients were thought to maintain an excellent quality of terminal life, 70 per cent a satisfactory, and only 1 per cent a poor quality of life at the end. In a more recent project concerning deaths from all causes in the same city, a survey as yet unpublished from the community nurses categorised the quality of terminal life as excellent in 16 per cent, satisfactory in 40 per cent, and poor in 44 per cent of cases. It seems therefore that the physical as well as the emotional sides both deal with problems as yet substantially unsolved.

A Validated Measurement

It is likely that, for cancer cases at any rate, Spitzer and his colleagues (1981) have delivered to us a simple, comprehensive and validated means of measuring the quality of life: and although based on panels of cancer patients, their relatives, healthy people and professionals in Sydney, this is likely to be of wide-ranging validity. This is likely indeed to be more relevant than many of the psychiatric scales in common clinical use.

It will be seen by the Quality of Life Index (Figure 1.1), reproduced by permission, that activity, daily living, aspects of health, support and outlook are all weighted and scored so as to include the variable confidence with which the observations are made. This will not do our work for us any more than the epidemiologists' findings can properly make our clinical decision. What a poor score can do, however, is to alert us to the need for deploying more non-medical or medical resources as seem indicated or available: and to remember Balint's phrase about the doctor himself being one of the most potent of treatments.

Yet it is important to remember that such support may involve not so much the mobilisation of medical care as its withdrawal. We see too much palliative chemotherapy in disseminated cancer that is a burden for the patient. This is meekly accepted by the family doctor because his patient is 'under the hospital'. A drive out in the car, or some form of work or diversional therapy, or just company may be far more relevant to the needs of some such patients.

And so we come back to the beginning, in emphasising the needs, despite the difficulties, to relate closely to our sick patients. Despite our previous criticisms, this relationship is likely to be good between patient and practitioner is nearly three-quarters of cases, although the doctors' poor ability to communicate is rated as a most important inhibiting factor in the remaining quarter.

What are the vital factors that the patient or the relatives so appreciate? They are kindness, willingness to spend time to visit, leaving their home telephone numbers and accepting out-of-hours calls as part of the commitment, sympathy, honesty, providing information and support, and having a real interest in the whole family. Such qualities are not the monopoly of any age-group. 'He has been our doctor for years, a real family doctor, more like a father' can be neutralised by 'the younger doctors have more time for you. You can talk to them better than the older ones.' It comes down in the end to a supportive relationship with

Figure 1.1: The quality of life index

QUALITY OF LIFE INDEX

Study No _____ / _____

Age _____

Sex M₁ F₂ (Ring appropriate letter) _____

Primary Problem or Diagnosis _____

SCORING FORM

Secondary Problem or Diagnosis, or complication (if appropriate) _____

Scorer's Specialty _____

Score each heading 2, 1 or 0 according to your most recent assessment of the patient.

ACTIVITY

During the last week, the patient
- has been working or studying full-time, or nearly so, in usual occupation; or managing own household; or participating in unpaid or voluntary activities, whether retired or not 2
- has been working or studying in usual occupation or managing own household or participating in unpaid or voluntary activities, but requiring major assistance or a significant reduction in hours worked or a sheltered situation or was on sick leave 1
- has not been working or studying in any capacity and not managing own household 0

DAILY LIVING

During the last week, the patient
- has been self-reliant in eating, washing, toileting and dressing; using public transport or driving own car 2
- has been requiring assistance (another person or special equipment) for daily activities and transport but performing light tasks 1
- has not been managing personal care nor light tasks and/or not leaving own home or institution at all 0

HEALTH

During the last week, the patient
- has been appearing to feel well or reporting feeling "great" most of the time 2
- has been lacking energy or not feeling entirely "up to par" more than just occasionally 1
- has been feeling very ill or "lousy", seeming weak and washed out most of the time or was unconscious 0

SUPPORT

During the last week
the patient has been having good relationships with others and receiving strong support from at least one family member and/or friend 2
support received or perceived has been limited from family and friends and/or by the patient's condition 1
support from family and friends occurred infrequently or only when absolutely necessary or patient was unconscious 0

OUTLOOK

During the past week the patient
- has usually been appearing calm and positive in outlook, accepting and in control of personal circumstances, including surroundings 2
- has sometimes been troubled because not fully in control of personal circumstances or has been having periods of obvious anxiety or depression 1
- has been seriously confused or very frightened or consistently anxious and depressed or unconscious 0

QL INDEX TOTAL

How confident are you that your scoring of the preceding dimensions is accurate? Please ring the appropriate category.

Absolutely Confident 1	Very Confident 2	Quite Confident 3	Not Very Confident 4	Very Doubtful 5	Not at all Confident 6

all those in need, to a sophisticated analysis of that need, to a training in the use of available medical and paramedical resources, and to personal commitment. These can, even in the most unpromising circumstances, permit us to protect the quality of the gift of life.

References

Cartwright, A. and Anderson, R. (1979) *Patients and their Doctors 1977*, Institute for Social Studies in Medical Care, published as Occasional Paper no. 8, *Journal of the Royal College of General Practitioners*

Spencer Jones, J. (1981) 'Telling the right patient', *British Medical Journal*, 283, pp. 191–2

Spitzer, W.O., Hall, J., Levi, J., Shepherd, R. and Catchlove, B.R. (1981) 'Measuring the quality of life in cancer patients', *Journal of Chronic Diseases*, 34, pp. 585–97

Wilkes, E. (ed.) (1982) *The Role of the Hospice in the Dying Patient*, MTP Press, Lancaster

2 PALLIATIVE CARE IN ADVANCED DIABETES MELLITUS

Ian Campbell

Introduction

Diabetes mellitus is a common disease with an incidence in Western countries of approximately 1 per cent: 0.5 per cent diagnosed and a similar percentage undiagnosed. As recently as 60 years ago, in the pre-insulin era, young insulin-dependent diabetics usually died within one or two years of the diagnosis from diabetic ketoacidosis. The advent of insulin dramatically changed this terrible prognosis. However, with the subsequent increase in longevity of the diabetic, the incidence of chronic complications increased considerably and has become the principal cause of morbidity and mortality in the diabetic. Various long-term studies have shown that in middle age the death rate among diabetics is two to six times that of the general population. Cardiovascular disease and renal failure in particular are responsible for this increased mortality. Figure 2.1 is taken from a prospective study of mortality in 3113 diabetics carried out in Edinburgh over eight years (1 January 1968 to 31 December 1975), during which time 1272 patients (41 per cent) died (Shenfield et al., 1979). It illustrates the increased death rate per thousand per year of diabetic males and females compared with those from a general population. In contrast to the general population, death rates amongst female diabetics are virtually equal to those for male diabetics, in accordance with other studies which similarly show that young diabetic women appear to lose their sex's 'protection' from cardiovascular disease.

Although younger insulin-dependent diabetics and older non-insulin-dependent diabetics are both prone to complications, the mortality rate rises with increasing duration of the disease, especially in the age-group of less than 50 years. The decisive factor for the mortality rate is the age of onset of diabetes mellitus; the highest mortality rate is seen among those individuals with an age of onset of 14 years or less. Patients from this group, who have had their disease for 15–20 years' duration, are especially prone to the various complications of diabetes. In addition, poorly controlled diabetics are reckoned to have a two to

Figure 2.1: Death rates of diabetic males and females compared with those from a general population

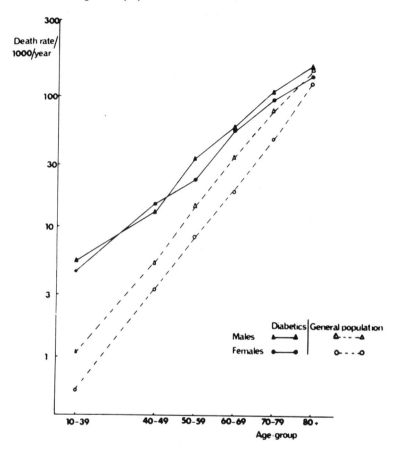

Source: G.M. Shenfield *et al*. 1979.

three times greater mortality than those who are well controlled. Those diabetics controlled with insulin and oral agents have a greater mortality rate than those treated with diet alone, but it must always be appreciated that the latter group may still develop complications. Recently the Medical Services Study Group of the Royal College of Physicians of London, in collaboration with the British Diabetic Association, examined factors contributing to the deaths of 448 diabetics under the age of 50 years who died in the UK in 1979 (Tunbridge, 1981). Although the major causes of death were myocardial infarction and other large-vessel disease (41 per cent), and diabetic renal disease (19 per cent), it was alarming to see that 74 deaths (15 per cent) were due to ketoacidosis, which was the commonest cause of death in those aged under 20 years. Delays in seeking and providing medical attention were the major contributing factors in those deaths. Thus, although the remainder of this chapter will consider the morbidity and mortality associated with chronic complications of diabetes, there must be no complacency with regard to ketoacidotic deaths, which should be avoidable in virtually all cases.

Background to Complications

Diabetics are prone to develop complications which may be classified as specific and non-specific (Table 2.1). The specific complications are due to a combination of microangiopathy and abnormal tissue meta-bolism. The microangiopathy is characterised by a thickening of the basement membranes of the capillary walls by glycoproteins which may cause ischaemia. The non-specific complications of atherosclerosis and cataract tend to occur earlier in diabetics than non-diabetics. Thus the morbidity seen, often in relatively young individuals, is that associated with blindness, renal failure, diverse neuropathic problems, gangrene and amputation, and premature coronary artery, peripheral and cere-brovascular disease.

Table 2.1: Complications of Diabetes

Specific	Non-specific
Retinopathy	Atherosclerosis
Nephropathy	(a)　coronary artery disease
Neuropathy	(b)　peripheral vascular disease
'Diabetic foot'	(c)　cerebrovascular disease
Skin lesions	Cataracts
	Infection

In younger diabetics, complications are not usually evident until 10–15 years after diagnosis. However, if diabetes develops in early childhood, these complications will be evident at a young age; for example, although diabetic retinopathy has not been seen in children younger than 10 years old, it has been reported in 5–15 per cent of teenage diabetics. In older diabetics, complications, especially vascular, may be present at diagnosis. The remainder of this chapter will consider principally those specific complications, apart from skin abnormalities, which give rise to little morbidity and have no effect on mortality, and finally mention will be made of the various atherosclerotic problems associated with coronary, peripheral and cerebrovascular disease. Cataract and infection will not be dealt with specifically, but will be referred to in those sections where impaired vision is discussed and where infection is associated with nephropathy, neuropathy and diabetic foot problems. Although the various complications will be discussed separately to highlight the problems associated with each, it must be remembered that many may coexist, adding more to the morbidity of the diabetic.

Diabetic Retinopathy

Incidence and Prognosis

Diabetes mellitus is the commonest cause of blindness in those under the age of 65 years in the UK and represents 10-20 per cent of all new blind registrations. A diabetic is ten to twenty times as likely to become blind as a non-diabetic. Although diabetics can become blind from glaucoma, optic neuropathy, cataract, etc., it is diabetic retinopathy which is the commonest cause. There are approximately 8000 diabetics blind from diabetic retinopathy in the UK. Diabetic retinopathy increases with duration of diabetes and about 80 per cent of all diabetics will develop retinopathy after 15-20 years of diabetes. Fortunately, the majority only show background changes, but about 10 per cent show proliferative features and, if untreated, half of this group will become blind within three to five years.

Clinical Features

The clinical features of diabetic retinopathy can be divided into three types (see Figure 2.2).

Mild Background Retinopathy. This is characterised by microaneurysms, deep round haemorrhages ('blots' or 'blobs') and a few scattered hard exudates. Occasionally the haemorrhages may be superficial and flame-shaped, even when there is no hypertension present. The hard exudates represent lipid and protein material which has leaked into the retinae through damaged capillary walls. These background changes are common and are not usually associated with visual impairment. They indicate the need for careful observation of the fundus for any progression to more serious changes.

Figure 2.2: Evolution of diabetic retinopathy (DR)

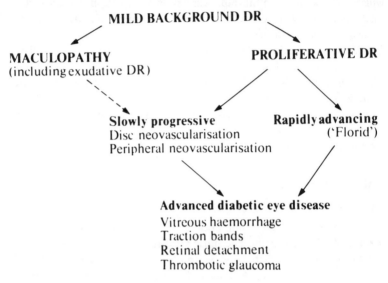

Source: From Toft, A.D., Campbell, I.W., and Seth, J. (1981) *Diagnosis and Management of Endocrine Diseases* (Blackwell Scientific Publications, Oxford).

Maculopathy. This is most common in diabetics treated by diet or oral hypoglycaemic agents, and is usually seen in the older age-group. Hard exudates, haemorrhages and oedema in the macular area result in severe visual loss. Patients with maculopathy usually have a slowly progressive impairment of visual activity.

Proliferative Retinopathy. This is common in all ages, but particularly affects long-standing insulin-dependent diabetics. New vessels, so-called neovascularisation, develop and are friable capillaries which can bleed with vitreous or pre-retinal haemorrhage causing sudden painless loss of vision in the affected eye. There is often accompanying change in the retinal veins, which become dilated and irregular with the potential to rupture, causing severe haemorrhage. Whenever haemorrhage occurs, secondary fibrosis occurs (retinitis proliferans) with irreversible damage to retinae and visual activity (Figure 2.3). A variety of severe advanced complications may ensue (Figure 2.2). All these eye problems can be aggravated by hypertension, which must be carefully controlled if present. In some instances, pregnancy may accelerate diabetic retino-pathy and the fundi of diabetic females must be carefully watched in

Figure 2.3: Fundal photograph of a 41-year-old insulin-dependent diabetic of 18 years' duration, blind due to diabetic retinopathy

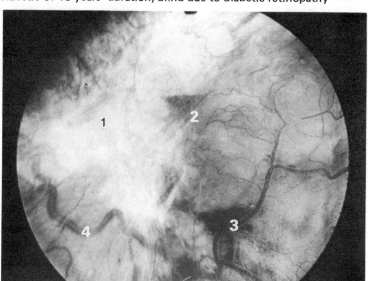

Notes: There is (1) extensive fibrosis, (2) new vessel formation, (3) haemorrhage and (4) venous irregularity. The fibrosis has destroyed a major part of the fundus with loss of visual acuity.

case treatment is necessary.

Impact of Retinopathy

Blindness is a dreaded complication of diabetes. Severe haemorrhage may potentially occur in up to 10 per cent of diabetics if they have not had their fundi checked regularly so that treatment may be given at an early stage to prevent bleeding and visual impairment (see below). The immediate psychological results of loss of vision are obvious both for patient and family. Many are often young patients in the 30-40 age-group. The longer-term social implications involve perhaps loss of employment and rehabilitation towards further suitable work. If the patient is registered blind, then the appropriate local authority Social Welfare Department can offer help in several ways. If the patient is still physically able to do some form of employment, then in the UK referral to the Blind Persons Resettlement Officer of the local labour exchange can be arranged and there assessment made as to whether the patient can go back with some basic training to his previous job or whether further training is required at one of the regional centres specifically designed for blind people. If the patient is not able to do any further work, there are centres available for social rehabilitation and in particular centres for training the individual with a guide dog. Further help in the form of 'talking book machines', learning braille, and in some instances attending various day centres for the blind, can all be organised to help the patient. These facilities are the same as for those patients blinded from causes other than diabetic retinopathy. However, proliferative-retinopathy changes are often associated with renal and cardiovascular complications of diabetes. In one Danish study of patients followed up after recognition of proliferative retinopathy, 10 per cent had died within five years (Deckert, Simonsen and Poulsen, 1967). Similar results have been reported from other studies from Europe and the USA.

Available Treatment

Diabetic maculopathy and proliferative retinopathy can be treated, particularly in their early stages. All diabetics should have their visual acuity and fundi examined annually. Various studies have shown that about 10 per cent of patients that attend a general diabetic clinic will have retinopathy requiring treatment. Retinal photocoagulation, usually done on an out-patient basis under local anaesthesia, can reduce the incidence of blindness in 60–80 per cent of cases. Two instruments are available. The first is the xenon-arc photocoagulator, which delivers an intense white light absorbed in the retinal pigment epithelium, the resulting burn destroys the surrounding leaking capillaries or fragile new vessels so that oedema and exudates are resolved and vitreous haemorr-hage prevented. The second instrument, a laser beam, produced by an argon, ruby or krypton laser, produces a more localised beam as its light is selectively absorbed by haemoglobin. The laser beam is best used for optic disc neovascularisation, for treatment of pre-retinal new vessels or for lesions near the macula.

Pituitary ablation has rarely been used in the past 10–12 years for treatment of proliferative retinopathy because of the advent of photo-coagulation, but it still has a place in the treatment of rapidly advancing florid types of proliferative retinopathy, often seen in teenage diabetics or those in their early twenties, many with a history of long-standing poor diabetic control, in which there are severe venous changes and extensive new vessel growth. The operation may cause a deterioration in already compromised renal function, and also makes the diabetic eventually prone to severe hypoglycaemic episodes, because of the destruction of pituitary-dependent insulin-antagonistic hormones such as ACTH and growth hormone. Few patients survive more than ten years after the operation.

Clofibrate may be used on a long-term basis to clear hard exudates in a dosage of 1 g twice daily. Especially in the presence of impaired renal function, clofibrate causes muscle weakness and tenderness with raised creatinine kinase and lactate dehydrogenase levels. It should not be used in diabetics with chronic renal failure.

Some diabetics with severe impairment of vision may benefit from very specialised ophthalmological surgery such as intravitreous injection of Urokinase or vitrectomy for vitreous haemorrhages, division of traction bands in the vitreous, or surgery for retinal detachment. It must be emphasised that this therapy is only of benefit to a few selected diabetic patients and cannot be regarded as a routine 'cure' for blindness. The pain of thrombotic glaucoma due to rubeosis iridis may be so severe that enucleation of the affected eye is the only means of affording pain relief.

Diabetic Nephropathy

Incidence

Diabetic nephropathy is a general term to describe the various pathological abnormalities in the kidney and their clinical sequelae (Figure 2.4). Chronic renal failure has become a major cause of death in young insulin-dependent diabetics. In earlier reviews it was estimated to be responsible for half of all the deaths in patients who had become diabetic before 20 years of age. However, in the UK study of factors contributing to deaths among diabetics under 50 years of age, 77 (19 per cent) of 448 deaths in 1979 were due to diabetic renal disease, this often being preceded by blindness (Tunbridge, 1981). Renal biopsy is the only reliable method of detecting diabetic nephropathy and thus the true incidence is difficult to assess. The risk of developing diabetic nephropathy in young insulin-dependent diabetics is as high as 30 per cent, but approximately 70 per cent will never develop diabetic nephropathy in spite of long-standing diabetes. The clinical hallmark of diabetic nephropathy is proteinuria. Persistent proteinuria develops after a mean duration of diabetes of fifteen years (very rarely less than ten years), with a mean survival thereafter of about seven years (Deckert *et al.*, 1981).

Figure 2.4: Various lesions of diabetic nephropathy leading to clinical features of renal failure

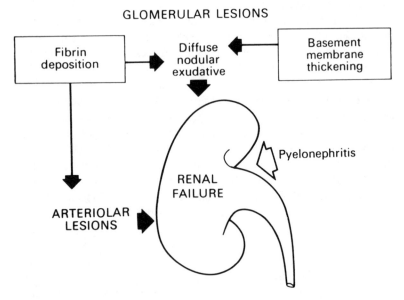

Source: From Cameron, J.S., Ireland, J.T. and Watkins, P.J. (1975) 'The kidney and renal tract', in H. Keen and J. Jarrett (eds.), *Complications of Diabetes*, Edward Arnold, London

Clinical Features

The pathological changes in the kidney in diabetes occur in the glomeruli and arterioles with damage to the interstitial tissue by infection and ischaemia. There is a thickening of the basement membrane of glomerular capillaries with resultant diffuse glomerulosclerosis, nodular hyalinised lobules in glomeruli in 30 per cent of cases (Kimmelsteil-Wilson nodules), exudation of protein and fibrinoid material from glomeruli and finally end-stage hyalinisation of glomeruli. There is also hyalinisation similar to that seen in hypertension in the afferent and efferent arterioles. The clinical progression of diabetic nephropathy is through three phases.

Asymptomatic Proteinuria. This appears after approximately 15 years' duration of diabetes mellitus. At first there may be intermittent proteinuria, separated by months of negative (Albustix) results.

Nephrotic Syndrome. After three to five years of persistent proteinuria, nephrotic syndrome, representing an advanced stage of diabetic nephropathy, results, with death occurring within two to four years of its onset. Clinically, the patient has peripheral oedema, hypoalbuminaemia (usually less than 30 g/l) and heavy proteinuria (usually greater than 3 g/day). Where there is heavy proteinuria, intravenous pyelography may precipitate acute renal failure.

Chronic Renal Failure. Once the plasma urea exceeds 10 mmol/l and serum creatinine is elevated, death usually results within two years. Anaemia and hypertension both commonly occur and pyelonephritis will be present, often severely, so-called papillary necrosis. Younger patients usually die in a uraemic coma, but in the older subjects the terminal event is more likely to be a myocardial infarction or cerebrovascular accident.

Impact of Nephropathy

There is no obvious morbidity to the patient when only symptomless proteinuria is present. Even in the early stages of nephrotic syndrome, there may only be mild ankle swelling. However, once this increases in severity and chronic renal failure ensues, the patient has all the features of the latter condition with tiredness, nausea, vomiting, diarrhoea and a general feeling of ill health. Work will be impossible unless it is a light sedentary job, and even then mental lethargy may prevent this. The patient and family now realise that death may be imminent unless measures are undertaken to restore renal function. These are basically the same as for the management of chronic renal failure in the non-diabetic (see Chapter 5), but an outline of those measures and their results of importance to the diabetic will be discussed here.

Available Treatment

The main aim, as with any of the diabetic complications, is to attempt to achieve as good control of the diabetes as possible, to prevent progression of the renal lesion. However, because insulin degradation is impaired in chronic renal failure, the daily requirement falls, and meticulous control may be associated with frequent hypoglycaemic reactions. If patients are controlled with a sulphonylurea, then those excreted mainly via the kidney (e.g. chlorpropamide, glibenclamide, glipizide) may accumulate and cause hypoglycaemia. In these circumstances, the newer sulphonylureas introduced in the past few years, such as gliquidone or gliclazide, may be recommended as less than 5 per cent of the dose is excreted in the urine. Biguanides, such as phenformin and metformin, are contra-indicated in the presence of chronic renal failure because of the risk of lactic acidosis.

Nephrotic Syndrome. Dietary protein is increased to 80–110 g daily and oedema is treated with large doses of diuretics. Rarely, intravenous salt-poor albumin may be necessary on a temporary basis to relieve severe oedema.

Chronic Renal Failure. Dietary protein should be reduced progressively to 40 g per day when plasma urea is greater than 20 mmol/l. When the creatinine clearance nears 20 ml/min or 0.33 ml/sec., thereafter a rapid deterioration may occur in the patient's condition and thus it is important that these diabetics should be assessed early for dialysis and transplantation before significant uraemia arises. The diabetic with end-stage renal failure faces the same choice as does the uraemic non-diabetic, namely, chronic haemodialysis, continuous ambulatory peritoneal dialysis (CAPD) or renal transplantation.

Chronic haemodialysis. Although a few centres have claimed good results for diabetics with chronic haemodialysis, most have experienced disappointing results. Survival rates for the first, second and third years are approximately 60 per cent, 50 per cent and 30 per cent, the last figure being less than half that for non-diabetics.

CAPD. This relatively new technique may prove useful in those diabetics with renal failure awaiting transplantation. It overcomes the difficulties of vascular access to maintain a shunt in diseased peripheral vessels. No heparinisation is required as with haemodialysis. This is important, as diabetics with renal failure often have associated diabetic proliferative retinopathy with increased danger of bleeding where heparin is used. Diabetics treated with CAPD seem to have better rehabilitation than those with haemodialysis, and have a tendency to show an increased haemoglobin and feeling of well-being. It has been possible to achieve good diabetic control by the use of intraperitoneal insulin. However, there are problems with peritonitis, obesity due to the excess of calories in concentrated glucose solution used for intraperitoneal infusion, acne and hypertriglyceridaemia (again because of the high glucose load).

Transplantation. This is the treatment of choice, but so far has been limited to a few specialised centres. The best figures in the USA are from the University of Minnesota, where diabetics have been offered renal transplants since 1969. Survival rates at one and four years for a diabetic receiving a transplant from a live related donor are 80 per cent and 60 per cent respectively compared with 90 per cent and 80 per cent for a non-diabetic recipient. The corresponding figures for cadaveric transplants are 60 per cent and 40 per cent respectively compared with 80 per cent and 75 per cent (Najarian *et al.*, 1979). It must be stressed that the experience for transplantation of diabetic kidneys in the US is very limited, simply because there is such a long waiting list for non-diabetics to have transplants. In the Minnesota Transplant Group series, with its excellent results, patients have been selected on an individual basis irrespective of age and degree of retinopathy, neuropathy and ischaemic heart disease. However, in Edinburgh over the past two years, the criteria for selection of diabetics for a dialysis/ transplantation programme have been set with the following exclusions:

1. blindness in both eyes;
2. severe ischaemic heart disease, i.e. several previous myocardial infarctions with poor left ventricular function (a previous myocardial infarction or angina in an otherwise fit person who enjoys reasonable quality of life would not exclude a diabetic for consideration);
3. severe peripheral vascular disease, i.e. generalised atherosclerosis with severe clinically detectable occlusions in subclavian, carotid and iliac circulation (patients with small vessel complications, e.g. gangrene toes, would not be excluded);
4. severe autonomic neuropathy, especially those patients with an atonic bladder or severe orthostatic hypotension (see below);
5. poor compliance with diabetic control or motivation for long-term treatment.

The aim is for early transplantation, where possible from a live donor and preferably before dialysis is required. If dialysis is necessary, then CAPD is preferred to haemodialysis.

Obviously there may be criticisms of such a selection policy, but it is up to each specialised dialysis/transplantation centre at the present time to decide what facilities they have to offer. The management of end-stage diabetic renal disease in the UK has been poor until now. In the 1979 survey of deaths under 50 years, of the 77 renal deaths, the attendant doctor regarded death as inevitable in most of these patients with only six (8 per cent) having undergone a renal transplant and only four others having either peritoneal or haemodialysis (Tunbridge, 1981). However, the good results from the Minnesota Transplant Group have stressed that diabetics must be offered transplantation, if possible at an early stage of their chronic renal failure (Najarian *et al.*, 1979). Some 82 per cent of the diabetics successfully transplanted were actively rehabilitated after transplantation, all of whom were unable to do any useful work before transplantation. In fact, 34 per cent were able to return to full-time employment. Despite the continuing risk of premature vascular death, there is evidence that there may be improvement in retinal and neuropathic complications.

Diabetic Neuropathy

Incidence and Prognosis

It is difficult to estimate the true incidence of diabetic neuropathy because it is a heterogeneous group of conditions with both somatic and autonomic abnormalities (Table 2.2). In addition, sophisticated electrophysiological tests can show abnormalities not obvious by routine clinical assessment. However, despite the different criteria that might be used to establish a diagnosis of diabetic neuropathy in the literature, if diabetic somatic neuropathy is considered as a loss of ankle-tendon reflexes with or without vibration sense or as symptoms and signs of mononeuropathy or neuritis, then up to 20–50 per cent patients will have evidence of this. In a prospective study of 4400 unselected out-patients observed in Brussels between 1947 and 1973, Pirart (1978) described the incidence and prevalence of diabetic neuropathy as being a function of the duration of diabetes, the prevalence being approximately 50 per cent after 25 years. Neuropathy is extremely rare in diabetic children. Autonomic neuropathy may be found in about 20 per cent of randomly selected diabetics if determined by abnormal non-invasive tests based on cardiovascular reflexes, but its true prevalence is difficult to determine, partly because of difficulty in assessing many of the vague symptoms associated with autonomic neuropathy (Ewing, Campbell and Clarke, 1980). Clinical features of autonomic neuropathy in the presence of abnormal cardiovascular reflex tests carry a poor prognosis, with the experience in Edinburgh showing 50 per cent of affected patients dead within three to five years of recognition of the neuropathy (Figure 2.5) (Ewing *et al.*, 1980). Many of the deaths are due to other complications of diabetes, especially chronic renal failure, but it must be stressed that sudden

Table 2.2: Classification of diabetic neuropathy

Somatic neuropathy	Chronic peripheral neuropathy
	Acute peripheral neuritis
	Mononeuropathy
	Amyotrophy
Autonomic neuropathy	Multiple visceral involvement

Figure 2.5: Five-year survival curves for age and sex-matched general population (from Registrar General of Scotland, 1970–6) (○), age and sex-matched diabetic population from survey of all diabetics in Edinburgh (1968–73) (▲), 33 diabetics with normal (□) and 40 diabetics with abnormal (■) autonomic function tests

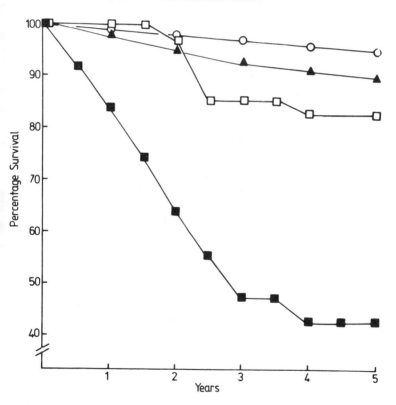

Source: From D.J. Ewing *et al*. (1980).

unexplained deaths can occur due to cardiorespiratory arrests especially in association with general anaesthesia, drugs which may suppress respiration (e.g. hypnotics), or chest infections. In some ways, the autonomic neuropathy may interfere with the control of respiration, but exactly how is not clear. It would appear from recent studies that the ventilatory response to hypoxia (carotid body chemoreceptor function) is intact and it may be that some central mechanism is implicated.

Clinical Features

Metabolic and microangiopathic factors are important in the development of diabetic neuropathy and, in addition, the affected nerves appear to be sensitive to damage to minor trauma, e.g. lateral popliteal nerve. Histologically the nerves show patchy segmental demyelination and axonal degeneration.

Somatic Neuropathy

Chronic Peripheral Neuropathy. This is the most common form of neuropathy and its prevalence increases with the duration of diabetes. The loss of appreciation of sensation, especially in the lower limbs, may result in repeated trauma leading to ulceration and infection (see the section below entitled 'diabetic foot'). In rare cases a Charcot arthropathy can develop with discomfort in walking if the mid-tarsal joint is affected. In severe cases there may be a wasting of the intrinsic muscles of the hand, but it is unusual for the patient to experience difficulty in fine hand movements. In occasional circumstances, the sensory neuropathy may be very severe in the upper limbs; if the patient is also blind from diabetic retinopathy, then the reading of braille may be difficult.

Treatment: There is no specific treatment for this painless form of neuropathy which follows a slowly progressive course. The patient should be advised about sensible footwear, avoidance of unnecessary trauma and visit a chiropodist regularly.

Acute Peripheral Neuritis. This principally causes symmetrical pain and paraesthesiae in the lower limbs, most often seen during poor control. In severe cases, especially in the older age-group, there can be marked weight loss and a carcinomatous neuropathy suspected, so-called diabetic neurogenic cachexia.

Treatment: The condition usually settles within a few months with good diabetic control. Excess alcohol should be avoided, as this aggravates the symptoms. Some form of analgesia is required and in a small number an antidepressant may help. Symptomatic relief may be variably obtained with drugs which directly 'influence neural tissue', e.g. quinine sulphate 600 mg at night, phenytoin 100 mg twice daily, or carbamazepine 100 mg three times daily.

Mononeuropathy. This can occur at any stage in the diabetic's lifetime and can affect either cranial or peripheral nerves. The lesions usually settle spontaneously, although occasionally surgical decompression may be necessary (e.g. for carpal tunnel syndrome or ulnar nerve compression at the elbow).

Amyotrophy. This is an uncommon condition of combined features of peripheral neuropathy and severe proximal muscle wasting. It is usually seen in newly diagnosed non-insulin-dependent patients, and is subsequently controlled as a rule without insulin treatment. Intensive physiotherapy over a period of months is required to restore muscle power.

Autonomic Neuropathy

Autonomic neuropathy may give rise to many symptom complexes affecting virtually all systems in the body (Figure 2.6). It is impossible to discuss all of these abnormalities in detail and for further information the reader is referred to a comprehensive review of this complication (Clarke, Ewing and Campbell, 1979). Many of these symptoms are distressing (e.g. postural hypotension, impotence, diabetic diarrhoea). The presence of autonomic neuropathy can now be confirmed by a simple test of the autonomic nerve function based on cardiovascular reflexes, for example, Valsalva manoeuvre, postural blood pressure fall and the variation in heart rate during deep breathing.

Treatment: The treatment of diabetic autonomic neuropathy is symptomatic as there is no single therapy to reverse the damage done to the autonomic nerve fibres. Table 2.3 lists the outline of management available for some of these distressing complications. They are in the main palliative procedures and in some cases the treatment for one complication may aggravate another, for example, probantheline used in sweating abnormalities may worsen gastric atony or urinary retention.

Figure 2.6: Syndromes of diabetic autonomic neuropathy

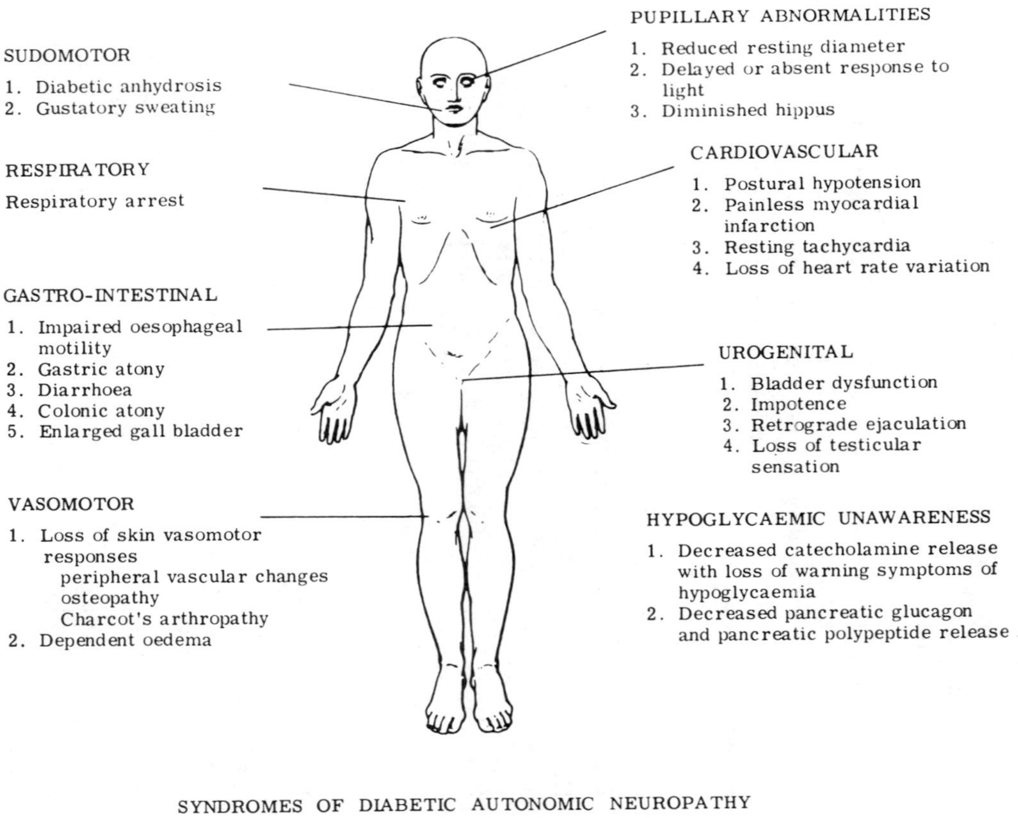

SUDOMOTOR
1. Diabetic anhydrosis
2. Gustatory sweating

RESPIRATORY
Respiratory arrest

GASTRO-INTESTINAL
1. Impaired oesophageal motility
2. Gastric atony
3. Diarrhoea
4. Colonic atony
5. Enlarged gall bladder

VASOMOTOR
1. Loss of skin vasomotor responses
   peripheral vascular changes
   osteopathy
   Charcot's arthropathy
2. Dependent oedema

PUPILLARY ABNORMALITIES
1. Reduced resting diameter
2. Delayed or absent response to light
3. Diminished hippus

CARDIOVASCULAR
1. Postural hypotension
2. Painless myocardial infarction
3. Resting tachycardia
4. Loss of heart rate variation

UROGENITAL
1. Bladder dysfunction
2. Impotence
3. Retrograde ejaculation
4. Loss of testicular sensation

HYPOGLYCAEMIC UNAWARENESS
1. Decreased catecholamine release with loss of warning symptoms of hypoglycaemia
2. Decreased pancreatic glucagon and pancreatic polypeptide release

SYNDROMES OF DIABETIC AUTONOMIC NEUROPATHY

Source: From Taft, A.D., Campbell, I.W. and Seth, J. (1981) Diagnosis and Management of Endocrine Diseases, Blackwell

Table 2.3: Treatment of symptom complexes seen in diabetic
autonomic neuropathy

Symptom	Treatment
1. Postural hypotension	Fludrocortisone 0.1–0.3 mg, daily
2. Bladder dysfunction	Regular voiding
	Antibiotics for infection
	Catheterise to decompress
	Carbachol or distigmine (stimulate detruser muscle)
	Bladder neck resection
3. Impotence (see text)	Discussion with patient
	Prosthetic implant (Figure 2.8)
4. Hypoglycaemic unawareness	Careful control, adjust insulin
5. Diabetic anhydrosis	Probantheline, 15 mg, four times daily
Gustatory sweating	Poldine, 4 mg, four times daily
6. Gastric atony	Metoclopramide, 10 mg, three times daily
7. Diabetic diarrhoea	Symptomatic: Codeine phosphate 60 mg, three times daily
	Lomotil, two tablets, four times daily
	Oxytetracycline, 250 mg, four times daily
	? Cholestyramine, 4 g, three times daily
8. Cardiorespiratory arrests	Close monitoring during 'at risk' situations, e.g. general anaesthesia, chest infections

Impact of Neuropathic Complications

The principal impact from somatic neuropathy is the ease with which simple, often unrecognised, trauma can cause foot ulceration. This is discussed below in the section dealing with diabetic foot problems.

Autonomic neuropathy may cause a great deal of morbidity and distress. Postural hypotension may cause such severe dizziness that the diabetic is unable to get out and about readily. Urogenital problems may cause a poor urinary stream, overflow incontinence and a predisposition to recurrent urinary infection. Impotence is discussed in more detail later. Hypoglycaemic unawareness is a frightening experience especially for the immediate family. Relatives should be instructed in the use of subcutaneous or intramuscular glucagon (1 mg, given by such injection) as this may reverse the hypoglycaemia in approximately 40 per cent of cases and the recovery of consciousness will allow further oral carbohydrate administration. Sudomotor abnormalities, especially gustatory sweating, may be very embarrassing in public if the diabetic is dining out, as the facial sweating may be profuse. Gastric atony may mimic the gastrointestinal symptoms of uraemia with nausea and vomiting. As a result of the delay in the passage of food from the stomach to the small intestine, recurrent hypoglycaemia may be a problem for the insulin-dependent patient. Diarrhoea can be extremely distressing with frequent fluid stools, especially troublesome at night with faecal incontinence. It is thus embarrassing for a relatively young diabetic to have to be prescribed incontinence pads. Vasomotor abnormalities may result in a loss of vasomotor response to both heating and cooling with the patient either complaining of cold painful feet or alternatively of a burning sensation in the feet. The abnormal dilatation of small blood vessels in the feet can cause disorganisation of bony structure, diabetic osteopathy, and be a factor in the development of a Charcot arthropathy.

Impotence in Diabetic Men

Impotence is three to five times as common in the diabetic as in the non-diabetic male. It has been variously reported that approximately 50 per cent of all diabetic males will develop impotence. In a recent Edinburgh survey of 541 diabetic men, aged 20 to 59 years, 190 (35 per cent) were found to have erectile impotence (McCulloch *et al.*, 1980). As can be seen from Figure 2.7, the prevalence is far in excess of that given by Kinsey and his colleagues (1948) for a non-diabetic population. Although the impotence may be transient at the time of diagnosis or during episodes of poor control, the usual problem is of chronic impotence, of gradual onset, in patients who have had diabetes for some years. The loss of penile erection with normal libido follows damage to parasympathetic innervation of the erectile tissue, but other factors may contribute (Campbell and McCulloch, 1979). In the author's present experience, psychogenic factors are not a prominent feature. Plasma levels of gonadotrophins and testosterone are normal.

Treatment of erectile impotence in the diabetic is difficult. It is vital to explain to the diabetic and his spouse the nature of the impotence, in particular that it is not due to any lack of virility on the male's part but it is caused in some way by the diabetes. Treatment with either gonadotrophins or testosterone preparations is without benefit; in fact they may make the matter worse by increasing libido. One possible form of treatment is the surgical implantation inside the corpora cavernosa of an artificial prosthesis (Figure 2.8) which makes the penis turgid and sufficiently erect to allow intromission during coitus. The penis can be folded downwards without breaking the prosthesis and can be kept in this downward position by well-fitting underpants. It should be stressed, however, that experience with this treatment in the UK is

Figure 2.7: Relationship of impotence to age in diabetic and normal male subjects

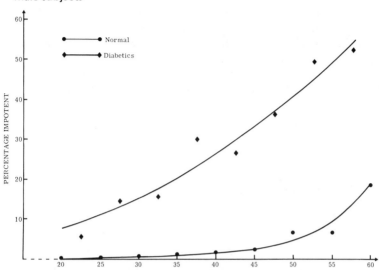

Source: The normal male data are derived from A.C. Kinsey *et al*. (1948). The diabetic male data are derived from D.K. McCulloch *et al*. (1980).

very limited, although it has been more widely used with success in several specialist centres in the USA.

Sexual Dysfunction in Diabetic Females

Although much more is known about sexual dysfunction in diabetic men, little is appreciated about it in the female diabetic. There are conflicting reports in several studies, some suggesting that about a third of diabetic women complained of 'non-orgasmic function' compared with 6 per cent in non-diabetic women; other studies have found no diminution in libido or fulfilment of the sex drive in female patients, irrespective of the presence or absence of neuropathy or other diabetic complications. In practice, this is a very difficult area to investigate and the female patient at the diabetic clinic rarely spontaneously complains of sexual dysfunction. However, patients with chronic renal failure and generalised atherosclerotic disease may very well have diminished libido because of the ill health associated with these problems.

Figure 2.8: Silicone prosthetic rods for implantation into penis (above) and a penis after implantation (below)

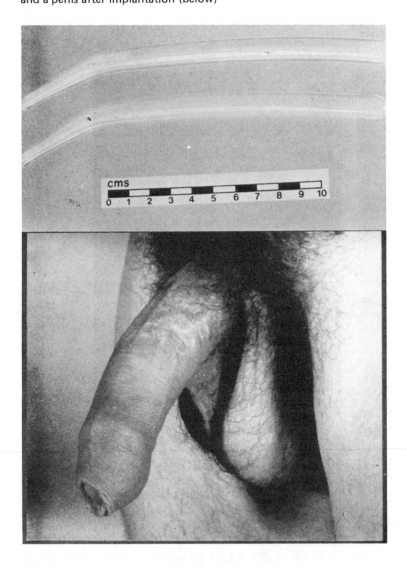

Source: From I.W. Campbell and D.K. McCulloch (1979).

The Diabetic Foot

Incidence and Prognosis

Gangrene of the foot and the threat of limb amputation is, as far as the diabetic patient is concerned, a dreaded complication of diabetes. Peripheral gangrene is much more common in diabetics than non-diabetics. Over the age of 40 years, one study showed it to be fifty times more common in diabetic males and seventy times more common in diabetic females. Approximately five out of every six lower-limb amputations are performed in diabetic patients.

It is difficult to estimate how common gangrene is in a diabetic population, but there are some facts as to its mortality and morbidity. In the Edinburgh mortality survey, it was a significant feature in the deaths of 29 male and 46 female diabetics (total deaths 1272) (Shenfield *et al.*, 1979). In another American series the in-hospital mortality following lower-limb amputation was 9 per cent, death being principally due to cardiovascular causes and septicaemia (Kahn, Wagner and Bessman, 1974). Even if this 1–2 month post-operative period is uneventful, the five-year survival rate for below-knee amputation in diabetics is about 35 per cent compared to 70 per cent in the non-diabetic (Cameron, Leonard-Jones and Robinson, 1964). This is simply a reflection that many diabetics who require a limb amputation have diffuse atherosclerotic disease and, in the few years following surgery, may die from myocardial infarction, congestive cardiac failure or cerebrovascular disease (see below).

Clinical Features

The diabetic foot represents a spectrum of disorders which may culminate in infection and gangrene. A combination of vascular insufficiency, neuropathy and infection is involved (Figure 2.9) to a variable extent from patient to patient, and it is important to determine the dominant factor in any particular case to plan effective treatment.

Vascular Insufficiency. Large blood vessels to the lower limbs may be atherosclerotic. In the diabetic this occurs at an earlier age, affects males and females equally, and tends to be more widespread than in non-diabetics with involvement often of the smaller peripheral leg arteries. However, 10 per cent of amputations in diabetics are performed in the presence of palpable foot pulses and the specific microangiopathy of diabetes, affecting small capillaries in the toes, can itself cause gangrene, ulceration and infection (Figure 2.9).

Figure 2.9: Interplay of vascular insufficiency, neuropathy and infection in the evolution of the diabetic foot

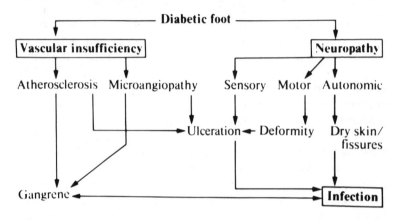

Source: From Toft, A.D., Campbell, I.W. and Seth, J. (1981) *Diagnosis and Management of Endocrine Disease*, Blackwell Scientific Publications, Oxford

Neuropathy. This affects the sensory, motor and autonomic fibres.

Sensory. Impairment of pain and temperature sensation results in unrecognised trauma, leading to ulceration and infection. The unappreciated trauma may result from ill-fitting shoes, a thread in a sock, hot-water bottles or electric-blanket burns, improper trimming of corns and calluses. All of these should be avoided with proper patient education. If sensory impairment is severe, there is also a loss of proprioception and, together with loss of pain appreciation, this contributes to the development of a Charcot's arthropathy.

Motor. Weakness and atrophy of the intrinsic muscles of the foot produce deformities such as clawing of the toes and prominent metatarsal heads.

Autonomic. Loss of the autonomic innervation of the skin causes the latter to become dry and brittle with resultant fissuring and infection. There is evidence that significant arterial venous shunting occurs in the diabetic foot, resulting in decreased capillary blood flow and this may be an important factor in the pathogenesis of indolent, neuropathic (or trophic) ulcers.

Infection. Ulceration caused by vascular insufficiency and neuropathy may become infected, resulting in local collections of pus or of spreading cellulitis. The characteristic odour of infected gangrene may be sensed. If the infection is untreated, it can result in further thrombosis in small blood vessels. If unchecked, the infection can spread deeply to cause osteomyelitis.

Available Treatment

This may be considered in three sections: prevention; medical management; and surgical management.

Prevention. All diabetic patients should be given advice regarding the care of feet. They should be instructed to wear socks of soft wool, well-fitting shoes and to avoid as far as possible walking in bare feet. Direct heat and cold should be avoided, for example, hot-water bottles and electric blankets. The feet should be washed in tepid water. Toe nails should be cut transversely and any corns and callosities treated by a chiropodist. If any inflammation or ulceration in the foot appears, then this should be reported immediately to the doctor or chiropodist. If the patient is a smoker, then advice should be given to stop smoking as this may lessen the risk of atherosclerotic damage.

Medical Management. If ulceration or gangrene develops, the diabetic will usually need to be admitted to hospital for treatment. Bed rest is important to relieve pressure areas and aid healing of neuropathic ulcers. A bed cage is often necessary to prevent friction of the sheets. On average, six to eight weeks in hospital is required to heal a neuropathic ulcer, but longer occasionally is necessary. If the ulcer is infected, a 'Eusol' dressing should be applied daily or twice daily. Once the area is clean, it should be left exposed to the air to granulate. Alternatively, a useful dressing regime is to apply porcine dermis. This need only be changed every two or three days in the early stages when the ulcer is dirty, but every five to ten days in the later stages of healing. This dressing initially cleans and desloughs the ulcer, and later promotes granulation. The relative infrequency of the dressing changes is also of value for nursing staff and lessens the discomfort to the patient (Bremner, Moffat and Lee, 1977). Antibiotics are important to treat any infection. As a deep-seated anaerobic infection may be present and difficult to identify bacteriologically, metronidazole should be added to other antibiotics which may be used, for example, flucloxacillin if a staphylococcal infection is present. 'Vasodilator' drugs have no proven value, but are worth a trial empirically if every measure is being undertaken to avoid amputation (for example, isoxsuprine, naftidrofuryl oxalate, oxpentifylline).

Surgical Management. If the sepsis is not satisfactorily controlled by antibiotics, then surgical drainage is necessary. A sympathectomy gives poor results in diabetics, possibly because many already have an 'auto-sympathectomy' due to pre-existing autonomic neuropathy. Bypass grafting may be of value for ischaemic foot reasons in diabetics if arteriography demonstrates localised disease in the femoral or popliteal arteries with patent vessels distal to the block. However, amputation becomes inevitable if well-established gangrene is present. Every effort should be made to preserve the knee-joint so that the prosthetic limb is fitted more easily. Even if the gangrene is confined to only one toe, local amputation only offers a one in three chance of immediate success and two-thirds of such diabetics presenting with a 'solitary black toe' go on to require a below-knee amputation within the next year.

In the absence of infection, amputation may be deferred for many months in the patient in whom gangrene is limited to one or two toes, as the diseased limb is preferable to an artificial leg provided the patient is not experiencing severe pain. In such patients, occasionally 'auto-amputation' may result: the devitalised toe(s) drop off from the foot and subsequently only minor surgical trimming of the proximal bone may be necessary. Figure 2.10 illustrates the extensive dry gangrene of the foot in a 66-year-old diabetic female with clinical evidence of vascular insufficiency and neuropathy. The lesion remained free of infection and the patient relatively pain-free for one year, after which the gangrene became even more extensive with infection, necessitating a below-knee amputation.

Impact of Diabetic Foot

The patient who is having medical treatment for a diabetic foot lesion is often aware that amputation may be necessary and often endures prolonged pain and discomfort without telling the nurses or doctors or even relatives for fear of amputation. Some patients with recurrent foot ulcers may lose a lot of time off work because of frequent hospital attendance or admission. In some cases employment may be impossible, for example, where driving is necessary for work and this is not feasible as the foot requires 'resting'. Sedentary work in offices is preferable in these circumstances. It should be stressed to the family and patient

Figure 2.10: Gangrene of the foot in a 66-year-old diabetic female showing extensive tissue necrosis of the forefoot

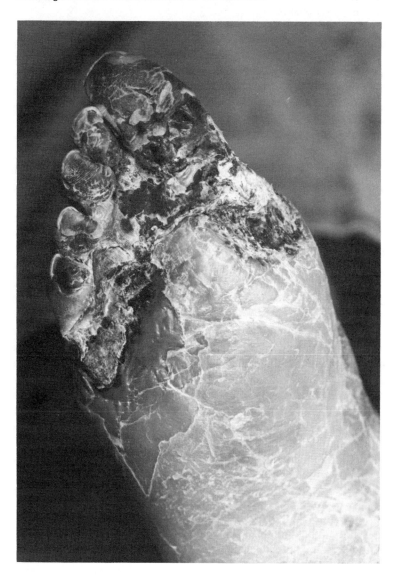

that, although conservative medical treatment of foot lesions is often time-consuming, the preservation of the foot wherever possible gives the best functional result.

Where amputation is required, even if only for a toe, then there is a lengthy hospital stay, on average two months and often longer (Cameron *et al.*, 1964). Thereafter, there follows the rehabilitation period during which a specialised artificial limb is fitted and regular visits are made to the appliance centre for the appropriate physiotherapy. Set-backs might include further amputations, often higher; the fitting of an above-knee prosthesis is more difficult than a below-knee appliance. Similarly, those patients with bilateral amputations have much greater rehabilitation problems. Some patients, albeit often elderly and generally frail, cannot adapt to a prosthesis and in these circumstances the prescription of a wheelchair is most appropriate to make the patient reasonably independent. Thus, it is important to stress to the diabetic and family that the amputation of the leg does not commonly lead to an early discharge from hospital, but rather is the first step in a prolonged rehabilitation programme.

Atherosclerosis in Diabetes Mellitus

Atherosclerosis is common among diabetics, and unlike non-diabetics affects males and females equally. The lesion is identical to that in the non-diabetic, but occurs at an earlier age and usually progresses more quickly. There is thus an increased prevalence of coronary artery disease compared with non-diabetics. Epidemiological studies have shown not only an increased mortality from atherosclerotic vascular disease in diabetics, but also an increased morbidity from angina, myocardial infarction, cardiac failure, intermittent claudication, ischaemic feet lesions and cerebrovascular accidents. In the Edinburgh mortality survey 335 males (66 per cent) and 561 females (73 per cent) died of vascular disease (Shenfield *et al.*, 1979). There was a predominance of myocardial infarction in the males and cerebrovascular disease in the females. In the UK survey of deaths of diabetics under 50 years of age, atherosclerotic vascular disease accounted for 41 per cent of all deaths (Tunbridge, 1981). The commonest death was ischaemic heart disease (31 per cent) with cerebrovascular accidents accounting for 7 per cent and other vascular disease 3 per cent.

Many factors have been implicated in the increased tendency to atherosclerosis in diabetics such as hyperglycaemia, hyperinsulinaemia and hyperlipidaemia; the latter occurs in 30-40 per cent of diabetics with an elevation in fasting VLDL triglycerides being the commonest abnormality. Obesity and hypertension are more common in the diabetic than general population. In addition, work in recent years has shown a diverse range of haematological abnormalities which may favour intravascular thrombosis in those already having atheroma. Some of these abnormalities include increased platelet adhesiveness and agglutinability, decreased fibrinolytic activity, increased blood viscosity at low and high shear rates, and abnormalities of various coagulation factors. Many of these are secondary to hyperglycaemia and return to normal with a correction of hyperglycaemia by improving diabetic control. It must be stressed also that in addition to atherosclerotic disease involving large and median-sized arteries being important in producing tissue ischaemia, diabetic microangiopathy is also an important contributory factor and this is invariably present in long-standing diabetics. Median-artery calcification (Mönckeberg's sclerosis) is also seen in long-standing diabetics, many with severe neuropathy, involving pelvic and limb vessels as well as smaller digital vessels. However, its presence does not necessarily imply impaired circulation of the blood flow.

In the remainder of this section on atherosclerotic disease there will be mention of specific points regarding morbidity and mortality of coronary artery disease, peripheral vascular disease and cerebrovascular disease in diabetics. In addition, special points in the management of coronary artery disease will be discussed. The epidemiological data for morbidity and mortality is taken principally from the sixteen-year follow-up study in the Framingham population (Garcia *et al.*, 1974). The impact to the immediate family of premature vascular disease and especially coronary artery disease will be dealt with in Chapters 7 and 17 below.

Coronary Artery Disease

Coronary artery disease is twice as common in diabetics as in non-diabetics. Angina, myocardial infarction, cardiac failure, arrhythmias and sudden death from myocardial infarction are all more frequent. The chances of a diabetic dying suddenly from a myocardial infarction are twice that of a non-diabetic, and there is a fourfold increase of death from cardiac failure. In addition to coronary artery disease, some cardiac deaths may be attributable to 'diabetic cardiomyopathy' with microangiopathy of the small vessels in the myocardium. The exact incidence of this is as yet unknown, but preliminary studies have shown in some diabetics abnormal myocardial function demonstrated by echocardiography, and histological changes have been described in small intramural vessels similar to the microangiography seen in the retina and kidney.

Special Points in the Management of Coronary Artery Disease in the Diabetic

Angina. The principles of treatment of angina are basically the same as those in the non-diabetic, but a number of points should be borne in mind:

Glyceral trinitrate. This and the vasodilator drugs must be used with care in patients with autonomic neuropathy as they may aggravate postural hypotension. Perhexilene maleate, also of value in the treatment of angina, may cause somatic or autonomic neuropathy.

β-Adrenoceptor antagonists. These drugs should be used with caution in diabetics. In patients receiving insulin or sulphonylureas, non-selective agents (e.g. propranolol, oxprenolol, sotalol) may mask the sympathomimetic effects of hypoglycaemia and may also delay recovery from hypoglycaemia by impairing gluconeogenesis and glycogenolysis. Thus, cardioselective drugs such as atenolol or metoprolol are preferred. All β-adrenoceptor antagonists, and especially the non-selective preparations, not only cause Raynaud's phenomena but also worsen the symptoms of peripheral vascular disease.

Coronary artery bypass surgery. This is not offered as often to diabetic patients because they often have other complications of diabetes such as nephropathy which preclude this operation. However, if the diabetic has severe angina uncontrolled by drugs and if there are not other complications of diabetes, coronary artery bypass surgery as a surgical relief of angina may be considered as with non-diabetics.

Acute Myocardial Infarction

Where autonomic neuropathy is present, myocardial infarction may sometimes be painless. Diabetic control may deteriorate due to the metabolic stress associated with an infarction, and it is usual practice to control non-insulin-dependent diabetics with insulin in the acute post-infarction phase. Patients with poor diabetic control show a higher mortality than those with good control.

Peripheral Vascular Disease

Intermittent claudication is four times as common in diabetics as non-diabetics. In a recent American survey, 8 per cent of diabetic patients had evidence of peripheral vascular disease at the time of diagnosis of diabetes (Melton *et al.*, 1980). It was estimated that the incidence of subsequent peripheral vascular disease at 10 years was 15 per cent rising to 45 per cent at 20 years after the diagnosis of diabetes.

The role of peripheral vascular disease in 'diabetic foot' lesions and the problem of the rehabilitation of the amputee has been discussed above. Unfortunately, various investigations such as arteriography and ultra-angiography usually show marked narrowing of vessels distal to the popliteal artery and arterial surgery is not feasible in these cases.

Cerebrovascular Disease

Cerebrovascular accidents, both fatal and non-fatal, are two to three times as common in diabetics. The postural hypotension of autonomic neuropathy may also increase the risk of cerebrovascular accidents by diminishing cerebral perfusion when the patient is in the erect position. In addition, it has been shown recently that insulin-dependent diabetics are prone to sudden unexplained reductions in cerebral blood flow (Dandona *et al.*, 1979). This may be an important aetiological factor in the development of cerebral infarction in those in whom perfusion is already marginal as a result of atherosclerosis.

Conclusion

Nearly all insulin-dependent diabetics are free of chronic complications when diagnosed and remain free for some years. There is now indisputable evidence that raised plasma–glucose concentrations over a period of years is a major factor in causing complications. It is thus very important to get as good control as possible of the blood-sugar levels to attempt to delay the onset of complications, slow down their rate of progression, or even reverse them. It can be seen that conventional insulin treatment does not always prevent the development of disabling or fatal complications. At the present time, much research is being made into new approaches to insulin therapy, such as assessing various mini-pumps for continuous subcutaneous or intravenous insulin delivery in an attempt to see if it is possible to achieve metabolic control with as near normal blood-glucose levels as possible. Whether it is possible to continue such treatment over a long period of years remains to be seen.

Finally, pancreatic transplantation, usually in association with renal transplantation, has been carried out in a few specialised centres, but this treatment is still regarded as experimental and not available routinely (leading article, *Lancet*, 1982). In the few successfully transplanted patients, there has been a return of normal carbohydrate tolerance and the diabetic no longer requires insulin and eats a normal diet. Little can be said as yet about the influence of pancreatic transplantation on diabetic complications, but preliminary studies have suggested an improvement in retinal and neuropathic abnormalities, and biopsy specimens of transplanted kidneys have not shown changes of diabetic glomerulosclerosis two years after transplantation.

Acknowledgements

I wish to thank Mr W.R.D. MacIntyre and Miss H. Clark of the Medical Photography Department, Victoria Hospital, Kirkcaldy, for their assistance in preparing the illustrations, and Miss Wilma Cairns and Mrs Margaret Frew for secretarial help.

References

Bremner, D.N., Moffat, L.E.F. and Lee, D. (1977) 'Porcine dermis as a temporary ulcer dressing', *Practitioner*, 218, 708–11

Cameron, H.C., Leonard-Jones, J.E. and Robinson, M.P. (1964) 'Amputations in the diabetic: outcome and survival', *Lancet*, ii, 605–7

Campbell, I.W. and McCulloch, D.K. (1979) 'Marital problems in diabetics', *Practitioner*, 223, 343–7

Clarke, B.F., Ewing, D.J. and Campbell, I.W. (1979) 'Diabetic autonomic neuropathy', *Diabetologia*, 17, 195–212

Dandona, P., James, I.M., Woolard, M.L., Newbury, P. and Beckett, A.G. (1979) 'Instability of cerebral blood-flow in insulin-dependent diabetics', *Lancet*, ii, 1203–5

Deckert, T., Simonsen, S.E. and Poulsen, J.E. (1967) 'Prognosis of proliferative retinopathy in juvenile diabetics', *Diabetes*, 16, 728–33

Deckert, T., Anderson, A.R., Christiansen, J.S. and Anderson, J.K. (1981) 'Courses of diabetic nephropathy. Factors related to development', *Acta Endocrinologica*, suppl. 242, 14–15

Ewing, D.J., Campbell, I.W. and Clarke, B.F. (1980) 'The natural history of diabetic autonomic neuropathy', *Quarterly Journal of Medicine*, 49, 95–108

Garcia, H.J., McNamara, P.M., Gordon, T. and Kannell, W.B. (1974) 'Morbidity and mortality in diabetics in the Framingham population: sixteen-year follow-up study', *Diabetes*, 23, 105–11

Kahn, O., Wagner, W. and Bessman, A.N. (1974) 'Mortality of diabetic patients treated surgically for lower limb infection and/or gangrene', *Diabetes*, 23, 287–92

Kinsey, A.C., Pomeroy, W.B. and Martin, C.E. (1948) 'Age and sexual outlet', in *Sexual Behaviour in the Human Male*, Saunders, Philadelphia, pp. 218–62

Leading article (1982) 'Transplantation of pancreas with kidney', *Lancet*, i, 720–1

McCulloch, D.K., Campbell, I.W., Wu, F.U., Prescott, R.J. and Clarke, B.F. (1980) 'The prevalence of diabetic impotence', *Diabetologia*, 18, 279–83

Melton, L.J., Macken, K.M., Palumbo, P.J. and Elveback, L.R. (1980) 'Incidence and prevalence of clinical peripheral vascular disease in a population-based cohort of diabetic patients', *Diabetes Care*, 3, 650–4

Najarian, J.W., Sutherland, D.E.R., Simmons, R.L., Howard, R.J., Kellstrand, C.M., Ramsay, R.C., Goetz, F.C., Fryd, D.S. and Sommer, B.G. (1979) 'Ten year experience with renal transplanation in juvenile onset diabetics', *Annals of Surgery*, 190, 487–500

Pirart, J. (1978) 'Diabetes mellitus and its degenerative complications: a prospective study of 4400 patients observed between 1947 and 1973', *Diabetes Care*, 1, 168–88

Shenfield, G.M., Elton, R.A., Bhalla, I.P. and Duncan, L.J.P. (1979) 'Diabetic mortality in Edinburgh', *Diabète et Métabolisme*, 5, 149–58

Tunbridge, W.M.G. (1981) 'Factors contributing to deaths of diabetics under fifty years of age', *Lancet*, ii, 569–72

3 PALLIATIVE CARE IN CHRONIC DISEASES OF THE LIVER AND BILIARY TRACT

Niall D.C. Finlayson

Chronic Liver Disease

Chronic hepatitis, cirrhosis and malignant disease are the three hepatic conditions which sooner or later lead to death, and they will be the subjects of this chapter.

Chronic Hepatitis

Chronic hepatitis is a well-recognised but nebulous entity which can only be diagnosed with certainty when clinical and/or biochemical evidence of liver disease has been present for more than six months. A definitive diagnosis requires that a liver biopsy be examined, and the clinical features, biochemical liver function tests and the liver biopsy findings are then used to determine which of two major forms of chronic hepatitis are present.

Chronic Persistent Hepatitis. Chronic persistent hepatitis is characterised by ill-defined malaise, anorexia and upper abdominal discomfort, and it may be discovered incidentally. There are no physical features of chronic liver disease, liver function tests are only mildly deranged and liver biopsy shows a normal hepatic lobular structure with a chronic inflammatory reaction confined to the portal tracts. The prognosis is excellent and no treatment is required; progression to cirrhosis is rare, but justifies a periodic review of these patients.

Chronic Active Hepatitis (CAH). This is a much more severe condition, although milder forms of the illness are being recognised increasingly.

CAH associated with autoantibodies. The most florid CAH usually occurs in young women, although it can occur in either sex and at any age. Half the patients are less than 30 years old and three-quarters are women. The disease can start suddenly or insidiously, and progresses with exacerbations, during which liver failure may occur, and remissions to the development of cirrhosis and its complications. Exacerbations are characterised by malaise, anorexia, jaundice and amenorrhoea in women, and clinical examination frequently reveals signs of chronic liver disease such as spider telangiectasia or hepatosplenomegaly. Systemic features are common and include a Cushingoid appearance, skin rashes, athralgia or arthritis and purpura. Associated disease may also be found including Hashimoto's disease, diabetes mellitus, renal tubular acidosis and autoimmune haemolytic anaemia.

Liver function tests in an exacerbation show particularly a very high serum transaminase activity, hyperbilirubinaemia, some increase of alkaline phosphatase activity, and a low serum albumin concentration and a prolonged prothrombin time due to poor liver function, and marked hyperglobulinaemia. Autoimmune abnormalities are characteristic of this disease; more than half the patients have antinuclear or smooth muscle antibodies in the blood, about a quarter have antimitochondrial antibodies and autoantibodies associated with other diseases, such as thyroid disorders, or autoimmune haemolytic anaemia may also be present. The LE cell phenomenon is found in 15-30 per cent of patients, especially during an exacerbation. On the other hand, this condition is not associated with hepatitis B virus infection and the hepatitis B surface antigen (HBsAg) test is negative.

These patients have a serious illness; 33–67 per cent die within five years of the onset and less than 20 per cent survive beyond ten years if treatment with corticosteroid drugs is not given. Treatment (see pp. 58-62 below) has reduced the early mortality substantially, but unfortunately it may not prevent the development of cirrhosis of the liver and its complications at a later date.

CAH without autoantibodies. Much milder clinical forms of chronic active hepatitis have become recognised with the increasing awareness of this condition. They come to attention when an episode of apparent viral hepatitis fails to resolve, from the development of cirrhosis or quite accidently. Physical evidence of liver disease is much less frequent, with hepatomegaly the most common sign, and systemic features other than arthralgia are uncommon. Liver function tests are usually not grossly deranged and autoimmune abnormalities are rare. A substantial proportion of these patients have the HBsAg in the blood, indicating a chronic hepatitis B virus infection. Corticosteroid therapy is of doubtful value for these patients, and may actually be harmful for those with chronic hepatitis B virus infection.

Hepatic Cirrhosis

Cirrhosis is a chronic condition in which hepatocellular necrosis and regeneration, inflammation and fibrosis over a prolonged period cause substantial and irreversible damage to the architecture of the whole of the liver. Liver-cell necrosis leads eventually to hepatic failure, damage to the hepatic vasculature leads to portal hypertension and abnormal liver-cell regeneration may give rise to hepatocellular carcinoma. Cirrhosis is a relatively common disease, although its frequency varies greatly between countries (Table 3.1), and it is a major cause of morbidity.

Table 3.1: Death rates from cirrhosis in adults in various countries (1971–2)

Country	Rate (per 100,000 population aged over 25 years per year)
France	57.2
Italy	52.1
West Germany	39.6
Spain	38.3
United States	28.6
Japan	21.8
Canada	19.6
Sweden	15.6
New Zealand	8.2
United Kingdom	5.7

Source: Data from *World Health Statistics Annual Volume 1: Vital Statistics and Causes of Death*, World Health Organisation, Geneva, 1972.

The clinical features of cirrhosis are many and varied, and they increase with the duration and severity of the disease. Initially, general health is good, but as the disease progresses lassitude and anorexia develop, episodic nausea may reduce the appetite further, and eventually weight loss and a deterioration in the general nutritional state occurs. Liver failure and portal hypertension eventually give rise to fluid retention, manifest as ascites or oedema, encephalopathy, bleeding from oesophagogastric varices and renal failure. The most common and important findings on physical examination are jaundice, hepatosplenomegaly (sometimes with dilated collateral vessels visible on the abdomen and chest reflecting portal hypertension), spider telangiectasia, palmar erythema and testicular atrophy in men. Skin pigmentation, Dupuytren's contracture and gynaecomastia may also be present. Kayser–Fleischer rings are very important manifestations of Wilson's disease, and diabetes mellitus should raise the suspicion of haemo-chromatosis.

Investigations are designed to substantiate the diagnosis of cirrhosis, usually by liver biopsy, to discover a cause (see p. 57 below), to detect any complication such as hepatocellular carcinoma, and to deter-mine the presence of portal hypertension and especially oesophago-gastric varices. Liver function tests do not show any characteristic feature. The serum bilirubin concentration, the serum albumin con-centration and the prothrombin time are rough measures of hepatic dysfunction, the serum transaminase is an indication of the activity of the liver disease and the serum alkaline phosphate gives a measure of cholestasis. The peripheral blood count frequently shows a mild anaemia, often macrocytic, and leucopoenia or (more often) throm-bocytopoenia is usually due to hypersplenism consequent on portal hypertension.

The overall prognosis for patients with cirrhosis is gloomy, for in large series more than three-quarters die within five years of diagnosis. However, this depressing picture should not be allowed to obscure the fact that certain patients do well. The mortality in cirrhosis is especially high in the first six months after diagnosis, as many patients present with severe complications such as bleeding from varices, ascites, en-cephalopathy or hepatocellular carcinoma. Patients without such com-plications who have liver function tests indicating good liver function can live for many years in good health. This is often the case in primary biliary cirrhosis, in which patients frequently present at an early stage on account of itching. Prolonged survival with a good quality of life can also result where the cause of the liver disease can be treated, even though the cirrhosis itself cannot be cured, as in chronic active hepatitis, haemochromatosis and Wilson's disease, and where a patient with alcoholic cirrhosis stops drinking.

Malignant Disease

Hepatocellular carcinoma is the most common malignant tumour in humans, owing to its high frequency in Africa and in certain parts of the Far East (Table 3.2). It is much less common in Europe and North America. Chronic hepatitis B virus infection has been recognised increasingly as an important cause of the tumour, especially in areas of high incidence where chronic carriage of the virus is common and where the tumours occurs at a relatively young age. Cirrhosis has also been recognised as an important antecedent to hepatocellular carcinoma throughout the world, and it is found in about three-quarters

Table 3.2: The frequency of hepatocellular carcinoma in young males (15–44 years) in various countries

Country	Rate (per 100 000/year)
Mozambique	164.6
Nigeria	10.2
Uganda	6.5
Singapore	4.1
Chile	1.1
Scotland	0.4
Australia	0.2
United States	0.2

Source: Data from R. Doll (1969) 'The geographical distribution of cancer', *British Journal of Cancer*, 23, 1.

of patients. Hepatocellular carcinoma can arise in any form of cirrhosis, but seems most frequent in haemochromatosis and least frequent in biliary cirrhosis and chronic active hepatitis not associated with chronic hepatitis B virus infection. Males predominate among patients with hepatocellular carcinoma, and hormonal factors may account for this.

Patients with hepatocellular carcinoma most often complain of weight loss, abdominal pain, anorexia and fatigue, and examination often shows hepatomegaly, sometimes with a bruit on auscultation over the liver which is virtually diagnostic, ascites, splenomegaly and deepening jaundice. About half the patients also have the clinical features of an underlying cirrhosis. Investigations are designed to identify the tumour in the liver, to determine whether it can be removed surgically, to detect concomitant cirrhosis and to assess overall liver function. Imaging, usually with radionuclides or ultrasound, liver biopsy and looking for an increased alphafetoprotein concentration in the blood are used to diagnose the tumour, imaging and angiography are used to determine the feasibility of surgery and liver function tests give a measure of the functional state of the liver (see p. 55 above). These investigations will also allow concomitant cirrhosis to be detected.

The prognosis for patients with hepatocellular carcinoma is poor, and in most patients the tumour cannot be resected (see p. 80 below).

Treating the Causes of Chronic Liver Disease

There are numerous causes of chronic liver disease (Table 3.3). It is important to determine the cause wherever possible, as withdrawal of a toxic agent or application of some other treatment may prevent progression to cirrhosis, slow the rate of progression in established

Table 3.3: Causes of chronic liver disease

Infection
    Viral hepatitis   Hepatitis B virus
                                       Non-A, non-B hepatitis virus (es)
    Other infections   Brucellosis
                                         Congenital syphilis

Drugs/toxins
    Alcohol
    Other drugs   Aspirin, datrolene, halothane, immuno-
                                       suppressive drugs, isoniazid, methyldopa,
                                       nitrofurantoin, perhexiline, phenylbutazone,
                                       propylthiouracil, sulphonamides

Biliary obstruction
    Primary biliary cirrhosis
    Secondary biliary cirrhosis
                                       Adults: strictures, stones, neoplasms,
                                       sclerosing cholangitis
                                       Children: biliary atresia, choledochal cyst,
                                       Caroli's syndrome

Hepatic congestion
    Budd-Chiari syndrome
    Veno-occlusive disease
    Cardiac failure

Metabolic disorders
    Haemochromatosis (primary and secondary)
    Wilson's disease
    α_1-Antitrypsin deficiency
    Fibrocystic disease
    Galactosaemia
    Glycogen storage disease
    Tyrosinosis
    Fructose intolerance
    β-Lipoproteinaemia
    Lipoatrophic diabetes

Nutritional
    Intestinal bypass operations for obesity

Granulomatous disease
    Sarcoidosis

Inflammation ('autoimmune')
    Chronic active hepatitis
    Cryptogenic cirrhosis
    Inflammatory bowel disease
    Indian childhood cirrhosis

Other
    Hereditary haemorrhagic telangiectasia

---

cirrhosis or be important in preventing disease in relatives where a hereditary disorder is found.

Alcohol (ethyl alcohol). Alcohol is the cause of a half or more of all the chronic liver disease in Europe and North America. The risk of developing cirrhosis increases in proportion to the amount and duration of drinking alcohol. The risk is clearly increased for males consuming 80 g of alcohol (4–6 normal drinks) daily for more than ten years, and the amount and duration of drinking required to produce disease in women is perhaps only one-half that for men. The value of abstinence once cirrhosis has developed has been disputed, but most investigators believe that patients who stop drinking have a better prognosis and the author takes this view. Abstinence also brings better general health and improved social conditions, which add immeasurably to the quality of life. Every effort should therefore be made to persuade patients to stop drinking altogether.

Corticosteroid Drugs. Chronic active hepatitis, especially when florid and associated with autoantibodies in the blood (see p. 52 above), is benefited greatly by treatment with corticosteroid and immunosuppressive drugs. Prednisolone or prednisone are the drugs of choice in an acute exacerbation. Prednisolone 40 mg/d should be given initially and reduced at not less than weekly intervals as the clinical condition and liver function tests improve. Long-term treatment is always needed, and most patients relapse within about three months when treatment is stopped, even after several years of therapy. The maintenance dose of prednisolone should be less than 15 mg/d if serious side-effects are to be avoided; where this cannot be achieved or where side-effects are a problem the addition of azathioprine 50–100 mg/d usually allows the dose of prednisolone to be reduced. Maintenance treatment should never be withdrawn within a year of achieving full remission, and a liver biopsy should be done first to ensure that the pathological abnormalities have regressed.

Metabolic Diseases. Idiopathic haemochromatosis and Wilson's disease are very important, as effective treatment is available for both, and asymptomatic but affected relatives need treatment as well as patients. Idiopathic haemochromatosis is suspected by finding a high serum iron concentration ($>$ 36 μmol/l; $>$ 200 μg/dl), a highly saturated serum iron-binding capacity ($>$ 70 per cent), and a high serum ferritin concentration ($>$ 1000 μg/l), and is confirmed by a liver biopsy showing a marked increase of hepatic iron for which no cause can be found. Treatment is by the weekly venesection of 500 ml of blood (250 mg) until the serum iron and ferritin concentrations are normal, and thereafter for life at intervals as required to keep these measurements normal. Wilson's disease should be suspected in any chronic liver disease starting before the age of 30 years. Neurological abnormalities, Kayser–Fleischer rings, a low serum ceruloplasmin concentration ($<$ 200 μg/l) and a family history of hepatic and/or neurological disease are usually sufficient to confirm the diagnosis. Sometimes, measures of serum copper ($<$ 70 μg/l), urine ($>$ 1.75 μmol/day; $>$ 100 μg/day) and liver copper ($>$ 250 μg/g of dry liver) are needed for diagnosis, and testing the ability to produce ceruloplasmin using radioactive copper (^{64}Cu) is occasionally necessary. Penicillamine (1.5 (range 1-4) g/day) in a dose to produce an adequate cupriuresis ($>$ 35 μmol/day; $>$ 2000 μg/day) is the treatment of choice, and this treatment needs to be continued for life, even during pregnancy, as the drug does not produce foetal abnormalities. Penicillamine can produce serious side-effects, but fortunately this is rare in Wilson's disease; triethylene tetramine dihydrochloride is the next drug of choice when penicillamine cannot be used.

Other Treatments. Other forms of cirrhosis may be susceptible to treatment. Drugs taken prior to the onset of liver disease should be reviewed and any that are not essential for the patient should be stopped, as some drugs have been suspected of causing chronic liver disease (Table 3.3). Biliary obstruction in the large extrahepatic bile ducts should be relieved whenever possible. Intestinal bypass operations for obesity should be reversed if evidence of liver disease occurs.

General Treatment of Chronic Liver Disease

The importance attached to general measures in acute diseases for which curative treatment is available has diminished greatly and often no more than lip-service is paid to them. However, general measures remain important in chronic disease for which there is no cure, because they emphasise the value of assisting the patient and his or her family in adjusting to the illness, the importance of paying attention to nutrition and the need to control the details of drug therapy so as to gain every possible advantage for the patient while minimising the undesirable effects of drugs and drug interactions. Good general treatment illustrates the dictum that attention to details leads to perfection and perfection is not a detail.

The Patient and the Family. Patients with chronic liver disease and their families need the continuing care of a kindly interested physician in the same way as do patients with any other form of chronic disease. They need continuing care from one or two physicians who know them well, and they need regular follow-up visits, even if every visit does not serve any specific 'medical' need, for such visits give encouragement and an opportunity to talk about problems which are not urgent enough to demand an immediate consultation. Hospital doctors are well advised to concentrate on patients with more advanced disease, who develop complications most often and who usually need several admissions to hospital. Such patients need at least 15 or 20 minutes at each out-patient visit, and they should as far as possible always be admitted to hospital under the care of the medical team to whom they are known. The patient's family also needs to know that the physician is interested in and cares about their difficulties, and they in turn contribute greatly to the success of the treatment by making the physician aware of failures of compliance by the patient and by helping more ill patients to keep to their treatment. The family may also need concrete help from available community services, such as domiciliary nursing or home helps, and the physician may need to initiate such help.

Nutrition. Malnutrition is common in cirrhosis, due mainly to in-adequate food intake resulting from anorexia and the unpalatable diets prescribed for some patients (see pp. 68 and 69 below). Alcoholics are at particular risk for they frequently suffer from dyspepsia, use their money to buy alcohol rather than food, and enjoy little or no orderly family life. Malabsorption is also common, especially where cholestasis (p. 74) is marked, and this may be made worse by drugs such as neomycin, lactulose and cholestyramine. Metabolic factors consequent on liver damage also contribute to malnutrition.

The physician should make a point of speaking to the patient and, more important, to the person who cooks the patient's food about the importance of diet. The diet should contain about 2500 cal/day and should comprise about 60–80 g of protein, provided there is no en-cephalopathy (p. 70) or fluid retention (p. 65), and adequate minerals and vitamins which may be given as supplements in the form of iron, calcium and vitamin D (p. 76), and multivitamin preparations. Fat should be reduced below 40 g/day in patients with steatorrhoea, which is particularly common when cholestasis is marked. Regular eating habits and food attractively presented to tempt the patient's appetite, in amounts which are not so large as to be immediately deterring, are important. Specific advice for the patient's cook from a dietician is of inestimable value. The diet has to be modified when encephalopathy (p. 71) or fluid retention (p. 77) is present or if the patient has diabetes mellitus (Chapter 2), which is relatively common in cirrhosis and especially haemochromatosis.

The Use of Drugs. Every patient with chronic liver disease will sooner or later require drug therapy, and the need for drugs becomes greater as the disease progresses. Unfortunately, the liver is the most important organ in drug metabolism and failing liver function impairs the patient's ability to metabolise drugs. Toxic reactions are consequently common, if the physician does not take special care. The general guidelines are to use as few drugs as possible in patients with liver disease, to start treatment at the lower end of the therapeutic range and to increase the dose slowly to the minimum effective dose. It is also important to recognise patients who are especially likely to have a limited ability to metabolise drugs by virtue of advanced liver damage. Jaundice, ascites, encephalopathy, hypoalbuminaemia and a prolonged prothrombin time are the best means of identifying such patients, and the need for caution in drug treatment increases in relation to the number of these features present. Patients who have had portalsystemic shunt operations also have striking limitations on their capacity to metabolise drugs, as the shunt allows a large proportion of orally administered drugs to bypass the liver. Such patients should always be given drugs with particular care. Finally, some drugs are more likely to produce toxic effects than others. Drugs can be classified roughly into those which are avidly removed from the blood by the normal liver and those which are not. The normal metabolism of the former is highly sensitive to alterations in blood flow, so that reduced blood flow and shunting of blood past the liver cause a marked increase in the amount of drug in the peripheral blood and increase the liability to toxic reactions. Examples of such drugs are pethidine, propranolol and heminevrin. Drugs which are less avidly removed from the blood by the normal liver are less likely to cause trouble.

Patients with chronic liver disease may need any of the numerous drugs used in medicine at some time so that a comprehensive discussion of individual drugs here is impossible. Some drugs used frequently are discussed elsewhere in this chapter. Analgesic and psychotropic drugs, however, are frequently needed to treat pain, depression and insomnia and are often used as premedication for various investigations.

Analgesics. Powerful analgesics such as morphine, pethidine and methadone are all liable to produce encephalopathy in patients with chronic liver disease. The author has found that pethidine (100 mg) can be given intramuscularly to patients without any of the features of liver failure noted above (pp. 54-5), that half that amount can be given initially to those with any one of the features noted and that a quarter can usually be given to those with the most severe disease. Subsequent doses should be given as required and not on a regular basis in order to prevent overdosage. Simple analgesics are often required for headaches and other aches and pains. Paracetamol (0.5-1.0 mg) six to eight hourly can be used for two or three days. Salicylates should be avoided as they may precipitate bleeding from varices.

Psychotropics. These drugs are potent causes of encephalopathy and need to be used cautiously. Diazepam can be given intravenously slowly prior to procedures such as endoscopy, but the dose required does not usually exceed 10 mg. Repeated oral doses for sedation or sleeping should use the smallest effective dose, and a benzodiazepine with a short half-life in the blood such as temazepam may be preferable.

Chlormethiazole is often given to alcoholics, but should be used very carefully in those with cirrhosis as its metabolism is much impaired and toxicity occurs readily. Phenothiazines also need to be given in minimal doses for the same reason. Depression is treated best with a tricyclic drug such as amitriptyline (25 mg thrice daily) as monoamine oxidase inhibitors readily produce drowsiness.

Treating Portal Hypertension (Bleeding)

Portal hypertension develops as a result of increased resistance to blood flow through the liver consequent on destruction and distortion of the hepatic vasculature, and it becomes increasingly common as chronic liver disease progresses. It causes gastrointestinal bleeding from varices, hypersplenism consequent on splenomegaly and it contributes to the development of ascites and possibly renal dysfunction. Gastrointestinal bleeding is much the most important effect, as it is a frequent cause of death in chronic liver disease; it alone will be discussed here. Hypersplenism is common, but is hardly ever of clinical significance as bleeding due to thrombocytopenia or recurrent infection from leucopenia is exceptional. Ascites and renal failure are discussed below (pp. 65 and 79 respectively).

Prognosis of Oesophageal Varices and Acute Variceal Bleeding. Gastrointestinal varices in cirrhosis are most common in the oesophagus and, to a lesser extent, the stomach, where they constitute an ever-present risk of acute bleeding; varices elsewhere in the gastrointestinal tract are uncommon, and acute bleeding from them is rare. The development of oesophagogastric varices in cirrhosis is therefore important, although where the liver function is good only one in four patients bleed in the five years after the varices are found and only a half of them die of that bleeding. Acute gastrointestinal bleeding in cirrhosis with varices is usually from the varices, but other sources of bleeding, usually gastric or duodenal erosions or ulcers, occur in about 20 per cent of patients, emphasising the need for diagnostic endoscopy in such bleeding patients. The precipitating factors for bleeding are poorly understood, but the most important are probably large varices, poor liver function and the ingestion of salicylate drugs. Acute bleeding from varices is usually severe and quickly leads to admission to hospital. The management of acute variceal bleeding is outside the scope of this chapter, but the important principles are rapid resuscitation, and measures to stop the varices bleeding including the use of vasopressin, balloon compression of the varices and occlusion of the varices by endoscopic sclerosis, or oesophageal transection transhepatic embolisation. The mortality of bleeding varices is high, and overall only a half of the patients survive; the severity of bleeding and the state of hepatic function determine the outcome. Three-quarters of patients requiring less than 5 l of blood survive, but only one-third of those needing more than 5 l of blood. Some 90 per cent of patients without jaundice, ascites or encephalopathy survive, a half with one of these features survive, a third with two survive and only a quarter with all three survive.

Preventing Recurrent Bleeding. Recurrent variceal bleeding is a major risk in patients who have bled from varices. Indeed, irrespective of the state of liver function, recurrent bleeding is the rule rather than the exception, although it occurs most frequently in those with poor liver function. It obviously constitutes a major threat to life, but it also means repeated hospital admissions for frightening and often uncomfortable treatment.

Portalsystemic Shunt Operations. The most certain way of preventing recurrent bleeding is an operation to construct a portalsystemic venous shunt, and several different operations have been described (Table 3.4). Unselective or total portalsystemic shunts divert all the portal blood away from the liver to the inferior vena cava and have been used for over thirty years. They give almost complete protection against

Table 3.4: Portalsystemic shunt operations

Unselective (total) shunts, i.e. divertion of all portal blood from the liver	Portacaval shunt end-to-side side-to-side Splenorenal shunt end-to-side side-to-side Mesenteric-caval shunt Interposition mesenterico-caval shunt
Selective shunts, i.e. only blood from variceal vessels diverted from the liver	Distal splenorenal shunt Coronary-caval shunt

rebleeding provided the shunt remains patent, which it does in all but a few per cent of cases in the hands of experienced surgeons. Unfortunately, patients need reasonably good liver function to undergo the operation; the mortality for those with good function is 2–5 per cent, for those with moderately impaired function 10–15 per cent and for those with poor function 30–50 per cent. Thus, only those with good or perhaps moderately impaired liver function can be considered. Furthermore, severe encephalopathy develops over about five years in a fifth or more of patients and this mars, and can ruin, the quality of a patient's life. Finally, recently completed controlled trials have shown that portacaval shunts do not prolong life.

These factors have led to a marked reduction in the use of unselective shunts, and have led to a search for better operations. Unselective shunts are thought to cause encephalopathy because they divert all the portal blood into the systemic circulation, thereby increasing the delivery of substances thought to cause encephalopathy from the gut to the brain (see p. 70) and decreasing liver blood flow with consequent impairment of liver function. Selective portalsystemic shunt operations have been devised to avoid this by decompressing the oesophagogastric varices through the spleen and distal part of the splenic vein to the left renal vein, or through the coronary (left gastric) vein to the inferior vena cava, while preserving the remaining portal blood flow to the liver. Selective portalsystemic shunts do achieve these aims, and they present rebleeding while avoiding the problem of severe encephalopathy at least in the early years after operation, but whether they prolong life is not yet known.

Endoscopic   Sclerotherapy. Endoscopic   sclerotherapy   aims   to obliterate the dangerous varices in the lower oesophagus without the risks of a major operation by repeated injection of sclerosant material into the variceal vessels. This can be done with a flexible endoscope and an average of 8–10 injections at two-weekly intervals is required. This treatment has been shown to reduce rebleeding significantly, although whether it prolongs life is not certain. Complications include oesophageal ulceration which generally heals well and oesophageal stricture which usually responds to endoscopic dilatation. It has the advantage of being applicable to all but those with markedly impaired blood coagulation.

Medical Therapy. Medical therapy aims to prevent rebleeding by reducing the portal pressure. This is done by β-receptor blockade of the mesenteric circulation with propranolol. The efficacy of this therapy remains to be proved.

There are currently conflicting views on the best treatment for patients with cirrhosis who have bled from varices. Portalsystemic shunt operations should probably be restricted to patients under 50 years of age with good liver function and a selective shunt should be done if possible. Endoscopic sclerotherapy can be recommended for other patients, and could also be used for those suitable for a shunt with the operation reserved for failure of sclerotherapy. Treatment with propranolol is not recommended until further evidence of its value is available.

Treating Fluid Retention (Ascites)

Liver failure causes marked retention of sodium by the kidneys, leading to a great increase in the total body sodium and water, and portal hypertension increases the mesenteric venous pressure which ensures that much of that sodium and water localises in the peritoneal cavity causing ascites. Hypoalbuminaemia is also common in such patients and it increases the tendency to ascites by reducing the colloid oncotic pressure of the blood. Patients with cirrhosis who develop ascites may also have peripheral oedema.

Diagnosis. Abdominal distension is the usual reason for patients presenting with ascites, although some also complain of abdominal discomfort or pain and a few with gross ascites may develop respiratory difficulty. Shifting dullness on abdominal percussion is the cardinal physical sign and it allows amounts of ascites exceeding 1–2 l to be detected. A fluid thrill can be elicited when ascites is marked and otherwise obvious. The umbilicus is often distorted or everted, a third to a half of patients have herniae — half of which are of the umbilical type — and some patients have peripheral oedema. Obesity is the most common cause of difficulty in diagnosing ascites, and in such cases an abdominal radiograph, ultrasonography or even paracentesis may be needed for diagnosis. Huge cysts, especially of the ovary, may also mimic ascites. Liver failure and portal hypertension are the usual reasons for ascites in patients with cirrhosis, but alternative causes should be considered, especially when features of these complications are not marked. Alternative causes related to cirrhosis include hepatocellular carcinoma and portal vein thrombosis, and others include any cause of ascites in patients without ascites. The possibility of spontaneous bacterial peritonitis in patients with cirrhosis and ascites should always be considered (p. 71) and the ascites fluid cultured.

Prognosis. The overall long-term outlook for patients with cirrhosis and ascites is poor; a half or more die within a year of first presentation and only about 10 per cent survive beyond five years. The prognosis is best when ascites is of rapid onset and due to a treatable cause (Table 3.5), when the response to treatment of the ascites is good and when diuretics are not required once the ascites is controlled.

Table 3.5: Precipitating causes of ascites in patients with cirrhosis

Gastrointestinal bleeding
Infection
Trauma (including surgery)
Portal venous thrombosis
Hepatocellular carcinoma
Alcohol abuse
Excessive sodium intake
    diet
      drugs (see Table 3.6)

General Principles of Treatment. Patients with marked ascites are treated best in hospital, for this facilitates the investigation of possible precipitating causes for the ascites (Table 3.5) and also allows better control over dietary and drug treatments. It is also the best way of stopping alcohol abuse, although it is not infallible in this regard!

The principles of treatment include the correction of causative factors, bed rest, restriction of sodium, and sometimes water, intake and the use of diuretic drugs. Most patients respond to this regimen, but other therapies are available for those who do not. Bed rest, sodium and water restriction and the correction of potassium depletion, with potassium chloride (100 mmol potassium daily) provided there is no uraemia, is the initial therapy, and this alone leads to diuresis in some 5-10 per cent of patients with good liver function. Patients who do not lose at least 2 kg in weight over four days are given diuretic drugs. These can sometimes be stopped once the ascites is controlled, but more often they are required on a long-term basis.

Bed Rest. Patients with ascites are most comfortable sitting up in bed, and slight elevation of the legs may facilitate the removal of peripheral oedema. There is no evidence, however, that bed rest is of any value for the ascites itself, and the patient must be encouraged to become mobile as soon as sufficient diuresis has occurred to make this feasible.

Sodium and Water Restriction. Patients with ascites do not generally lose more than 10 mmol of sodium daily in the urine, and other sodium losses amount to only about 1 mmol daily. In practice, a daily intake of 22 mmol usually suffices to produce a negative sodium balance once diuresis is established, but a daily intake of 10 mmol may sometimes be required. Hyponatraemia is common in cirrhosis with ascites, but it is not a sign of sodium depletion. Mild hyponatraemia (130-135 mmol/l) can be ignored, and moderate hyponatraemia (125-130 mmol/l) treated by restricting water intake to 1 l daily. Severe hyponatraemia, especially associated with other electrolyte abnormalities and uraemia, is a serious prognostic sign and is often a terminal condition.

Dietary Sodium. It is important for doctors to realise the difficulties faced by a patient advised to take a 'low sodium diet'. A normal diet contains more than 100 mmol of sodium daily, and this can be reduced to around 60-70 mmol by avoiding obviously salty food and by adding no salt at table. Moderate salt restriction can be achieved by adding no salt in cooking as well and this will reduce sodium intake to 40-50 mmol daily. More severe salt restriction requires a knowledge of the sodium content of foods themselves and is achieved best with the help of a dietician. A diet containing 2000 cal and 50 g protein daily with a sodium content of 22 mmol can be devised readily.

Drugs and Sodium. Certain drugs contain relatively large amounts of sodium or cause sodium retention by the body (Table 3.6). These drugs

Table 3.6: Drugs containing relatively large amounts of sodium or causing sodium retention

High sodium content	Sodium retention
Antacids (liquid)*	Carbenoxolone
Magnesium trisilicate mixture	Caved-S
Magnesium carbonate mixture	Phenylbutazone
Gaviscon	Indomethacin
Alginates	Propionic acid derivatives
Fucidin	Corticosteroids
Para-aminosalicytate	Oestrogen
Effervescent calcium	Diazoxide
Phenytoin	
Valproate	
Fybogel	

Notes: Large parenteral doses of penicillins, cephalosporins and chloramphenicol contain considerable quantities of sodium.
* Self-medication with baking soda (sodium bicarbonate) and several over-the-counter preparations (e.g. Andrews Liver Salts, Eno Fruit Salts) are also important.

have to be avoided by the doctor, and the patient also needs to be warned about drugs often taken by the public without medical advice.

Diuretic Drugs. Most patients require diuretic drugs, and these are now so effective that intractable ascites is relatively uncommon. They do not, however, prolong life and they readily cause serious side-effects resulting from their diuretic actions. These side-effects can be minimised by restricting diuresis to that necessary to produce a weight loss of 0.5–1.0 kg daily, and ascites should be reduced only to the extent necessary to relieve the patient of symptoms. The blood urea and electrolyte concentrations should be measured twice or thrice weekly initially to detect increasing uraemia or electrolyte disturbance at an early stage.

The aldosterone antagonist, spironolactone, is a safe and effective diuretic; it produces a moderate diuresis after three to four days of treatment by competitive antagonism of the action of aldosterone on the distal renal tubule, allowing more sodium to pass to the urine. This action also reduces potassium loss in the urine and hyperkalaemia can occur if potassium supplements are not reduced or if uraemia is present. Side-effects are uncommon and include gastrointestinal symptoms, headache, drowsiness, skin rashes, impotence and painful gynaecomastia. Most patients require 200 mg/day to produce a diuresis, and if this is not effective the dose can be increased to 400 mg/day or a powerful diuretic can be added. The powerful diuretics include fruse-mide, ethacrynic acid and butmetanide, which produce natriuresis primarily by preventing sodium and chloride resorption in the ascend-ing loop of Henle. The natriuretic effect they produce is about ten times greater than that due to spironolactone, and their short duration of action (8 hours) allows for great flexibility in using them. They are given orally (frusemide 40 mg, ethacrynic acid 50 mg, bumetamide 1 mg), and the dose is increased gradually until diuresis is producing a weight loss of 0.5–1.0 kg or toxic effects ensue. Fluid and electrolyte imbalances are the most common toxic effects, and uraemia and hyponatraemia are particularly common. Gastrointestinal symptoms, blood dyscrasias, skin rashes, parasthesia and hepatic or renal dys-function have been reported but are rare, and ethacrynic acid may occasionally cause deafness. Thiazides are diuretic drugs with a natri-urectic potency between that of spironolactone and the powerful diuretics. Bendrofluazide (5–10 mg/day) is used most commonly and toxic effects are uncommon, provided hypokalaemia is avoided by giving potassium supplements.

The author usually starts diuretic therapy with spironolactone (200 mg/day), and then adds frusemide if the response to spirono-lactone is inadequate. The dose of frusemide is increased by 40 mg/day on alternate days until the minimum effective dose is reached. Treat-ment is then continued until sufficient ascites has been removed and the sodium intake in the diet has been increased to a 'no added salt at table' level before the dose of frusemide is reduced to the minimum required to prevent recurrence of ascites. A few patients with good liver function find that they no longer need diuretic drugs once the ascites has resolved.

Intractable Ascites. Intractable ascites is ascites which fails to respond to the measures described above. The first step in such cases is to review the treatment given. This may reveal that the diet has contained more salt than realised, usually because the patient is taking salt-containing foods in addition to the prescribed diet. Any patient who finds the diet palatable is likely to be receiving more salt than is desirable. Some-times salt-containing or salt-retaining drugs may be being given in-advertently, and occasionally diuretic drugs are not being taken. These patients often appear relatively well in spite of the failure of therapy, and the important steps are those needed to correct deficiencies in their treatment.

Other patients with intractable ascites have failed to have a diuresis in spite of adequately applied therapy. They are usually obviously ill with poor liver function, and as the doses of diuretic drugs are increased they frequently develop oliguric renal failure and marked hyponatraemia with or without some diuresis. Many, perhaps most, of these patients have reached the end of the natural history of their disease and they are dying. They have suffered a gradual deterioration of liver function, they have spent increasing amounts of time in hospital and the quality of their lives at home has been steadily eroded. Examination has showed them to be ill and often malnourished, and renal failure is frequently present as well as liver failure. Further treatment of ascites is nothing more than an affliction for these patients; their care should centre on their physical, mental and spiritual comfort, part of which involves continuing regular visits from their attending physician, who thereby assures the patient of his or her continuing importance and value as a person.

Some patients, however, may be less ill and for them further treatment of ascites may be tried. Albumin infusions (salt-poor albumin 50 g over 4 hours with frusemide 80 mg intravenously) can be given on alternate days to a total of 150–300 g or the ascites itself can be reinfused intravenously, either directly or after concentration through a dialysis membrane, along with a similar dose of frusemide. These treatments expand the plasma volume, increase the renal blood flow and can initiate a continuing diuresis. More useful in the longer term is the insertion of a LeVeen shunt which connects the ascites to the central veins via a one-way valve which only allows ascites fluid to flow into the central vein. This is not a major operation and it can be tolerated by ill patients. Portalsystemic shunt operations have been advocated to relieve intractable ascites, but few, if any, suitable patients are well enough to tolerate such operations.

Treating Encephalopathy

Hepatic encephalopathy is a neuropsychiatric syndrome of altered brain function resulting from liver failure. Most believe its manifestations are due to toxins which interfere with brain function without necessarily producing structural brain damage. No single toxin has been found to account for hepatic encephalopathy. Several potential toxins have been proposed, however, and some of them may act synergistically. It is likely that the most important toxins are nitrogenous substances, as encephalopathy is worsened by increasing the intake of protein or other nitrogenous material and is improved by reducing nitrogen intake. Furthermore, some of these substances are likely to be produced in the bowel by bacterial action, as oral treatment with antibiotics which are poorly absorbed from the gut improves encephalopathy. Experimental work in animals, however, shows that toxins from the gut are unlikely to be derived solely from bacterial action, and toxins may also originate in organs other than the gut. It is likely that many of the toxins are products of normal metabolism which are metabolised further by the healthy liver. The diseased liver, however, fails to metabolise them fully and they reach the systemic circulation in large amounts. Ammonia has long been considered important in encephalopathy and it continues to be thought an important neurotoxin. Amino acids have been considered increasingly as neurotoxins in liver disease, as some are important precursors of cerebral neurotransmitters and their metabolism and blood concentrations are grossly disturbed in liver disease. Several amino acids or their metabolites may be able to combine with normal neurotransmitter receptors in brain cells owing to their structural similarity to the true neurotransmitters, but they do not have normal neurotransmitter function. They therefore interfere with normal neurotransmitters and have been called false neurotransmitters. Other substances suggested as toxins in hepatic encephalopathy include short-chain fatty acids and mercaptans.

Clinical Features. Hepatic encephalopathy causes abnormalities of the intellect, the personality, the emotions and alteration of consciousness with or without neurological abnormalities. Intellectual changes usually develop first and are associated with apathy, poor concentration and deterioration of the memory. Irritability, childishness, restlessness, anxiety and depression can all occur. Disorientation leads to confusion, and as encephalopathy becomes more severe somnolence, slurred speech, perseveration and occasionally convulsions develop. Severe encephalopathy leads to coma, hypothermia, hyperventilation and sweating. Examination may show a flapping tremor (asterixis), hyperreflexia, extensor plantar responses and sometimes a stiff neck. Simple clinical tests show an impaired constructional ability, illustrated by drawing such objects as clocks and stars, and an impaired ability to connect numbers or letters sequentially.

Acquired Hepatocerebral Degeneration. This rare condition is characterised by irreversible neurological damage in patients with chronic liver disease and extensive portalsystemic shunting of blood. The features are those of damage to the basal ganglia and cerebellum, spastic paraplegia, dementia, paranoid states and epilepsy.

Table 3.7: Differential diagnosis of the electroencephalographic changes seen in hepatic encephalopathy

---

Uraemia
Hypercapnia
Hypoglycaemia
Vitamin B_{12} deficiency

Investigations. Electroencephalography can be helpful in diagnosing hepatic encephalopathy and in following its progress, although the electroencephalographic changes it causes are not specific for hepatic encephalopathy (Table 3.7), and this emphasises the need to interpret the encephalogram in the light of the patient's clinical features. Electroencephalography is most useful when the diagnosis of encephalopathy is uncertain, for revealing minor degrees of encephalopathy prior to portalsystemic shunt operations and for following the treatment of encephalopathy. The blood ammonia is usually increased, but its measurement is not necessary for diagnosis.

Treatment. The first step in treatment is to look for factors which may have precipitated the encephalopathy (Table 3.8) and to correct these wherever possible. Otherwise, the treatment of the encephalopathy itself is based on measures designed to correct those factors believed to cause the syndrome (p. 70). This primarily involves reducing nitrogen intake, inhibiting bacterial action in the bowel and increasing the removal of nitrogenous material and bacteria from the bowel. Other treatments have been advocated for patients who do not respond to these measures, but their efficacy is open to doubt.

Nitrogen Restriction. Very severe encephalopathy requires that all nitrogen intake be stopped. Such patients are fed on glucose given through a fine-bore nasogastric tube or, more frequently, into a large central vein as 20 per cent dextrose (glucose). Less severe encephalopathy can usually be treated by restricting protein intake to 20 g/day. The nitrogen intake is increased once the encephalopathy has improved by increasing the dietary protein by 10 g/day every three days provided that no worsening of the encephalopathy occurs. Electroencephalography is a useful adjunct to clinical means of assessing encephalopathy as the protein intake is increased. Protein intake should be increased steadily until a normal intake (60-80 g/day) is reached; long-term health requires that eventually the dietary protein intake should exceed 25-30 g/day.

Table 3.8: Factors precipitating encephalopathy in hepatic cirrhosis

Uraemia	— spontaneous	Constipation
	— diuretic drugs	Infection
Drugs	— sedatives	Liver failure
	— analgesics	Trauma — surgery
	— anaesthetics	Paracentesis — abdominal
Alcohol		
Gastrointestinal bleeding		
Hypokalaemic alkalosis		
Excess nitrogen intake		

Antibiotics. Broad spectrum antibiotics are important and effective drugs for treating hepatic encephalopathy; they probably act by destroying enteric bacteria capable of producing cerebral toxins from nitrogenous material in the bowel. The aminoglycoside neomycin, which is absorbed poorly from the bowel, is the drug of choice and it is given in a dose of 1–2 g/6 h. It can be given as an elixir by mouth or rectally when patients have difficulty swallowing. Serious toxic effects are fortunately few and include damage to the inner ear and kidney, malabsorption and bowel superinfection. Renal damage and deafness are most likely to occur in uraemic patients who should be given smaller doses (1–4 g/day) if protein restriction and lactulose are insufficient to control encephalopathy.

Lactulose. Lactulose is a synthetic disaccharide which is not absorbed from the small intestine and which is then hydrolysed by bacteria in the colon. Hydrolysis leads to the production of lactic acid and acetic acid and these cause an osmotic catharsis associated with a reduction in stool pH. The means whereby lactulose alleviates hepatic encephalopathy is uncertain, but reduced ammonia production by bacteria due to the lowered pH and increased nitrogen excretion due to the catharsis are probably important. Lactulose syrup 30 ml three times daily with meals is given initially and the dose adjusted so that two to three soft stools are produced daily. The needs of individual patients vary greatly (20–200 ml/day), and it is important not to cause diarrhoea which can quickly lead to serious losses of fluid and electrolyte.

Combined Therapy. Protein restriction, neomycin and lactulose can be used together to treat hepatic encephalopathy. Long-term treatment requires that the patient be allowed at least 30 g protein per day, and uraemic patients should be managed as far as possible by protein restriction and lactulose.

Other Treatments. Levodopa and bromocriptine have been used in hepatic encephalopathy as they increase dopamine activity in the brain, and the oral administration of lactobacilli to displace urease-producing bacteria or acetohydroxamic acid to inhibit urease activity have been used to reduce ammonia production in the gut. None of these measures is as effective as those described above. Ileosigmoidostomy or even colectomy have been advocated as a means of limiting or preventing the access of nitrogen to the colonic bacteria in those who fail to respond to conservative treatment, but such patients are generally quite unsuitable for such major surgery.

Treating Cholestasis

Cholestasis occurs in many chronic liver diseases, but is most characteristic of biliary forms of cirrhosis.

Biliary Cirrhosis. Primary biliary cirrhosis, the most common form of biliary cirrhosis, is predominantly a disease of women characterised by a chronic inflammation in the portal tracts leading to progressive destruction of the medium-sized and small intrahepatic bile ducts and associated with autoantibodies to mitochondria in the blood. Liver function remains good for several years, but continuing inflammatory damage leads eventually to cirrhosis, with all the usual complications of that condition (p. 54 above). The average survival from the onset of symptoms is five or six years (survival ranges from one to fifteen years), and ominous signs include the development of jaundice, a rising serum bilirubin concentration, the appearance of oesophageal varices and the development of ascites. Secondary biliary cirrhosis results from prolonged obstruction of large bile ducts, particularly of the extrahepatic biliary tree, and is caused by biliary strictures due to surgical trauma, gallstones or sclerosing cholangitis. It is rare in adults because these conditions are either uncommon or effectively treated, and because malignant biliary strictures are usually fatal before cirrhosis can develop. Secondary biliary cirrhosis is associated with more marked and often fluctuating jaundice, abdominal pain and recurrent attacks of cholangitis. The prognosis is dependent on the extent to which biliary obstruction can be relieved.

Clinical Features. Cholestasis gives rise to certain clinical features irrespective of its cause. The most characteristic are pruritus, jaundice, dark frothy urine and pale stools. Pigmentation, due to an increase of melanin in the skin, and xanthelasmas become more frequent as the condition continues. Degenerative disease of the skeleton (hepatic osteodystrophy) due to a combination of osteoporosis and osteomalacia also occurs in prolonged cholestasis. Hepatomegaly is often a feature of the underlying liver disease.

Treating Causes of Cholestasis. This is obviously most important in secondary biliary cirrhosis, where surgical relief of obstruction may be possible. Episodes of cholestasis in nonbiliary forms of liver disease may be caused by drugs, and stopping the drug relieves the cholestasis. No specific treatment is available for primary biliary cirrhosis; azathioprine and penicillamine have both been tried recently, but neither gives consistent benefit and both can cause serious side-effects.

Treating the Results of Cholestasis. The most important consequences of cholestasis needing treatment are pruritus, bone disease, malabsorption and, occasionally, neuropathy.

Pruritus occurs frequently and may be disabling, but it can usually be relieved by giving the ion-binding agent cholestyramine orally, provided that biliary obstruction is not complete. The cause of pruritus in cholestasis is unknown, but most still attribute it to the effects of bile acids in the skin and its relief by cholestyramine is in turn attributed to the ability of this agent to bind bile salts in the gut and prevent their reabsorption. One sachet (4 g) of cholestyramine powder daily is given initially and increased by one sachet daily every fifth day until pruritus is clearly being relieved or a total of four sachets (16 g) daily is being taken. The first two sachets should be taken with breakfast and the second two sachets, if needed, can be taken with lunch. Cholestyramine is not pleasant to take, but otherwise its side-effects are few; it may cause diarrhoea or abdominal discomfort initially, and hypochloraemic acidosis can occur in uraemic patients. It can interfere with the absorption of drugs, which are best given later in the day whenever possible, and it also reduces vitamin K absorption, which can be offset by giving vitamin K_1 10 mg intramuscularly each month. Cholestyramine does not relieve pruritus where there is total biliary obstruction, but in such patients norethandrolone 20-30 mg/day in women or methyl testosterone 25 mg/day in men usually brings substantial relief. The minimum effective dose should be used, as both these drugs increase jaundice. The increase in jaundice is not in itself harmful, but patients need to be warned that it may occur.

Osteoporosis and osteomalacia can occur in any chronic liver disease (hepatic osteodystrophy), but they occur most frequently and in greatest severity in patients with prolonged cholestasis. Hepatic osteo-dystrophy causes pain, especially backache, bone deformity and pre-disposes to fractures, and is diagnosed by bone biopsy. Several factors probably contribute to the development of hepatic osteodystrophy, but vitamin D deficiency is important and it probably results principally from a poor diet, malabsorption and perhaps insufficient exposure to sunlight. Hepatic osteodystrophy should be treated by giving vitamin D and calcium. Vitamin D can be given as calciferol 100 000 (2.5 mg) intravenously every month or as a vitamin D metabolite such as 1,25-dihydroxyvitamin D 5-15 μg/day orally. Serum calcium and phosphate concentrations must be measured regularly to detect hypercalcaemia, and in this respect vitamin D metabolites have the advantage of short half-lives (2-4 days) compared to calciferol (30 days), making it easier to reverse hypercalcaemia. Calcium supplments (1-4 g/day) should be given separated from cholestyramine, and calcium gluconate, effer-vescent calcium or Ossopan can be used. Effervescent calcium should be avoided in patients requiring sodium restriction (Table 3.7). Severe bone pain afflicts a few patients, but this can usually be relieved by calcium infusions (1.5 mg/kg body weight in 500 ml of 5 per cent dextrose) daily for 12 days. This treatment may need to be repeated at intervals of a few months. Malabsorption of fat and fat-soluble vitamins probably results from reduced delivery of bile to the small bowel. Dietary fat should be limited to 40 g/day and vitamin A (100 000 i.u.) and vitamin K_1 (10 mg) given intramuscularly monthly. Vitamin D has already been discussed above.

Neuropathy in cholestasis is rare and results from infiltration of peripheral nerves by fat in patients with prolonged hyperlipidaemia. It can be relieved by repeated plasmaphoresis.

Treating Infection

Patients with chronic liver disease are very susceptible to infection. The infections can occur at any site, but it is worth remembering that bacteriaemia is particularly common and that it is not necessarily associated with fever, rigors or leucocytosis. There are several reasons for the susceptibility to infection of patients with chronic liver disease, including their frequently poor nutritional state, impaired reticulo-endothelial function of the liver in removing bacteria from the blood, impaired production of complement factors by the liver and more specific deficiencies of leucokyte function. Other factors include the effects of alcohol abuse, anaemia and uraemia.

The manifestations of particular infections, such as pneumonia, are similar to those occurring in patients without liver disease. It is, however, important to bear in mind that bacteraemia often presents purely as a general deterioration of health, so that the doctor is faced with a patient who is ill for no obvious reason with the development or worsening of hepatic encephalopathy. In addition, patients with cirrhosis are especially liable to infection in ascites (spontaneous bacterial peritonitis). This usually presents with sudden abdominal pain, rebound abdominal tenderness and absent bowel sounds with fever, possibly rigors and hepatic encephalopathy. Again, however, the patient may simply become ill for no obvious reason, which emphasises the importance of culturing ascitic fluid whenever deterioration occurs in a patient with ascites. Infection may also localise in other fluid collections giving rise to empyema, purulent pericarditis or meningitis.

The susceptibility of patients with chronic liver disease to infection emphasises the importance of looking for infection whenever patients deteriorate in health, and blood culture and ascites culture are always important. Early antibiotic treatment is advisable as about half the patients die even when bacteraemia is recognised and the responsible organism is known.

Treating Renal Failure

Any form of renal failure can arise in patients with chronic liver disease, but in addition there is a form of renal failure in such patients which develops as a consequence of liver failure. This renal failure is not due to any primary abnormality of the kidney, but is a failure of renal function consequent on failure of liver function. Thus, it has been shown that kidneys from patients with cirrhosis dying in hepatorenal failure work well when transplanted into patients with end-stage renal failure, and liver transplantation in patients with cirrhosis and hepatorenal syndrome results in a restoration of renal function. This form of renal failure has been termed the hepatorenal syndrome or functional renal failure of cirrhosis. The mechanisms causing the hepatorenal syndrome are controversial, but ultimately they lead to a marked increase in renal vascular resistance with a reduction in renal blood flow and consequently of glomerular filtration. Renal tubular function remains good. Consequently, investigations in functional renal failure reveal kidneys of normal size, an absence of proteinuria or abnormal urinary sediments, a low urine sodium excretion (10 mmol/day) and a high urine/plasma osmolality ratio (> 1.5).

Patients with functional renal failure almost always have advanced cirrhosis. The onset may be sudden or gradual, and precipitating factors include gastrointestinal bleeding, infection, the removal of large amounts of ascitic fluid, excessive diuretic therapy and surgical procedures. The patients are weak, anorectic and apathetic, and as uraemia advances they develop nausea, vomiting, thirst and drowsiness and tremor, which is probably both hepatic and renal in origin. Examination reveals advanced cirrhosis with muscle wasting, jaundice and ascites which has often proved resistant to therapy. Bruising is common, the systolic blood pressure is frequently less than 100 mmHg, and as the condition worsens oliguria and encephalopathy become more severe. Investigations usually confirm hyperbilirubinaemia, serum enzyme activities (alanine aminotransferase, alkaline phosphatase) are variable and plasma protein analyses show hypoalbuminaemia with hyperglobulinaemia and a prolonged prothrombin time, reflecting poor liver function. The blood urea and creatinine concentrations are increased. Hypoatraemia is the rule and it becomes more severe as the illness progresses. Hypokalaemia and acidosis only develop terminally. The findings in the urine are given above (p. 77).

The prognosis in functional renal failure of cirrhosis is governed wholly by liver function, and renal function will improve only when liver function improves. The possible precipitants of functional renal failure given above (p. 77) should be sought and treated, and consideration should be given to the possibility of some independent cause of renal failure such as urinary tract obstruction or infection needing treatment in its own right. Otherwise, the object of therapy is to keep the patient alive in the hope that liver function will improve spontaneously. This involves recognising that in some patients there is no realistic hope of improvement, let alone a return to a worthwhile life, and in such instances peace and comfort alone should be aimed at. This applies particularly to elderly patients, those who have had gradually deteriorating liver function for which no cause other than the liver disease itself can be found, and those with other serious associated diseases. General measures in the treatment of functional renal failure include limiting uraemia and encephalopathy by restricting protein intake to 20 g/day and by providing 200 g/day of carbohydrate to limit endogenous protein breakdown. Hepatic encephalopathy is treated with neomycin and lactulose (p. 73), although care should be exercised with neomycin in the fear of uraemia by using a restricted dose (2-4 g/day). Almost all patients are overhydrated, as evidenced by ascites and oedema, and hyponatraemia·should therefore be treated by restricting water intake to 500 ml/day. Occasionally, renal failure has been precipitated by excessive fluid loss by vomiting, aspiration, diarrhoea; paracentesis of ascites or excessive diuretic therapy, and in such patients there is no ascites or oedema. They require treatment with saline. Potassium deficiency is very common and should be corrected, as it affects renal function adversely and worsens hepatic encephalopathy (p. 70). A serum potassium concentration below 3.5 mmol/l always indicates potassium deficiency, but a normal serum concentration does not exclude deficiency. Potassium can be given intravenously provided that the serum concentration is checked twice daily initially, but not in amounts exceeding 10 mmol/h or in concentrations above 40 mmol/l. Magnesium deficiency occasionally needs to be corrected.

The promotion of improved renal function is achieved most logically by expanding the intravascular volume to improve renal blood flow and by using diuretics as required. Regular measurements of pulse rate, blood pressure, hourly urine output for which catheterisation is needed and central venous pressure should be made during this therapy. The intravascular volume can be expanded with blood, plasma, salt-poor albumin or dextra 70, or by reinfusing ascitic fluid intravenously under aseptic conditions; of these the author uses fresh-frozen plasma most often. Several drugs have been advocated to improve renal blood flow further, but the only one used by the author is dopamine 1–5 µg/kg/w intravenously. Diuretics such as frusemide are given as required to try and maintain a urine flow about 30 ml/h. Patients who respond reasonably well to this treatment but who continue to have considerable ascites may benefit from the insertion of a LeVeen shunt. Hepatic transplantation should not be forgotten in young, reasonably fit patients.

Renal Tubular Dysfunction in Chronic Liver Disease. Marked sodium retention by the renal tubules is the commonest renal tubular dysfunction in cirrhosis and is central to sodium and water retention leading to ascites (p. 67). Water excretion may also be impaired and contributes to hyponatraemia. Metabolic acidosis is uncommon; but paradoxically incomplete renal tubular acidosis is quite common. It can aggravate hepatic encephalopathy by increasing potassium loss in the urine and impairing ammonia excretion, and is treated by giving potassium bicarbonate orally.

Treating Malignant Hepatic Tumours

Primary Tumours. Hepatocellular carcinoma is one of the commonest human tumours in the world. Most patients with chronic liver disease are particularly susceptible to it, especially those with chronic hepatitis B virus infection. Resection is the only treatment to give prolonged survival, but unfortunately this is hardly ever possible in patients with cirrhosis. Hepatocellular carcinomas are difficult to diagnose in patients with cirrhosis and are often advanced by the time they are recognised. In addition, tumours in the right lobe of the liver cannot be removed in cirrhosis, as the remaining cirrhotic left lobe usually cannot support life, and often overall liver function is such as to preclude any operation at all. The most valuable investigations in determining the operability of a tumour are a liver scan, usually with the radionuclide ^{99M}Tc sulphur colloid, angiographic examination of the hepatic tree, the portal vein and the inferior vena cava, a peritoneoscopy and a chest radiography and radionuclide bone scan to detect distant metastases. Other methods of treatment are purely palliative, but a combination of embolisation of the hepatic artery via a catheter introduced under radiological control and/or chemotherapy may give good relief from local pain and even improve the quality of survival. Adriamycin is probably the best drug in current use.

Overall, the prognosis for patients with cirrhosis and hepatocellular carcinoma is poor; the great majority die of the disease within 3-6 months, although a few survive for a year or more.

Secondary Tumours. The liver is affected by metastatic tumour more frequently than any other organ, and is involved in a third of cases of malignant disease coming to autopsy. The prognosis for patients with metastatic tumour in the liver is in general poor and for the most part only symptomatic treatment can be offered (Ch. 13). It is, however, important to investigate patients whose general health is good as they may have metastases confined to a part of the liver which can be resected. The investigations required in these patients are those described above for primary tumours. It is also important to identify hepatic involvement in lymphoproliferative diseases, such as Hodgkin's disease, as these are amenable to chemotherapy.

Chronic Biliary Disease

Chronic biliary disease is fortunately rare and the only conditions which will be referred to briefly here are benign and malignant biliary strictures and sclerosing cholangitis. The aims of therapy are to obtain as good biliary drainage as possible, to prevent and treat infection and to treat the consequences of chronic cholestasis.

Benign Biliary Strictures

Postoperative Strictures. Postoperative biliary strictures usually follow cholecystectomy. Their incidence has fallen, and they probably now occur after about one in every thousand gallstone operations. Early skilled reconstruction of the strictured bile duct is of the utmost importance in preventing chronic liver damage, and more than one operation may be needed. The most frequent injury involves the common hepatic duct and this usually requires a hepaticojejunostomy Roux-en-Y using a transhepatic tube as a splint for a period after the operation (Figure 3.1) but end-to-end anastomosis of the bile duct is done if possible.

Figure 3.1: Reconstruction of a high bile duct stricture by a hepatico-jejunostomy Roux-en-Y with a transhepatic tube

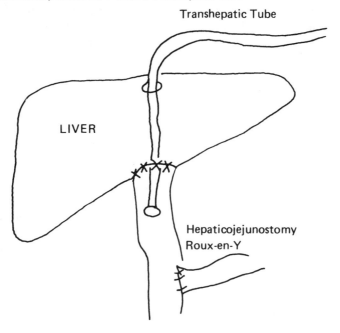

Transhepatic Tube

LIVER

Hepaticojejunostomy
Roux-en-Y

Failure to effect an adequate repair of a biliary stricture results in chronic cholestatis jaundice; episodes of abdominal pain and cholangitis lead eventually to secondary biliary cirrhosis with liver failure, causing ascites and encephalopathy and portal hypertension which in turn causes oesophagogastric varices and bleeding. Treatment at this stage includes consideration of the placement of a catheter across the stricture to improve biliary drainage by either the percutaneous transhepatic route or the endoscopic retrograde route, relief of the consequences of chronic cholestasis (p. 75) and the treatment of episodes of cholangitis. Episodes of cholangitis are treated by relieving abdominal pain with morphine (15-20 mg) or pethidine (100-150 mg) intramuscularly, by treating shock and by giving antibiotics. Suitable antibiotics include ampicillin, a cephalosporin such as cefuroxime and cotrimoxazole. Seriously ill patients should be given gentamycin and ampicillin, cotrimoxazole or lincomycin. Metronidazole is the drug of choice for anaerobic infections. Antibiotics can be given on a long-term basis and in rotation if frequent attacks of cholangitis occur.

Choledocholithiasis. Chronic biliary obstruction due to untreated stones in the common bile duct with or without stricture is rare. The clinical features are the same as in postoperative strictures, although abdominal pain is more frequent and often more severe. Treatment involves removing the stones and repairing any stricture. Endoscopic papillotomy and removal of common bile duct stones which are less than 15-20 mm in diameter should be done in elderly or otherwise infirm patients.

Primary Sclerosing Cholangitis

This rare condition is characterised by chronic inflammation of the extrahepatic and sometimes the intrahepatic bile ducts for unknown reasons. It is usually a diffuse process, but segmental lesions can occur. It has to be distinguished from biliary stricture due to stones or trauma and from a slow-growing biliary carcinoma (Table 3.9). Half the patients have ulcerative colitis, and occasional associated diseases include thyroid disorders such as thyroiditis, hypothyroidism and Riedel's stroma, Crohn's disease, retroperitoneal fibrosis and pancreatitis.

The clinical features of primary sclerosing cholangitis are those of chronic cholestasis (p. 74) with fluctuating jaundice, abdominal pain and recurrent cholangitis. Cirrhosis develops eventually, and physical examination reveals hepatomegaly and sometimes splenomegaly. Liver

Table 3.9: Criteria for the diagnosis of primary sclerosing cholangitis

Diffuse thickening of the extrahepatic bile ducts
No previous biliary surgery
No biliary tract calculi
Exclusion of sclerosing carcinoma of the bile ducts by five-year follow-up

function tests reflect cholestasis, autoantibodies are not found in the blood, and percutaneous transhepatic or endoscopic retrograde cholangiography shows diffuse, or rarely segmental, narrowing of the large bile ducts. Laparotomy and bile duct biopsy may be needed to exclude biliary carcinoma. Treatment is unsatisfactory and includes the use of antibiotics to control cholangitis, if necessary on a long-term basis (p. 82), and measures to treat the results of cholestasis (p. 75). Corticosteroid drugs and azathiorpine have been used, but there is no evidence that they are beneficial. Surgical treatment for localised forms of the disease are as for other localised strictures (p. 81); the place of surgery in diffuse disease is controversial and limited, and several forms of temporary external or internal biliary drainage have been advocated.

Malignant Biliary Strictures

Malignant disease can cause biliary obstruction in the liver, in the porta hepatitis where biliary carcinoma frequently arises at the junction of the left and right hepatic duct or from invasion from locally affected lymph nodes, or in the common bile ducts due to carcinoma of the bile duct itself, the pancreas or the papilla of Vater. Intrahepatic biliary obstruction due to lymphoproliferation disease, such as Hodgkin's disease, may respond to appropriate chemotherapy; other tumours of the bile duct should be investigated carefully with a view to surgical treatment, particularly in respect of carcinomas at the papilla of Vater in younger patients.

Most tumours cannot be removed surgically, particularly pancreatic carcinomas, and the major problems they cause are pain, pruritus caused by cholestasis and malabsorption. The management of pain is considered elsewhere (p. 62), and diarrhoea from malabsorption can be treated by reducing dietary fat below 40 g/day. Pruritus can be treated with cholestyramine (p. 322) or anabolic steroids (p. 322), but these agents become ineffective once biliary obstruction is complete, which is frequent in these patients. The most effective way of relieving pruritus is to drain the bile into the bowel. This can be done by operations such

as choledochoduodenostomy or, less effectively, by cholecystentero-
stomy, when the tumours are in the distal common bile duct or in the
pancreas, and in patients with pancreatic carcinoma a gastrojejuno-
stomy will prevent the consequences of later duodenal obstruction.
Biliary carcinomas at the junction of the left and right hepatic ducts
may be amenable to a hepaticojejunostomy Roux-en-Y. Many patients,
however, are in poor health or have tumours which are unsuitable for
surgical treatment. These patients can be relieved of pruritus by placing
a drainage tube across the malignant stricture using a percutaneous
transhepatic or endoscopic retrograde approach. The aim should be to
effect drainage into the duodenum rather than to the exterior, and although cholangitis or tube blockage may develop, good palliation is
frequently achieved.

4 PALLIATIVE CARE IN HAEMATOLOGICAL DISORDERS

Norman C. Allan

Haematological Disorders

Almost all patients with haematological disorders which will require palliative care suffer from some form of haematological malignancy. These are relatively uncommon conditions compared with some other malignant diseases, but are of considerable importance because they have proved remarkably susceptible to treatment with the possibility of cure for some sufferers. The majority of cases progress with varying periods of remission to death and in the later stages require much palliative care. This is the stage when forms of treatment designed to control the disease no longer do so and further active management is deemed not to be in the patient's best interests.

The disorders in question include the various forms of leukaemia, both acute and chronic, lymphomas — both Hodgkin and non-Hodgkin varieties — myeloma, polycythaemia, myelofibrosis, essential thrombocythaemia and other rarities. A brief description of these disorders will be given to set the scene for a discussion of the palliative care they are likely to require.

Leukaemias

There are many types of leukaemia. In general terms they can be divided in two ways. They may be described as acute or chronic, depending on the rapidity of progression of the disease, although these categories can also be largely recognised by the types of cells which characterise them. Acute leukaemias occur at all ages, whereas chronic leukaemias are generally found in middle-aged and old patients, although they can occur rarely in the young. A division into leukaemias which are associated with the lymphocytic lineage of cells, lymphoblastic/lymphocytic and those associated with the granulocyte 'series' (neutrophils, eosinophils and basophils) and the monocyte, so-called 'myeloid' leukaemias, is also made. This latter distinction is important, as it strongly influences treatment, general management and prognosis.

Table 4.1: Summary of description of haematological disorders

Disease	Age-range	Prognosis untreated (mean)	Responsiveness to treatment	Principal problems in terminal phase	Page reference in text
Acute lymphatic leukaemia	All ages	8 weeks	Very good; 50% 'cure' in children	Anaemia Bleeding	88
Acute myeloid leukaemia	All ages	5 weeks	Temporary remission for 60%. 'Cure' very rare	Infections Pain Anorexia	88
Chronic myeloid leukaemia	Adult: mostly > 35	2½ years	Control of disease for a while. Cure only by success-ful transplantation	As for acute leukaemia Discomfort of massive splenomegaly	89
Chronic lymphatic leukaemia	Middle to old age: mostly > 40	4 years	Fairly good; may not require treatment for years	Recurrent infection Anaemia	88
Hodgkin's lymphoma	All ages, especially teenagers and young adults as well as older	2 years	Good response; many cured	Cachexia Skeletal pain Infections	89
Non-Hodgkin's lymphoma	All ages	Low-grade malignancy: 4 years	Good response; no cures	Increase susceptibility to infections Side-effects of local tumour formation	89
		High-grade malignancy: 9 months	Good response in 50%; possible cure in some		
Myeloma	Middle to old age	9 months	Good response in up to 80%	Skeletal pain Renal failure Bleeding Infections Anaemia	90

Table 4.1: Summary of description of haematological disorders *(contd)*

Disease	Age-range	Prognosis untreated (mean)	Responsiveness to treatment	Principal problems in terminal phase	Page reference in text
Polycythaemia rubra vera	Middle to old age	1.5 years	Very good; not curable	As for acute leukaemia or myelofibrosis	99
Myelofibrosis	Middle to old age	3 years	Poor	Weight loss Massive splenomegaly Severe anaemia Infection and bleeding	91
Essential thrombo-cythaemia	Middle to old age	4–5 years	Very good	Often die of something else	91

Acute Lymphoblastic Leukaemias. The common variety of this disorder is remarkably susceptible to drug therapy and about half the patients can expect long remission and possibly cure of the disease. This is particularly so in young children, in whom this is the most common type of leukaemia. The less common varieties (B cell, T cell and Null cell) may show good responses to treatment initially, but usually relapse with progressive resistance to therapy. Initial drug therapy using vincristine and prednisolone frequently induces a very rapid remission and this is consolidated with further chemotherapy, intrathecal drug therapy and cranial irradiation to eradicate residual disease. If good remission is obtained, a cycle of maintenance therapy is continued for up to two years. Once relapse has occurred the chance of cure is remote unless successful bone-marrow transplantation can be performed.

Acute Myeloid Leukaemias. The acute myeloid leukaemias, which include myelomonocytic, monocytic and a number of other variants, are much more common than lymphoblastic leukaemias and unfortunately much less responsive to treatment. At best, only about 60 per cent obtain an initial remission and this is all too frequently brief. Cure is very rare. Nevertheless, the prospect for these patients has improved, compared with the dismal outlook of, on average, five-week survival after diagnosis before any form of effective therapy was available. Treatment aimed at induction of remission involves aggressive chemotherapy regimes usually employing a combination of daunorubicin, cytosine arabinoside and 6-thioguanine. Ablation of the marrow is undertaken with the hope of allowing normal haemopoietic elements to repopulate the marrow. If successful, remission may last for variable periods. After relapse further remission can sometimes be obtained. Eventually the disease becomes therapy-resistant.

Chronic Lymphocytic Leukaemia. This occurs mainly in middle and old age, although some of its variants occur in younger patients. In its classical form it is the most chronic of the leukaemias, sometimes requiring no active treatment for years. Other forms are less chronic, but usually with treatment allow several years of reasonable life. It commonly presents with vague ill health, swollen lymph nodes and sometimes splenomegaly. Not infrequently it is discovered as an incidental finding, either following a routine check-up or during the treatment of an infection. The younger the patient, the more aggressive the course of the disease tends to be.

This is the form of leukaemia most closely related to the non-Hodgkin type of lymphoma. The disease is rare among the Chinese, Japanese and related races.

Hairy cell leukaemia (leukaemic reticuloendotheliosis) is a variant that can carry a very good prognosis of many years of life, although in some cases, for reasons unknown, the progression may be rapid. Most therapeutic benefit is obtained from splenectomy. Steroid therapy may also help. Results with chemotherapy are usually disappointing.

Chronic Myeloid Leukaemia. This is usually diagnosed in the middle-aged and its common form (Philadelphia chromosome positive) carries a 50 per cent survival of three to four years. Patients usually present with general ill health and are found to have marked splenomegaly, moderate anaemia and very high white cell counts. The disease is not curable other than by successful bone-marrow transplantation. Drug therapy can achieve good remission of the symptoms by keeping the disease under control for varying periods of time. Occasionally patients survive for lengthy periods (15-18 years). In the uncommon variety (Philadelphia chromosome negative) treatment is less successful and survival is often less than one year. The disease terminates in the majority of cases by transforming to an acute form of leukaemia which is usually very resistant to therapy.

Hodgkin's Lymphoma

This is a malignant disorder of the reticulo endothelial system characteristically affecting the lymphoid tissues of the body, often presenting with swollen lymph nodes in the neck. It occurs in young people, particularly in the age-range 15-30, but also in older patients. Four varieties exist — lymphocyte predominant, nodular sclerosing, mixed cellularity, and lymphocyte depleted — and in this order range from the most benign to the most malignant. By careful and extensive staging of the disease and the use of either radiotherapy for early disease or chemotherapy for more widespread disease, or a combination of both, the condition can be effectively treated in many cases with possible cure. In others the disease proves relatively refractory to treatment and is progressive with a fatal outcome sooner or later. Such patients suffer from a progressive loss of effective immunity to infection and from infiltration of the organs of the body by Hodgkin's tissue.

Non-Hodgkin's Lymphomas

With few exceptions these are malignancies of the lymphocyte cell lineage. A wide variety of lymphomas are included in this group and the progression of the disease is very variable. They occur at all ages, but the more chronic, 'good prognosis', forms tend not to occur in younger persons. Some of the highly malignant varieties, so called 'histiocytic' or large cell types may be very sensitive to chemotherapy with induction of long-term remission and even cure. The more benign forms may require little or no treatment for varying periods up to years, but eventually prove fatal. The majority respond well to treatment for a variable time.

Myeloma (Multiple Myeloma)

Myeloma is a malignant disorder of the plasma cell. The plasma cell derives from lymphocytes by transformation in response to antigenic stimuli and is the producer of most of the antibodies found in the body. In most cases the disease is confined to the bone marrow and causes rarefaction and erosion of bone with pathological fractures and collapse of weight-bearing bones. The normal bone-marrow elements also suffer, producing anaemia and thrombocytopenia. Damage to the renal tissue is also common due to the abnormal proteins produced, The malignant cells cease to be immunologically competent and the patient suffers progressive impairment of humoral immunity with increasing susceptibility to infection, which is often the terminal event. The disease presents in a wide variety of ways. There is usually general ill health and aches and pains in bones, acute pain due to pathological fracture, pneumonia or other infections that direct attention to the problem. Treatment with radiotherapy for localised bone problems and chemotherapy for generalised disease is often successful in controlling the problems for varying periods of time. Despite serious and debilitating disease at diagnosis, considerable progress can be made by many patients with re-establishment of satisfactory life.

Waldenstrom's macroglobulinaemia is a rare disease similar to myeloma, but with less drastic erosion of the bone. It is associated with reduced immunity, increasing susceptibility to infection and problems of hyperviscosity.

Polycythaemia Vera

This is a relatively benign malignant disorder affecting mainly the red blood cell precursors with overproduction of red cells. This produces a very high haemoglobin and the patient often looks plethoric. Patients complain of headaches, lassitude and irritability. Vascular disease is commonly associated, particularly in men, and the frequency of duodenal ulcer is high. White cell counts and platelet counts may also be raised. The disorder grumbles on for years and can be controlled by venesection, radioactive phosphorus or drug therapy. Eventually it becomes refractory to treatment and may transform to myelofibrosis, acute leukaemia or an erythemic myelosis.

Myelofibrosis

In this condition the marrow is increasingly replaced by fibrous tissue and there is myeloid metaplasia with primitive blood cells in the blood, spleen and liver. The course is very variable, but there is progressive failure of blood cell production, weight loss and characteristically massive splenomegaly. There is no known treatment other than supportive measures. Drugs are generally not very helpful. Sometimes the spleen requires to be removed to relieve abdominal discomfort.

Essential Thrombocythaemia

This is a malignant disorder of platelet production associated with very high platelet counts, bleeding and thrombotic problems. Most patients are elderly. The disease is usually easily controlled for long periods with radioactive phosphorus or cytotoxic drugs. The patients often die of other disorders.

Palliation

Palliation is required for patients with these disorders when the disease has reached the state at which no further active treatment aimed at either cure or achievement of remission is reasonable or possible. In some cases this may be before any treatment is given, because active treatment would be inappropriate. However, it is true that some forms of gentle single-agent chemotherapy have been used in a palliative manner with some success.

Palliation in Acute Leukaemias

Once acute leukaemia becomes refractory to treatment, the prognosis is usually poor and often mercifully brief. The problems created by the illness come to the fore. The normal bone marrow functions are largely eliminated by overgrowth of leukaemic tissues. The result is a loss of normal blood production which causes anaemia, bleeding because of a lack of platelets, and infection due to lack of white cells.

Table 4.2: Summary of management of problems associated with haematological disorders

Problem	Management	Other comments	Page references in text
Symptomatic anaemia	Transfuse with red cell concentrate using diuretic and anti-histamine cover		93
Transfusion reactions			
allergic	Antihistamines Corticosteroids		93–94
pyrexial	Antipyretics Stop transfusion if associated pain at site, backache or rigors Antibiotics	Future transfusions — washed or filtered blood	
incompatibility	Stop transfusions Mannitol diuresis Treat for shock		
Oral candida	Nystatin lozenges Amphotericin Miconazole Gentian violet Ketoconazole	Very mild, asymptomatic infection may require no treatment	97–98
Herpes simplex (labialis)	Acyclovir Ice cube to lip for 2 minutes	Must be used early in infection	97
Herpes Zoster	Acyclovir Herpid (topical) Calamine lotion Analgesics	Corneal protection	98
Urinary tract infections	Co-trimoxazole Prophylaxis	Almost always present if patient catheterised	96
Neutropenia	Aseptic precautions Avoid toothbrushes Avoid rectal examinations		96
Skeletal pain	Radiotherapy Nerve blocks Analgesics Indomethacin Mithramycin in myeloma		98–99
Confusional state	Treat hypercalcaemia Treat thrombocytopenia, if appropriate		95, 99
Anorexia	Corticosteroids Home cooking Anti-emetics Alcoholic drinks		100

Table 4.2 *(contd.)*

Sore mouths	Frequent mouth toilet	96-97
	Benzydamine H11	
	Chlorhexidine gluconate	
	Fizzy drinks	
	Pineapple	
	Soft foods, liquidised food	
Alopecia	Wigs	
	Head coverings	
Thrombocytopenia		
Skin rash	No treatment needed	95
Mouth bleeding	Frequent mouth toilet	
Epistaxis	Debridement and nasal packing	
Clouding of consciousness	Platelet transfusion if deemed necessary	95

Anaemia

Anaemia causes problems mainly for those who remain fairly active. Breathlessness, dizziness, lassitude and weakness may be troublesome. The patient tires easily and life is a drag. This anaemia is relatively easily treated with blood transfusion, which should not be spared if there is the possibility of giving the patient a better quality of life, however brief. Transfusion, however, may not be without problems, such as reactions with attendant fever and malaise. The repeated need for hospital visits may also be a burden. Patients themselves can usually assess whether transfusions are worth while. Often the early dramatic response to transfusion wears off and the law of diminishing returns seems to apply.

Patients at rest may tolerate quite low haemoglobin levels without discomfort or distress and do not necessarily require donations of blood. Indeed anaemia may induce a pleasant tranquil state, which can be beneficial in the terminal phase of the disease. A low haemoglobin is not in itself a good reason to transfuse. There should be justification such as symptoms which are distressing and which transfusion may relieve, for example, angina.

Blood Transfusions

The use of red cell concentrate (packed cells) rather than whole blood is preferred when treating anaemia. It provides a maximum number of red blood cells with minimum volume. Cover of the transfusion with an antihistamine such as chlorpheniramine maleate, 4 mg orally or 10 mg by subcutaneous intramuscular or slow intravenous injection, is worth while as it will help to suppress allergic phenomena that accompany some units of blood and which are of no serious consequence to the patient. This practice will not mask reactions due to incompatibility, nor will it suppress pyrogenic reactions. The latter are often due to the development of antibodies to white cells and platelet antigens infused during previous transfusions. Stored blood does not contain viable white cells or platelets, but does have the remnants of these cells and it is these that stimulate the immune response and, in turn, the reactions. If reactions are proving a nuisance and antileuco-cyte and antiplatelet antibodies are demonstrated, blood in which these antigenic substances are removed by special filtration techniques can be obtained, usually be negotiation with the Blood Transfusion Service.

Pyrogenic reactions are generally not of serious import, but are un-pleasant and exhausting to the patient. Antipyretics can be used to control them, if necessary.

Availability of blood for patients who have a relatively uncommon blood group sometimes poses a problem. For example, the patient may be group O, Rhesus negative and no blood of this type may be available because it is heavily in demand for obstetric and other areas of medical practice. In this event the use of group O, Rhesus positive blood may be ethically acceptable, especially in older patients and when the reci-pient's prognosis is poor. Patients receiving such donations do not necessarily develop anti-Rhesus antibodies. If they do, they may take weeks or months to appear and transfusion thereafter would have to be with Rhesus negative blood. The use of blood which is not strictly the correct blood group should only be undertaken after consultation with the local Blood Transfusion Service who, in any event, will probably request its use in the first place.

Overloading of the circulation may occur despite the use of red cell concentrates. It is common practice to administer a diuretic such as frusemide at the beginning of a transfusion. Usually three to four units of red cell concentrate can be given at a time in this way, at a rate of one unit every two to three hours. If more is required, it is better practice to divide the transfusion and give a second after a break of one or two days. Patients with problems of renal failure may require special care and often are best not transfused. Renal function may be impaired if the haematocrit is raised too much and the protein load given by a transfusion may exacerbate uraemia.

Thrombocytopenic Bleeding

A lack of platelets is the most common reason for bleeding in patients with haematological malignancies. However, other factors may contribute, the most important being infection. Infections may cause local bleeding at the site. Also toxaemia arising from infection may damage the microvasculature, making the vessels more susceptible to bleeding. Sensitivity reactions to drugs also damage the capillaries and when associated with thrombocytopenia can cause extensive purpura.

Bleeding from thrombocytopenia is seen mainly in the skin, mucous membranes and eyes. The same capillary bleeding may occur internally and be extensive, but it tends not to produce much symptomatology. Purpura in the skin, while disfiguring, is seldom a clinical problem. Patients should be reassured that the rash is not serious. Bleeding into mucous membranes, however, can promote ulcer formation, infection and a very sore mouth.

Nose bleeds are a common and distressing complication. They require all blood clots to be removed from the nose and nasal packs inserted and left for two or three days. The expertise of an ENT specialist is often required. Cautery is not often beneficial in this type of bleeding.

Bleeding into the retina and aqueous humour is very distressing, causing varying degrees of loss of vision and being slow to clear. Other problems that arise include haematuria, gastrointestinal bleeding and clouding of consciousness due to purpuric intracranial bleeding. Not infrequently a massive intracranial haemorrhage occurs, which is usually terminal.

At the stage at which palliation is required, management of thrombocytopenic problems is largely symptomatic. Active therapy to bring the disease under control and allow the recovery of endogenous platelet production is not usually planned. Platelet transfusions may be administered, but are of evanescent value producing amelioration of the problems for a few hours only. One platelet pack is harvested from six fresh donations of blood and is therefore expensive and may be difficult to obtain. The decision to use platelet transfusion as a palliative procedure therefore depends on the individual circumstances of the case and should be employed only when there are very good reasons, such as the extreme distress caused by intraocular bleeding.

One major reason for thrombocytopenia in these patients is the drug therapy used to treat the disease. Once the stage of palliation has been reached, this is usually withdrawn and a surprising recovery of endogenous blood production, including platelets, may occur for a while.

If this can be even in part anticipated, supportive measures to carry the patient into such a phase may be worth while. However, the basic philosophy of palliation is to allow nature to take its course while controlling as far as possible, any unpleasantness in the process. Such a course of action or inaction may bring pleasant surprises. Patients have been known to go into clinical remission lasting months once cytotoxic therapy is withdrawn.

Infection

Infection which reflects the deterioration in the immune mechanisms of the patients is a common and often terminal event. A lack of neutrophils is associated with bacterial and fungal infections. Loss of functional lymphocyte activity, as in the lymphocytic leukaemias and lymphomas, renders the patients very susceptible to viral infections. Massive and overwhelming infections — either septicaemic or respiratory — are common terminal events. Before the phase of palliation, such infections would be vigorously treated with intravenous antibiotics such as a combination of gentamycin, or one of its analogues, and mezlocillin. If streptococcal infection is suspected, flucloxicillin should be used and metronidazole for anaerobic infections. Also, intravenous support therapy, in addition to intensive nursing support, would be required. Such measures are largely irrelevant — other than the good nursing — during the palliative phase, unless the infection is seen to be robbing the patient of a period of reasonable life. Urinary tract infections (UTIs) are often worth treating actively to reduce the discomfort to the patient. Likewise, cellulitis and local abscess formation may require active antibiotic and surgical management as a means of pain relief. If UTIs recur, long-term oral co-trimoxazole — available either as tablets, of which there are water-dispersable forms, or suspension — may be given as a prophylactic.

Oral infections give rise to much distress. They are often associated with painful ulceration, which makes chewing and swallowing a misery. Patients with infected mouths are often self-conscious and aware that their breath may be smelly. Edentulous patients usually have less trouble than those with teeth, particularly those with bad teeth. Fortunately, these problems tend to be more troublesome during periods of active chemotherapy than in the terminal stages. Careful mouth toilet is also worth giving to patients, even if they have not yet developed symptomatic problems. Debilitated patients often have dry mouths from sleeping with their mouths open or mouth breathing. A clean mouth can have a distinctly morale-boosting effect.

Frequent gentle mouth toilet is required. Neutropenic patients should not be allowed to use toothbrushes, as they may induce local cellulitis by aiding invasion of bacteria. When neutropenia is not severe only 'soft' toothbrushes, preferably previously soaked in hot water, should be used. The action of the brush is then very gentle, but should be adequate to dislodge debris between teeth. Dentures should always be removed and thoroughly cleaned during mouth toilet.

Many patients resort to using antiseptic mouthwashes, gargles, lozenges and sprays. Some of these cause more harm than good and should be discouraged. Simple mouthwashes containing glycerine of thymol are probably harmless, but may not be very effective. An oral rinse containing benzydamine hydrochloride is useful for painful mouths and can be gargled. It may be used as frequently as every 1½ hours, but every 3 hours is usually adequate. It is recommended that its use should not be continued for more than one week. Mouthwashes containing chlorhexidine gluconate are effective. These are used to prevent the formation of plaque on teeth and treat gingivitis. If the neat solution proves too strong, it may be diluted in an equal volume of water. Hydrogen peroxide mouthwashes have a cleansing effect due to frothing, but many patients dislike the preparations. Simple fizzy drinks containing carbon dioxide may have a similar effect and be more palatable to the patients. However, some of these may be nauseatingly sweet. Drinks containing quinine offset this by introducing the bitter taste element which is refreshing. Pineapple has a cleansing effect in the mouth by providing proteolytic enzymes. These are particularly active in fresh, uncooked pineapple, but this may prove too drastic. Tinned pineapple is moderately effective. If the patient is unable to chew, the pineapple can be broken up or liquidised.

Herpes simplex (labialis, cold sores) infections occur very frequently. When complicated by bleeding, huge bloody crusts may form on the lips and nose. If these are more than a trivial lesion, treatment with acyclovir may be worth giving. At the first sign of a lesion, application of an ice cube to the affected part for two minutes may abort the problem and is worth trying.

Patients vary in their likes and dislikes and it is useful to have a variety of possible preparations so that something to the patient's liking can be found. The patient is then much more likely to accept and use the preparation.

Candida albicans infection (thrush) is a ubiquitous problem and a cause of very sore mouths and throats. Severe heartburn should alert the clinician to the possibility of candida oesophagitis, which usually affects the lower third of the oesophagus; this can be diagnosed by barium swallow as the appearances are characteristic. Hoarseness may be caused by candida laryngitis. Patients on corticosteroid therapy are particularly prone, as the steroid inhibits neutrophil function. Neutropenia itself also allows candida to flourish. Since corticosteroids are often employed in the palliative phase to induce a feeling of well-being, improve the appetite and suppress malaise, its attendant problems cannot be ignored.

A number of preparations are available to treat candida infections. Suspensions containing nystatin and amphotericin may be used, and the latter as lozenges to suck. The patient should be encouraged to hold these in the mouth for as long as possible. Miconazole 2 per cent (w/w) may be applied as an oral gel. Regular use of these preparations every six hours is required. Often patients find them distasteful and in the palliative phase minor candida infections may not be worth treating if the patient is little troubled. Topical gentian violet, though messy, sometimes controls severe candida infection when all else fails and should not be ignored as a possible line of treatment. In some patients the relief can be quite dramatic and gratifying. Some of the dye is swallowed and is harmless. It may discourage oesophageal infection.

Ketoconizol is also a very effective treatment for candidiasis, but is usually reserved for cases where other forms of treatment have failed. Vaginal candida is a cause of several vulval itch and should be treated with pessaries and cream containing nystatin.

Herpes Zoster (Shingles)

Shingles is a common complication of haematological malignancies. Most patients succumb sooner or later. It is worth treating in the phase of palliation in order to control the symptoms. Unilateral pain in the skin with redness going on to vesicle formation should alert the clinician. Topical idoxuridine should be applied and calamine lotion is also soothing. If caught in the early stage, administer acyclovir IV and hyperimmune globulin, particularly if there is evidence of dissemination. Once the lesions start to crust, these treatments will not have much effect. Associated pain may require opiate. If the ophthalmic division of the trigeminal nerve is involved, watch for corneal involvement, and if necessary close the eyelids with strapping or stitching.

Pain

In the terminal phase of haematological malignancies pain is common. Patients with myeloma are particularly susceptible to skeletal pain, but other disorders such as the lymphomas may give rise to bony deposits and local pain. More widespread aching due to subperiosteal infiltration and pressure due to expanding tissue in the bone marrow is common, often difficult to localise and frequently shifting position. It can be very severe. Where pain and its cause can be localised, local radiotherapy, if available, is usually effective within a few days. This is particularly useful in myeloma, as it is unlikely that pain will recur in the site treated during the patient's life, unless there is associated structural damage. Similar beneficial effects may be seen in cases of lymphoma and leukaemia with localised problems. Such management does not infer an abandonment of the palliative approach, as it will not significantly alter the course of the disease. The cytotoxic antibiotic mithramycin can also be used to obtain pain relief in myeloma, as it inhibits tumour-induced activation of osteoclasts. Osteoclasts are responsible for the bone erosion. Mithramycin also decreases the mobilisation of calcium from the skeleton and is used to treat hypercalcaemia. Disadvantages of this form of treatment are that it tends to be of evanescent value and can exacerbate or cause thrombocytopenia.

Where radiotherapy cannot be used for local lesions, a nerve block may be of benefit as a means of inducing temporary relief. It is particularly valuable for severe sharp pain, often poorly relieved by the most potent analgesic. Strangely, pain produced by local lesions is often severe for a limited period unless it is associated with structural damage as occurs in the vertebrae and other weight-bearing bones. If the patient can be tided through the painful phase, the severity dies down to a point where it is easily controlled and in some cases the pain may disappear altogether without any specific local therapy.

Inevitably analgesics play a large part in pain relief and should be used appropriately. Simple non-addictive analgesics such as paracetamol are useful only for relatively mild pain. Prostaglandin-suppressing drugs such as indomethacin (25-50 mg three times daily) can be dramatically effective in some cases, but should be avoided if gastrointestinal problems liable to bleeding are present. Aspirin is often avoided for similar reasons and because it interferes with platelet function, but in practice it is often well tolerated and liked by patients.

For rather more severe pain, dihydrocodeine tartrate, alone or in combination with paracetamol, and likewise dextropropoxyphene (when combined with paracetamol, Distalgesic) are commonly used. Constipation tends to be a problem and nausea, dizziness and excessive sleepiness may prove unacceptable. Patients vary greatly in their ability to use and accept these drugs and effective use can only be by trial and error. Pentazocin is generally disliked because of its tendency to cause hallucinations. Methadone hydrochloride is a very useful analgesic and can be given either orally or intravenously.

It is important to realise that pain may be caused or exacerbated by anxiety and stress. Anxiolytic drugs therefore play a part in pain control. They should not, however, be used without analgesics or confusional states will result in which the patient is disturbed by pain although is not necessarily fully aware of it. These drugs should be used additionally. Phenytoin sodium may also be of benefit in a similar role.

Eventually the full power of the morphine group of potent analgesics should be used and indeed will be required to control severe pain at any time. These drugs have anxiolytic qualities as well, which are very helpful. Diamorphine hydrochloride is probably the most widely used. Long-acting preparations are available. Dosage should be adequate and frequent enough for satisfactory pain relief, but not so excessive as to render the patient unrousable. The most common mistake is to give inadequate doses.

Nausea is often associated with analgesic therapy, but may be present for other reasons. Chlorpromazine is a useful anti-emetic to combine with analgesics. If this causes excessive sedation, other anti-emetics such as metochlopramide hydrochloride orally or intravenously up to 10 mg three times daily, or cyclizine hydrochloride 50 mg three times daily may be tried. When nausea is very severe, it is worth combining more than one of these anti-emetics.

However, nausea is often an element of anorexia and some patients may feel the nausea only when they are presented with food. Anorexia is a very difficult symptom to treat. Institutional food very often exacerbates the problem, which may be considerably relieved when the patient is returned to his or her own home surroundings and is provided with food to which he or she is accustomed. Strong psychological factors operate in this area and it is important to remember that dietary modifications may have little or no effect if what the patient really desires is a change of surroundings or a return to home. Unfortunately, this is not always possible. In this area the judicious use of alcohol in its various forms may be very beneficial, if acceptable to the patient.

The majority of patients with leukaemia and related disorders know their diagnosis and its implications to a greater or lesser extent. If they are not told, they discover through talking to other patients or by putting two and two together. The degree of trust the patient has in his or her medical adviser usually relates to the honesty with which they have been dealt. When patients know what they want to know, they can usually face up to the terminal stages of their illness with dignity and fortitude. Their chance to do so is enhanced if they know that the discomforts and problems of the terminal stages will be handled effectively.

Patients who have one or other form of lymphoma, myeloma or one of the other disorders already discussed may not have such a clear understanding of their disease or its import as those who have leukaemia. Few patients, however, reach the terminal stages of these diseases without appreciating that they have an incurable disorder which will be lethal eventually. A number do, however, reach the terminal stage without an understanding of their disease and its prognosis.

Patients should be regarded as having a fundamental right to know the nature of their illness and its outlook. Not every patient wishes to know, some preferring the 'bliss of ignorance'. Nothing can be more distressing to the majority of patients than uncertainty. It therefore behoves the physician caring for these patients to ensure that they know and understand what they want to know.

A suggested approach which can generally be used at any time in the patient's illness, but is best used at the first encounter, is as follows. The first step is to indicate to the patient that you will not withhold anything from them they might wish to know and that to the best of your ability you will not intentionally tell them any untruths. Naturally this will be possible only if you have followed this line in your dealings with them in the past. In response to this, the patient usually gives an indication of how much he or she wants to know. The manner of the response gives further clues about how genuinely they mean what they say. Some express great satisfaction and indicate that they would be very pleased to be kept fully informed. At the other extreme, the response may be that they do not wish to be burdened with information and would be happy to leave the whole matter to their physician's hands.

If the patient has indicated that they would like to know, the truth should be unfolded carefully, gently and compassionately. It is often useful to ask the patient initially what he or she knows and understands. This may be quite revealing and some patients know a great deal more than they are given credit for. Some may know, but pretend ignorance in order to compare what you will say to them with what they have been told elsewhere. Others will genuinely say that they do not know. After a certain amount of information has been divulged, the patient may indicate that that is enough. Others press for the whole story. They want 'to know where they stand'. For a start, it is often helpful to indicate that the patient has an incurable problem and in the terminal stages the proposition has to be made that active treatment has lost its effect or that the body cannot take any more. To give more would make the patient even more ill. Patients generally understand this and may then seek to evaluate the prospects of future treatment. Patients should not be told that nothing more can be done for them. That would destroy hope and be unnecessarily unkind. In any case, much can be done to make their remaining life easier with pain relief and other supportive measures. In some cases gentle chemotherapy may be continued as a palliative measure.

Time has to be given to patients to ask what they want in an un-hurried way. Inevitably they will pose the same questions to other people and will compare the answers. In this respect the great value of being honest with patients comes through. Untruths will be found out and will destroy trust.

The response to a clearer understanding of their prognosis varies and often produces distress, grief and even anger. This is a natural response which may last for a few hours or even a few days and some-times longer. Most patients, however, go through this phase and at the end of it reach a stage of acceptance and even resignation and are able to bear their terminal phase with dignity. Many patients are apprecia-tive of the fact that they may have had a number of extra years of life as a result of the treatment given for the blood disorder.

The age of the patient clearly bears heavily on the type of response to a bad prognosis. A considerable number of patients with acute leukaemia and Hodgkin's disease are young and some are children. Unfortunately, there is often distress at the shortness of life, a feeling of having been treated unfairly, of anger and resentment. Some become intolerably depressed and may need a lot of skilled and sympathetic support and even psychiatric assistance. Many of these reactions, how-ever, are muted by the severity of the illness from which they are suffering.

Problems sometimes arise in persuading either the patients or their relatives that further active therapy will not be beneficial. Generally a careful explanation that the disease has become resistant to the treat-ment, a concept remarkably well understood by patients and relatives, is enough. If this does not satisfy, it can often be truthfully pointed out that the body is not capable of tolerating further treatment which, if given, could be lethal. Faced with this position, the patient may well ask bluntly: 'How long have I got then?' It is usually true to reply that it is difficult to give an accurate answer and vague phrases such as 'not very long', said in the right way, may then prompt a suggestion of a length of time from the patient. Often the patient's estimate can be accepted, unless it is quite unrealistic. With relatives the answer should be more specific, but should always be covered by the caveat that surprises can happen.

The final phase of most haematological disorders, if not terminated by an acute bleeding or infective episode, is best controlled by adequate pain relief and, if necessary, sedation. Some patients become very absorbed with the details of how they are going to die. They should be reassured that it need not be unpleasant.

Further Reading

Winthorpe, M.M. (1981) *Clinical Haematology*, 8th edn, Lea and Febiger, Philadelphia

5 PALLIATIVE CARE IN CHRONIC RENAL FAILURE

Robin Winney

Introduction

Until the early 1960s chronic renal failure was a progressive and fatal disorder, so that for most patients traditional palliative care was necessary in the later stages. The development of dialysis and transplantation, however, has resulted in a unique form of palliative care by means of an artificial organ or replacement organ. The initial success of these treatments in the early 1960s has been followed by a dramatic growth in the number of patients maintained alive beyond the natural end-point. In Europe at the end of 1980 there were 48 408 patients alive on haemodialysis treatment, 2749 alive on peritoneal dialysis treatment and 12 394 alive with a functioning transplant. In 1980, 14 084 new patients started treatment in Europe (Jacobs *et al.*, 1981). With improvement in techniques, the majority of patients will now benefit from treatment. Only in the past three years the development of continuous ambulatory peritoneal dialysis (CAPD) has improved the quality of life which can be achieved for patients for whom in the past haemodialysis and transplantation were either difficult or impossible — the very young, the elderly, patients with cardiovascular disease and patients with diabetes mellitus. Unfortunately, dialysis is expensive and this has significantly influenced the application of treatment. In countries with economic restrictions, patients who would benefit from treatment may be deprived of such an opportunity (Knapp, 1982; Office of Health Economics, 1978). By contrast, in an affluent society, where a financial incentive to treat patients may be present, there may result the inappropriate treatment of some patients (Waterfall, 1981).

The type of palliative care needed in patients with end-stage renal failure is variable. For some patients treated by dialysis and transplantation, one achieves almost a cure. However, although for the majority of patients one falls well short of this ideal, nevertheless a good quality of life can be achieved. In a minority of patients, including some for whom dialysis and transplantation are not feasible, the success is less good and the form of treatment is similar to traditional palliative care.

Availability of treatment for end-stage renal failure should not allow one to forget that good medical management of chronic renal failure may delay the time when such treatment is needed and may also enable a worthwhile prolongation of life for patients for whom such treatment is not appropriate.

Incidence

The incidence of chronic renal failure has been well defined in the United Kingdom (Pendreigh *et al.*, 1972). Some 38 patients per million population under the age of 55 and without any other serious disease will develop end-stage chronic renal failure each year. All such patients, with the possible exception of the very young, will benefit from treatment by dialysis and transplantation. If one extends the upper age to include patients up to the age of 65, without any other serious disease, the figure rises to 52 per million population per year; indeed, it rises further to 96 per million population per year if one includes all patients with end-stage chronic renal failure under the age of 65, with or without other significant disease – included in this figure will be some who will not benefit from dialysis and transplantation and others where the benefit is marginal.

Figure 5.1: Age distribution of patients commencing hospital haemodialysis in Europe in 1978

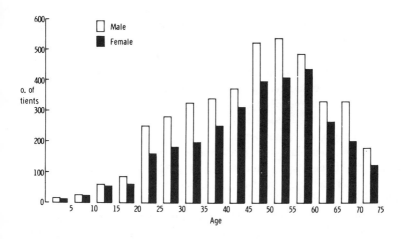

Source: *Proceedings of the European Dialysis and Transplant Association* (1979) vol. 16, p. 11, Pitman Medical, Tunbridge Wells

Table 5.1: Aetiology of chronic renal failure in patients commencing haemodialysis in Europe in 1978

	Percentage of total
Chronic renal failure (aetiology uncertain)	10.5
Glomerulonephritis	32.7
Pyelonephritis and interstitial nephritis (including obstructive uropathy)	20.9
Drug nephropathy (including analgesic nephropathy)	3.0
Cystic kidney disease	9.2
Heredo-familial (Alport's syndrome particularly)	2.8
Renal vascular disease (including hypertension and polyarteritis)	8.3
Multi-system disease (diabetes, amyloid, systemic lupus erythomatosis)	8.5
Other (including tuberculosis, nephrocalcinosis)	4.2

Source: *Proceedings of the European Dialysis and Transplant Association.*

Chronic renal failure affects all age-groups (Figure 5.1) and may involve the young, the teenager, the breadwinner and the elderly. It therefore has major implications for family groups, societies and health planners.

Aetiology

The causes of chronic renal failure and their relative importance are shown in Table 5.1. The advances in the treatment of end-stage chronic renal failure have not been accompanied by the same rate of progress in prevention or specific treatment. For the majority of disorders, there is either no treatment available or the treatment has no significant effect on the outcome. Important exceptions are, however, drug-induced interstitial nephritis and obstructive uropathy. Early detection of both conditions, followed by cessation of drug therapy or relief of obstructive uropathy, may arrest or significantly delay progress of the disease. In particular, the recognition of the association between phenacetin-containing compounds and analgesic nephropathy has resulted in a restricted availability of these compounds to the general public and, hopefully, should result in a reduced incidence of this condition. By contrast, in glomerulonephritis, the most important cause of end-stage renal failure, increased understanding of the pathogenesis has not yet led to a major therapeutic breakthrough. Nevertheless, for a limited number of patients with an acute glomerulonephritis resulting in rapid deterioration in renal function, treatment by immunosuppression and plasma exchange may result in a striking improvement in renal function. Similarly, the development of new potent anti-hypertensive drugs such as captopril and minoxidil may enable improvement in renal function in patients presenting with malignant hypertension associated with severe renal failure. Other important conditions where treatment may have a significant effect on the outcome of renal disease are connective tissue disorders and myeloma.

Although specific treatment will be of little value in the majority of disorders, early investigation is still essential. Specific treatment is of little value if the kidneys are irreversibly damaged — experience indicates that this may happen in as short a space of time as one or two weeks in some types of glomerulonephritis, myeloma and polyarteritis. Early referral also enables a diagnosis to be made and an indication of prognosis to be given to the patient — various histological types of glomerulonephritis have, for instance, a varying prognosis. Finally, the introduction of the general management of renal failure may slow down the progress of the disease.

Disturbance of renal function indirectly influences the function of many organs. As a result, the manifestations of renal disease are extremely variable. Presenting symptoms may range from urinary symptoms to tiredness, breathlessness, oedema, cramp and bone pain. In patients presenting with vague symptoms, simple investigations such as urinalysis and the estimation of blood urea and electrolytes will help early referral.

Inherited Renal Disease

Most renal disease does not have an inherited basis. Patients should be informed of this, since many continue to worry that the condition will be passed to their children. There are two inherited disorders which are important causes of chronic renal failure: the adult form of polycystic kidney disease and Alport's syndrome (Editorial, *British Medical Journal*, 1981).

Polycystic kidney disease is inherited as an autosomal dominant, but the severity of the disease varies between and within families, so that not all affected members develop renal failure. The peak prevalence of end-stage renal disease in this condition is in the age-range 35-45 and it is uncommon for patients to develop end-stage renal disease before the age of 30.

Alport's syndrome results in inherited nephritis and nerve deafness.

It is also inherited as an autosomal dominant, but the exact mode of inheritance is not clear and it is in some way sex-linked. The condition is passed on by affected females, but only affected males develop severe renal failure. In this condition, end-stage renal disease often occurs in young people in their twenties.

When one of these diagnoses is made, the patient's relatives and family should be informed. This enables other members of the family to be screened and enables genetic counselling, so that affected members can make a rational decision about having children.

Conservative Management

With the knowledge that dialysis and transplantation are available in the future, it is easy to neglect the medical management of chronic renal failure. Good medical management may, however, delay progress of the renal disease and put off the time when dialysis and transplantation are required. No patient wishes this form of treatment unless it is absolutely necessary. In addition, good management in this phase is necessary if the patient is to receive maximum benefit from dialysis and transplantation therapy in the future.

Pathophysiology of Chronic Renal Failure

An understanding of the pathophysiology of chronic renal failure is an absolute necessity to manage the patient correctly, and a brief description is therefore indicated.

All functions of the kidney are affected to some degree, sooner or later. Current understanding of chronic renal disease indicates that the individual nephrons (glomerulus and convoluted tubule) either remain functionally intact or become non-functioning — the so-called intact nephron hypothesis. The excretory functions of the kidney fail in the expected manner so that progressive accumulation of waste metabolites occurs in direct proportion to the degree of renal failure. By contrast, the failing kidney adapts to fluid and electrolyte disturbance almost completely until the glomerular filtration rate falls to 1-2 ml/minute. This adaptation consists of the excretion of a greater proportion of the filtered load than normal. Adaptation is, however, limited. In the face of a reduced intake of sodium and water, the kidney is unable to conserve sodium and water normally and behaves as if under the influence of an osmotic diuresis. This results in a higher obligatory sodium and water loss, with impaired urine concentration. In the face of reduced intake, the patient with chronic renal failure is therefore at risk of sodium and water depletion, which will result in hypovolaemia, a further reduction of the glomerular filtration rate, and exacerbation of renal failure. In general, it is only in the later stages that salt and water retention become a problem. Sodium and water retention may occur at an earlier stage, particularly in the presence of cardiac failure, hypertension or nephrotic syndrome, and severe sodium loss occurs with some tubular disorders. Day-to-day regulation of potassium by the kidney remains normal until a late stage, but the ability to deal with an acute rise in plasma potassium is impaired. For other substances, regulation is partial and the most important example is phosphate. Phosphate retention secondary to renal failure results in stimulation of parathyroid hormone secretion, which results in reduced renal tubular reabsorption of phosphate. The plasma phosphate is by this mechanism maintained normal, but at the expense of secondary hyperparathyroidism. This regulation is only completely effective, however, until a glomerular filtration rate of 40 ml/minute, when the plasma phosphate rises despite this regulation.

The acidosis of chronic renal failure results mainly from impaired ammonia production; in the later stages, reduced filtration of phosphate also contributes. Patients with predominantly tubular disease tend to have a more severe acidosis than patients with glomerular disease, as a result of defective distal tubular acidification. The acidosis in chronic renal disease is usually not progressive, and this is thought to be a consequence of bone buffering which occurs at the expense of demineralisation of bone.

The hormonal functions fail in a variable fashion. Hypertension is usually due to a combination of salt and water retention and excess renin production, but either factor may be more important. Anaemia results from a shortened red-cell survival, impaired production of erythropoietin and bone marrow suppression by uraemia. In the later stages, it is an important factor contributing to tiredness. Some patients, particularly those with polycystic kidney disease, retain significant erythropoietin production and are therefore less severely anaemic. Vitamin D resistance in chronic renal failure results from impaired hydroxylation of vitamin D by the kidney. Below a glomerular filtration rate of 40 ml/minute, hydroxylation of vitamin D by the kidney stops and leads to impaired production of the active vitamin D metabolite 1,25-dihydroxycholecalciferol. This results in malabsorption of calcium, hypocalcaemia, rickets or osteomalacia and secondary hyperparathyroidism.

The Uraemic Syndrome

Classically, the uraemic syndrome has been ascribed to an accumulation of small molecular weight substances, characterised by urea and creatinine. Recent doubt has been cast on the toxicity of such compounds, mainly on the basis of their lack of toxicity in experimental animals. Rather more emphasis has been placed on the toxicity of larger molecular weight substances, the so-called 'middle molecules', as well as on other substances which accumulate as part of the adaptation to renal failure, for example, parathyroid hormone. The uraemic syndrome seems likely to be much more complex than was originally thought and this has implications for the treatment of patients, particularly since most haemodialysis membranes are relatively impermeable to these larger molecular weight substances. Nevertheless, despite these doubts, symptoms of uraemia bear a good relationship to plasma concentrations of urea and creatinine and, with dialysis therapy, improvement in uraemic symptoms occur with a reduction in concentration of the classical toxins.

Whereas in acute renal failure uraemic symptoms may arise rapidly, in chronic renal failure man adapts to the uraemic environment and symptoms are of insidious onset. At a blood urea of 30 mmol/l (180 mg/dl), symptoms first arise and consist of tiredness, anorexia and difficulty coping with daily tasks. By the time the blood urea rises to 40 mmol/l (240 mg/dl), in addition to progression of these symptoms, anorexia, nausea, vomiting, pruritus, difficulty in concentrating and looseness of the bowels may occur. Above this level, the most severe complications may arise and consist of pericarditis, drowsiness and convulsions as well as a bleeding tendency. These latter symptoms indicate the terminal phase of renal failure. The aims of treatment should be to minimise symptoms and maintain uraemic toxicity at the level of the earliest complications.

Treatment

Treatment aims to delay progress of the disease, compensate for disturbances arising as a result of renal failure, treat symptoms occurring and ensure that the regulatory mechanisms are enabled to operate optimally.

Uraemia. The aims of treatment are to minimise symptoms, while ensuring that the patient does not become malnourished as a result of treatment. This is achieved by restricting protein intake and increasing calorie intake to maintain energy balance. Failure to increase the calorie intake will result in muscle wasting and a weak, debilitated patient. For this reason, inappropriate use of protein restriction can contribute to ill health, rather than improving it.

Protein restriction is commenced when symptoms interfere with the normal life-style. This is usually around a blood urea of 30 mmol/l (180 mg/dl). The degree of restriction will depend on the intake, but is usually 40 g daily with the calorie intake being maintained around 2500 daily. Protein restriction limits the intake of bread, and low-protein flour and bread are available on prescription to act as substitutes. In deciding the level of protein restriction one must remember that protein intake varies — an active young man may eat 100 g of protein, whereas a middle-aged lady may only eat 40 g. Thus a more moderate reduction in protein intake may be all that is required if the protein intake is higher than the average of 70 g daily. With modern-day management, protein intake is not reduced below 40 g daily if the patient is a candidate for dialysis or transplantation, as by this stage nausea from uraemia limits the ability to increase the calorie intake and the patient is, as a result, likely to become malnourished and unable to work. The aims of treatment are to maintain rehabilitation so that when symptoms of uraemia recur on a 40 g protein diet, this is an indication to commence dialysis treatment.

For patients who will not be treated by dialysis, further restriction of protein intake to 20 g daily may improve uraemic symptoms when they have occurred on a 40 g intake. With this level of restriction, one accepts that muscle wasting is a price that has to be paid, but this can be minimised by encouraging as high a calorie intake as can be tolerated.

There are a number of useful calorie preparations which can be obtained on prescription and which can supplement the carbohydrate intake in the diet in patients on a protein-restricted intake. Hycal is a flavoured drink available in various flavours, which contains 410 calories in a 171 ml bottle. Maxijul and Caloreen powders are white tasteless carbohydrate sources which contain 4 calories per gram and can be added to a variety of foods.

Water. As a general rule, a high fluid intake of 2.5-3.0 litres daily should be maintained to ensure that water depletion does not arise as a consequence of the impaired concentrating ability. In addition, a high urine flow rate increases urea clearance by the kidneys. One should encourage the patient to utilise this high fluid intake to increase the calorie intake, for example, by taking some of the fluid as Hycal.

Exceptions may occur, and if hyponatraemia arises without evidence of sodium depletion, then the fluid intake may have to be restricted to 500 ml plus the previous day's urine output. This is most likely to happen in patients with cardiac failure.

Impaired ability to excrete water only arises in the very late stages, usually when the glomerular filtration rate is 1–2 ml/minute and can be detected by a falling urine output with a rise in weight and hyponatraemia. At this stage, fluid restriction to 500 ml plus the urine volume should be given. By this time, most patients will be on dialysis treatment or requiring it.

Sodium. For the majority of patients, a normal intake of sodium is desirable because of the inability to conserve sodium normally. The requirements for sodium may change as the disease advances and restriction to a no-added-salt (avoidance of added salt at the table), strict no-added-salt (avoidance of added salt at table, plus avoidance of salty food), or – rarely – a 50 mmol sodium intake (previous restrictions with no salt in the cooking) may be needed at some stage. There are exceptions to this general guideline. Sodium retention will occur in patients with cardiac disease, nephrotic syndrome or hypertension. In these patients, sodium restriction to a strict no-added-salt level will be required. By contrast, in some patients with tubular disease, excessive sodium loss may occur. In these patients, additional sodium supplements, sometimes large amounts, may be required and are important since significant improvement in renal function may occur as a result.

Assessment of the sodium requirements of a patient with chronic renal failure is an important part of the management. Clinical examination may give some indication, there either being evidence of salt and water overload or an indication that the patient is salt and water depleted, for example, the presence of postural hypotension. Daily weighing of the patient will also give some guide – a falling weight indicates an inadequate intake and a rising weight accumulation. Alternatively, measurement of the 24-hour urine sodium when the dietary intake of sodium is known will give an approximate guide to the level of sodium intake required. If there is any doubt that the dietary sodium intake is insufficient to maintain sodium balance, then one should give sodium chloride, 1 g three times daily and continue to weigh on a regular basis, adjusting the sodium chloride until either weight is stable or there is evidence of salt and water overload. Such an approach ensures that the renal blood flow is maintained at a maximal level.

Table 5.2: Causes of hyperkalaemia in chronic renal failure

Dietary, including I.V. administration of potassium	
Acidosis	
Increased tissue catabolism	— infection
	— shock
Increased red-cell breakdown	— haemolysis
	— gastrointestinal haemorrhage
'Potassium-sparing' diuretics, e.g. spironolactone, triamterene	

Table 5.3: Treatment of acute hyperkalaemia

Immediate	1.	50 ml 50% dextrose mixed with 8 units soluble insulin I.V.
	2.	10 ml 10% calcium gluconate I.V. Repeat 1 and 2 if necessary
Followed by	3.	If acidotic I.V. infusion of 500 ml 1.26% sodium bicarbonate over 4–6 hours
or	4.	I.V. infusion of 500 ml 10% dextrose with 8 units soluble insulin over 6 hours
	5.	Calcium resonium 30 g. orally and/or rectally
	6.	Oxygen if hypoxic
Followed by	7.	Dialysis if necessary
Monitor electrocardiogram and measure plasma potassium at regular intervals.		

Potassium. It is commonly thought that chronic renal failure is accompanied by hyperkalaemia, but this is not usually a problem until the later stages (glomerular filtration rate < 10 ml/minute). Until this stage, patients may have a normal potassium intake. In the later stages, when hyperkalaemia indicates the need for restriction, instruction to avoid an excess of potassium-containing foods is normally all that is required.

Patients with chronic renal failure are unable to excrete an acute potassium load so that an acute rise in plasma potassium may arise under certain circumstances (Table 5.2). Under these circumstances, the underlying cause must be corrected. Provided the plasma potassium is below 6 mmol/l, the potassium can be monitored at regular intervals with no immediate action being taken. If the potassium exceeds 6 mmol/l, then urgent treatment is required because of the risk of cardiac arrest (Table 5.3). During the acute episode, restriction of potassium intake may be required and calcium resonium (an exchange resin) in a dosage of 30 g orally or rectally can be given once to twice daily. The use of such resins should, however, be limited, since they are extremely unpleasant and constipating, and no patient with chronic renal failure requires to take such resins on a regular basis. In addition to these measures, the plasma potassium must be monitored frequently and in some patients dialysis therapy may be necessary on a temporary basis because of hyperkalaemia.

In a stable patient in whom the plasma potassium is between 5–6 mmol/l, the correction of mild acidosis is often all that is required to lower the plasma potassium to a satisfactory level.

Acidosis. When the plasma bicarbonate falls below 20 mmol/l, this should be treated with bicarbonate supplements as bone buffering may contribute to skeletal demineralisation. Normally one gives sodium bicarbonate 1 g three times daily and this is usually sufficient in patients with glomerular disease. Some patients with tubular disease may require larger doses than this – up to 6 g daily. The sodium bicarbonate increases the sodium intake and may result in sodium overload and hypertension. One therefore requires to see the patient more frequently initially, monitor the weight, and it may be necessary either to restrict the sodium intake to a strict no-added-salt level or to add a diuretic.

Occasionally, if the patient is hypokalaemic as well as acidotic, one may give potassium bicarbonate 1–2 g three times daily, but this will apply to a minority of patients.

Monitoring of the Patient with Chronic Renal Failure

Patients with chronic renal failure are in a changing situation, proceeding down a path of declining renal function. Below a glomerular filtration rate (GFR) of 60 ml/minute, any small change in renal function will result in an acute rise in the degree of uraemia. They therefore require to be reviewed at regular intervals in order that treatment can be appropriately altered at each stage, residual function maximised and symptoms minimised. Detection of complications at an early stage is always much better for the patient than dealing with an established problem which may result in irreversible deterioration in renal function.

The severity of uraemia can be assessed by monitoring urea and creatinine, and below a GFR of 60 ml/minute these also are a reasonable index of renal function. However, the blood urea is also influenced by dietary protein intake and tissue catabolism as well as by changes in renal function, so it may give a false guide to renal function. Particularly when the patient is on a low-protein diet, measurement of creatinine as well as urea is important in indicating the degree of renal impairment.

Table 5.4: Reversible factors in chronic renal failure

Fluid and electrolyte disturbance, particularly depletion
Cardiac failure
Urinary tract obstruction
Infection
Urinary tract infection
Hypertension
Drugs adversely affecting renal function
Atheromatous occlusion of renal arteries

Reversible Deterioration in Renal Function

Whenever one assesses a new patient with chronic renal failure, or when the patient becomes ill, or even during a routine review, one should be constantly looking for reversible factors, attention to which may preserve or improve renal function (Table 5.4). All of these factors may give rise to deterioration in renal function which may improve if they are corrected. Particularly with an intercurrent illness, the patient may not be able to maintain a normal intake of water and sodium, which may result in worsening of uraemia, with nausea, vomiting and the creation of a vicious circle. Infection results in increased urea production, so the patient requires maximum renal function to cope with the increased load of urea. One should therefore never hesitate to hospitalise these patients during any intercurrent illness, since intravenous fluids may be required. Attention to all of these reversible factors is underestimated in delaying the progress of renal disease.

Obstruction of the upper urinary tract is now simple to exclude by renal ultrasound and this should always be performed on a new patient with chronic renal failure or a patient in whom there is a suggestion of urinary tract obstruction. When performing intravenous pyelography, it is important to remember that a high dose will be required to adequately visualise the renal tract. The radiological contrast medium used for intravenous pyelography is potentially nephrotoxic and the risk of this can be minimised by ensuring that the patient with chronic renal failure is not fasted before this examination. A reasonable index of obstruction in the lower urinary tract in a patient with suggestive symptoms is the presence of a residual urine volume of over 200 ml after micturition.

Complications

Important Complications due to Uraemia

Pruritus. The specific cause of pruritus is unclear. It occurs with un-controlled uraemia, hyperphosphataemia and in association with hyper-parathyroidism. It can be one of the most disturbing symptoms of uraemia, particularly since it is characteristically made worse by heat and therefore occurs particularly in bed at night and disturbs sleep. In most patients severe pruritus can be minimised by adequate control of uraemia and hyperphosphataemia with treatment of secondary hyperparathyroidism, if this is a factor. While the cause is being treated, symptomatic relief can be attempted with calamine lotion or anti-histamine creams. Relief at night can be obtained by the use of an oral antihistamine, either trimeprazine 10 mg or chlorpheniramine 4 mg. These agents should not be used on a regular basis, since they accumu-late in renal failure and cause drowsiness. If pruritus is intractable despite these measures (this is extremely unusual), then a course of ultraviolet light therapy may be of benefit. In the majority of patients, pruritus becomes troublesome around the stage at which dialysis is indicated and normally improves with dialysis therapy.

Nausea and Vomiting. When these are sufficiently severe to cause symptoms and are not controlled by protein restriction, this usually indicates the need for dialysis or is an indication of terminal renal failure. These symptoms will be uncommon with a blood urea below 35 mmol/l (220 mg/dl). It is important to remember that the symptoms may not be due to uraemia, but there may be another cause, for example, peptic ulceration. Drug accumulation in the presence of renal failure is another important cause of nausea and vomiting. Codeine derivatives are particularly important as causes of nausea and vomiting and such preparations should be used with extreme caution in patients with renal impairment. If there is no other cause except for uraemia, the symptoms may be controlled with metoclopramide 10 mg before meals or cyclizine. Metoclopramide should be used with caution, since it may accumulate and cause extrapyramidal movements.

Pericarditis. This may be an incidental finding or present with chest pain which may mimic myocardial infarction, but is characteristically eased by sitting forward. Unless precipitated by an intercurrent illness with acute reversible deterioration in uraemia, the onset of pericarditis indicates the need for dialysis or is a terminal event. If unassociated with pain, it requires no symptomatic treatment. Relief from pain may be obtained with indomethacin 25 mg three times daily. The only specific treatment for pericarditis is to improve the degree of uraemia, and this usually means dialysis therapy. The main risk of pericarditis is the development of a pericardial effusion and cardiac tamponade. Patients with pericarditis should be monitored for evidence of cardiac tamponade by frequent clinical examinations, observation of the heart size on X-ray and by ultrasound of the heart.

Peripheral Neuropathy. This complication of uraemia is rarely seen with the early use of dialysis and avoidance of severe protein restriction. It seems likely that it is as much a consequence of poor nutrition as of uraemia. If it occurs, the only treatment is dialysis and adequate nutrition, but it may take some months to improve. The antibiotic nitrofurantoin can induce a peripheral neuropathy and should not be used in chronic renal failure.

Infection. Uraemia depresses the cellular and the humeral defences against infection, so patients with chronic renal failure are both more susceptible to infection and are likely to develop more severe manifestations of infection than healthy people. Patients should be aware of this so that appropriate antibiotic treatment can be given early. Since infection may result in reversible deterioration in the degree of uraemia, treatment of this is also likely to be required.

Salt and Water Retention (Peripheral Oedema and Pulmonary Oedema)

In addition to the expected symptoms of fluid retention, a persistent cough, particularly at night, may be the only clinical manifestation of pulmonary oedema in chronic renal failure.

Fluid overload should be treated by restriction of dietary sodium to 100 mmol (no added salt, with avoidance of salty food) and diuretics. Thiazide diuretics are ineffective with impaired renal function and one has to rely on the more potent loop diuretics, frusemide or bumetanide. Even with these agents, there is likely to be considerable resistance and large doses may be required. However, one should start with a small dose (40 mg frusemide or 1 mg bumetanide) and double the dose every few days until an effect is achieved, as evidenced by a reduction in weight. The dose may require to be increased to a maximum of 1 g frusemide or 20 mg bumetanide to achieve an effect. It is useful to remember that there is a 500 mg tablet of frusemide, which is of value when one is prescribing large doses. In general, when used in high dosage, these diuretics are more effective as a single dose than when given in divided doses. Once an effect has been achieved, the patient must be monitored closely with frequent weighing and assessment of renal function. A rise in blood urea may indicate an excessively rapid diuresis and be an indication to reduce the dose. Once the diuresis has been achieved, the patient may become more sensitive and continued diuresis may occur with a lower dosage than that used initially. Once the patient is free of evidence of pulmonary oedema and/or peripheral oedema has almost cleared, the dosage should be reduced until the weight has stabilised, ensuring that the blood urea does not begin to rise. If the patient is grossly oedematous initially, one may not achieve a response with oral diuretics since they may not be adequately absorbed from a congested gastrointestinal tract and the diuretics may require to be given intravenously initially, with the oral route being used at a later stage. When using diuretics in large doses intravenously, they should be given slowly (over approximately 30 minutes) to avoid transient deafness due to ototoxicity. If the patient is resistant to maximum doses of loop diuretics, then addition of metolazone in a dosage of 5-20 mg daily may achieve a diuresis, since this diuretic acts synergistically with loop diuretics. This combination of diuretics should be commenced in hospital and the dosage of loop diuretic may require to be reduced, since occasionally a large diuresis may result. If the patient has cardiac disease, then treatment of this may also be required to improve fluid overload, since diuretics may simply result in a rise in blood urea without much improvement in the symptoms of fluid overload.

In patients with advanced chronic renal failure, treatment with diuretics is best commenced in hospital. Fluid overload is the only indication for diuretics in chronic renal failure, and if wrongly used may result in exacerbation of renal failure. Diuretics are not a treatment of hyperkalaemia.

When using diuretics in renal failure, one initially would not give potassium supplements unless the plasma potassium falls. Potassium-sparing diuretics — spironolactone, triamterene and amiloride — should be avoided, since they may result in potassium retention and precipitate hyperkalaemia.

In the absence of cardiac disease, resistance to large doses of diuretics indicates the need for dialysis therapy. In some patients with cardiac disease, fluid overload may necessitate the use of dialysis before it is required to treat uraemia.

Hypertension

Hypertension may be the cause or a consequence of renal failure and is an important factor aggravating renal failure. Control of hypertension may delay progress of the disease as well as preventing other complications of hypertension. The blood pressure should not be rapidly lowered and care should be taken not to overtreat hypertension resulting in postural hypotension, since these may both result in deterioration in renal function. One therefore aims to maintain the diastolic blood pressure around 95-100 mmHg in the supine and erect positions.

The drugs used to treat hypertension are no different from those in regular usage and can, in general, be given in normal dosage. Treatment would normally be commenced with a vasodilator (prazosin or hydrallazine) with a β-adrenergic blocker being added if necessary. If there is evidence of fluid overload, a diuretic should be given. These drugs are sufficient to control hypertension in the majority of patients.

Caution should be exercised in the use of β-adrenergic blockers, since there is concern, but no proof, that by depressing cardiac output they may decrease renal blood flow. Sensitivity to β-blockers is very variable and a small dose should be used initially. This may, by suppressing renin production, be sufficient to produce improvement in hypertension and a larger dose may not be required.

It is important to remember that the side-effects of antihypertensive drugs, particularly tiredness and impotence, may exacerbate existing uraemic symptoms. This applies particularly to methyl dopa.

Occasionally hypertension is more severe and resistant to the above drug regime. The recent availability of captopril and minoxidil has enabled control of hypertension in such patients. However, these drugs should be used only by physicians familiar with them and they require combination with a loop diuretic for effectiveness. Patients are more sensitive to captopril when not fluid overloaded, and this allows use of a lower doage, which minimises the risk of a deterioration in renal function due to the drug. Minoxidil causes fluid retention and hirsutism and requires combination with a diuretic. When these drugs are initially introduced, other antihypertensive drugs should be stopped and only reintroduced if blood pressure is not adequately controlled.

Anaemia

This is an important factor contributing to tiredness in the later stages. There is no specific therapy but, since it is of gradual onset, adaptation occurs and it is usually much less disabling than would be expected. Regular blood transfusion is not advocated, as there is a risk of transmitting hepatitis which may influence future management, and of sensitisation to transplantation antigens, which may make future transplantation difficult. In addition, regular blood transfusion creates dependency on blood transfusion by depressing residual erythropoetic production by the kidney. Thus, although the patient's symptoms might be improved temporarily, the risks outweigh the advantages. If the haemoglobin is below 5 g/dl, transfusion should be given to produce a rise to 7 g/dl. If there is severe cardiovascular disease, for example, severe angina, which is being made worse by anaemia, then transfusion to a level of 8 g/dl may be of benefit. There is no indication to transfuse to a normal haemoglobin.

One must be aware that other causes of anaemia may co-exist and must be looked for in the event of an acute fall in haemoglobin, or if anaemia is out of proportion to the degree of renal failure. If the patient is on a protein-restricted diet, he may be at risk of deficiency in haemotinics, including iron, and this can be prevented by supplying a vitamin preparation containing B vitamins, ascorbic acid, folic acid and iron. Vitamin preparations containing vitamin D should be avoided.

Renal Osteodystrophy

Disturbance of calcium, phosphate and vitamin D metabolism in chronic renal failure may result in hypocalcaemia, osteomalacia or rickets, secondary hyperparathyroidism, as well as vascular and metastatic calcification. Osteoporosis may also occur, but is not an important cause of symptoms.

Metastatic calcification can be peri-articular or in soft tissues, particularly the myocardium. When it develops around joints, it induces acute pseudo-gout with a painful, swollen, hot, tender joint. This may result from hypercalcaemia, hyperphosphataemia or a combination of both, but hyperphosphataemia is probably the most important factor. The risk of this complication can be minimised by maintaining the plasma phosphate below 2 mmol/l (6.2 mg/dl) with restriction of dietary phosphate intake (protein restriction achieves this) as well as the use of aluminium hydroxide before meals, which acts as a phosphate-binding agent, preventing absorption. Aluminium hydroxide is available either as a liquid gel or in tablet or capsule form. Magnesium-containing preparations should not be used, because of the risk of hypermagnesaemia. The dosage is either 5 ml of the gel three times daily, or 1 tablet/capsule three times daily, five minutes before meals, increasing to 10 ml three times daily or 2 tablets/capsules three times daily if indicated. Caution should be exercised in increasing the dosage further because of the risk of aluminium accumulation. If this dosage is not effective, it is likely that the patient is either not taking the preparation, not taking them immediately before meals, or the phosphate intake is excessive. Compliance is greatly improved by explaining the reason for the use of these agents. Over treatment is not desirable, since hypophosphataemia may induce osteomalacia.

If acute pseudo-gout develops, this can be treated symptomatically with indomethacin 25 mg three times daily, which often obviates the need for analgesics. At the same time the cause must be identified and treated. If the cause is hypercalcaemia, this is usually a result of tertiary hyperparathyroidism, requiring parathyroidectomy, or is induced by excessive vitamin D therapy, necessitating cessation of treatment. Prevention of hyperphosphataemia is also of importance in preventing secondary hyperparathyroidism.

The pathogenesis of vascular calcification in chronic renal failure is ill understood, but may be the result both of hyperphosphataemia and secondary hyperparathyroidism. There is no known treatment and the emphasis must be on prevention by controlling hyperphosphataemia and secondary hyperparathyroidism.

Hypocalcaemia may result in tetany. If the plasma calcium is below 2 mmol/l (8 mg/dl) when corrected for protein, this should be treated either with calcium supplements, alfacalcidol or calcitriol. Calcium supplements may be given as Sandocal, three tablets daily, which provides 30 mmol (1200 mg) calcium. This, however, provides 13 mmol of potassium and may induce hyperkalaemia. For this reason, Calcium Sandos syrup, 15 ml three times daily, providing 24 mmol (960 mg) of calcium, is preferable. Calcium carbonate acts both as a phosphate-binding agent and as a calcium source, so that if the patient is hypocalcaemic and hyperphosphataemic, this may be of value in an initial dose of 2 tablets three times a day before meals, providing 24 mmol (960 mg) of calcium. It is a less effective phosphate-binding agent, however, than aluminium hydroxide. If the plasma calcium does not rise, a further increase in dose of calcium carbonate can be given.

Alternatively, hypocalcaemia can be treated with alfacalcidol or calcitriol in an initial dose of 0.25 µg daily, increase by 0.25 µg increments up to 2 µg daily if needed. If there is no response, one should ensure that the dietary intake of calcium is normal and one may have to give calcium supplements in addition. While the patient is being treated, the plasma calcium should be monitored every two or three weeks; once the plasma calcium is normal, a maintenance dose of 0.25–0.5 µg daily should maintain the plasma calcium normal, provided the dietary calcium intake is normal. In the treatment of renal osteo-dystrophy, there is now no place for calciferol, since it is ineffective, is stored, and induced hypercalcaemia may persist for some time after stopping vitamin D. The synthetic vitamin D metabolites both have a short half-life, so that the plasma calcium will return to normal with-in a few days of stopping if hypercalcaemia is induced.

Osteomalacia and rickets may result in diffuse bone pain and a proximal myopathy with fractures (particularly of the ribs) and failure to grow in children. Secondary hyperparathyroidism may also result in proximal myopathy and fractures, with pain, particularly around the knee and ankle joints. Both conditions may significantly reduce the mobility of the patient. Any child with renal disease is at risk of rickets, while in the adult osteomalacia is most likely to occur when nutritional deficiency of vitamin D and calcium is superimposed on renal disease. Secondary hyperparathyroidism is most likely to be a clinical problem in patients who have had renal disease for a long time. Bone disease may present as predominantly one condition or the other, but is often a combination of both. The diagnosis may be confirmed by the finding of a high alkaline phosphatase of bone origin and by X-ray features. If there are no specific features on X-ray, bone histology will confirm the diagnosis. Treatment of either condition is with 1–2 μg daily of either calcitriol or alfacalcidol, together with calcium supplements, if the patient is hypocalcaemic. These vitamin D metabolites increase phosphate absorption so that the introduction of a phosphate-binding agent may be required if the patient is not already taking this. Failure to control the plasma phosphate with vitamin D treatment may result in failure of response and metastatic calcification. A clinical response, with resolution of bone pain, and improvement in proximal myopathy, is usually dramatic within a month or so and precedes bone healing. During treatment, the plasma calcium, phosphate and alkaline phos-phatase must be monitored every two or three weeks. A return of alkaline phosphatase to normal indicates bone healing and at this stage hypercalcaemia is most likely. At this stage, a reduction in dose to a maintenance level of 0.25–1 μg daily is required, aiming for the low-est dose possible to control bone disease. Monitoring must then con-tinue.

If hypercalcaemia is induced by the vitamin D metabolites, the drug should be stopped and the plasma calcium will normally return rapidly to normal. A smaller dose may then be reintroduced.

If hypercalcaemia co-exists with secondary hyperparathyroidism, or if hypercalcaemia is precipitated by vitamin D treatment in a patient with secondary hyperparathyroidism, then the patient requires parathyroidectomy. The diagnosis should be confirmed by the finding of subperiosteal erosions on X-ray and by a high plasma parathyroid hormone, before proceeding to surgery.

There has been concern that treatment with synthetic vitamin D metabolites may be associated with deterioration in renal function. The evidence available indicates that this is not a significant risk, provided that hypercalcaemia and hyperphosphataemia are avoided. Nevertheless, renal function must be carefully monitored during vitamin D treatment.

Sexual Disturbance

Impotence, menstrual disturbance, particularly amenorrhoea, and reduced libido may all develop in association with severe uraemia. Amenorrhoea is unlikely to improve without improvement of uraemia by dialysis or transplantation. Impotence and reduced libido may either be a result of uraemia or be a psychological reaction to the illness. It is not uncommon for both factors to be important. In addition, reduced libido and impotence may occur in the spouse because of psychological disturbance. If it is of organic basis, the treatment is to improve uraemia. If it is of psychological origin, then simple discussion with the patient and spouse may be all that is required. Sexual counselling and sexual therapy may be of benefit to some patients.

Severe uraemia is associated with reduced fertility and it is commonly thought that contraception is not necessary. However, conception may still occur, and in patients of child-bearing age contraceptive advice should be given, since an undesired pregnancy in a family with one member affected by severe chronic renal failure may cause severe disruption.

Use of Drugs in Patients with Chronic Renal Failure

Perhaps in no other branch of medicine can drugs potentially cause so much harm to patients as in the presence of renal impairment, for the following reasons. First, drugs may cause renal disease. Second, patients with renal disease are possibly more susceptible to the nephrotoxic effects of drugs. Third, accumulation of drugs may arise in renal failure, with not only the risk of direct nephrotoxic effects but other toxic effects such as nausea and vomiting, which may indirectly affect renal function. This applies not only to drugs excreted directly by the kidney,

Table 5.5: Drug dosage modification in renal failure

---

1. Avoid   tetracyclines except doxycycline (increase tissue catabolism)
            nitrofurantoin (causes peripheral neuropathy)
            cephaloridine (nephrotoxic)
            clofibrate (metabolised to active metabolite and accumulation may
            result in myopathy and deterioration in renal function)
            combination of cephalosporin, aminoglycoside and frusemide
            (increased risk of toxicity)

2. Antibiotics   Dose reduction
   Penicillins   no
   Cephalosporins   yes
   Aminoglycosides   yes (measure plasma level)
   Chloramphenicol   no
   Erythromycin   no
   Metronidazole   no
   Carbenicillin   yes (has high sodium content)
   Co-trimoxazole   yes

3. Analgesics, antihistamines, narcotics, sedatives, hypnotics, tranquillisers,
   anti-emetics:
   use cautiously if needed, using the lowest dose possible
   particular problems are respiratory depression from codeine derivatives and
   extrapyramidal effects from metoclopramide

4. Cardiovascular and antihypertensive drugs
   Digoxin: reduce dose
   Antihypertensive drugs: normal dosage
   β-Adrenoreceptor blocking drugs:
       reduce dose of atenolol, nadolol, pindolol and sotalol
       start with a small dose of metoprolol and propanolol

5. Miscellaneous
   Cimetidine: reduce dose (produces confusional state)
   Allopurinol: reduce dose (metabolised to active metabolite)
   Anti-inflammatory drugs: avoid if possible (cause fluid retention and may
       produce deterioration in renal function)

---

but also to drugs metabolised by the liver, since the metabolites may be active, be dependent on renal excretion and accumulate. Understanding of drug metabolism in renal failure is still at a very early stage and use of drugs should therefore be minimised in patients with renal disease. Before using any drugs, the following questions should be answered: 'Is it needed? Should it be avoided in renal failure? What dosage can I give? How can I monitor for adverse effects? Is it implicated in causing renal disease? — in which case it should not be used. Adherence to these guidelines should minimise the risk associated with use of drugs in renal failure. Table 5.5 indicates examples of drugs to avoid in renal disease, and alteration in dosage of important drugs (Editorial, *British National Formulary*, 1982).

Communication with Patient and Family

Patients adjust better to any chronic illness if they understand the implications for the future. Explanation of the symptoms, the effect the illness is likely to have, and the importance of treatment are required at all stages, both with the patient and the family. This is likely to increase compliance with treatment and to enable acceptance of the illness and adjustment of life-style. The emphasis should be on how to do things in the light of the illness, rather than what they will not be able to do. Since the family are also involved, one has also to consider the implications for them. Help may be required at home in order that other members of the family may continue to support the family financially. Many patients and families require help in discussing the illness in order to adjust adequately, and many members of medical and paramedical teams as well as other members of society can help with this.

Preparation for Dialysis

Patients must be prepared for dialysis as long as possible *before* it is needed, and should be referred to a specialist unit when the glomerular filtration rate is 20 ml/minute. If possible, they should be under the care of the specialist unit for a year before dialysis is likely to be required, thus enabling the patient and family gradually to come to terms with the future and incorporate the treatment into their life-style. It also enables the start of treatment to be planned and an assessment of which treatment is most likely to be appropriate. Vascular access is required for haemodialysis and this takes time to develop before being able to be used; a Cimino fistula should be created three or four months before dialysis is needed. It is now possible to consider a live-related donor transplant before dialysis, but it takes six months to prepare for this.

All such preparation is important if the transition to dialysis is to be smooth, with minimal interruption of life-style. particularly since the aims of treatment are to continue rehabilitation so that time off work is minimised — nowadays if a job is lost it is unlikely to be available again, and this may have a disastrous effect on the family. Early referral is perhaps most important when there is doubt about suitability. All too often, such patients are referred in the terminal stages of their illness for assessment. Assessment takes time and is not possible in a patient who is severely uraemic. Early referral is not always possible, particularly if the patient does not present until a late stage. These patients usually have a difficult initiation to dialysis with major psychological disturbance and family distress. Such problems can be avoided in patients known to have renal disease at an early stage.

Patients not to be Treated by Dialysis

For such patients, a worthwhile prolongation of life can be achieved by good conservative management with continued protein restriction. Particularly in patients with other major incapacitating disease, dialysis and transplantation may simply add to the burden of the patient and family with a deterioration in the quality of life. Since a patient whose activities are severely restricted by some other disease (for example, cardiac disease) may be unaware of tiredness and lack of energy, conservative management may be possible for a much longer period of time than in a patient in whom renal disease is the only problem.

Terminal Care

The terminal care of the patient with chronic renal failure is no different from the care of any patient in the terminal phase of any illness. The emphasis must be on patient comfort, physical and spiritual, with the application of drug therapy as necessary. Since fluid overload and nausea will be prominent symptoms, the use of opiates and anti-emetics will normally be required at some stage.

Treatment by Dialysis and Transplantation

Aims of Treatment

The aims of treatment are to compensate for the normal functions of the kidneys, prevent the complications of renal failure and rehabilitate the patient and family in society. The level of rehabilitation achieved will depend on the physical and psychological state of the patient and family, and in particular on the patient's ability to adapt to, and accept, the treatment. Adequate rehabilitation is critically dependent on finding the most appropriate treatment for the individual and adapting the treatment as much as possible to suit the individual needs. Careful assessment of each patient and family is therefore required, if the aims are to be achieved. Doctors (as well as patients) often have unrealistic objectives, and awareness of the limitations, both physical and emotional, of individual patients will help their appropriate rehabilitation.

When to Start Treatment

Treatment should be started when uraemic symptoms are not controlled on a 40 g protein diet and are interfering with rehabilitation of the patient. Normally this occurs when the blood urea is 30-40 mmol/l (180-240 mg/dl) and creatinine 1200-1400 μmol/l (13.5-16 mg/dl). Since symptoms are progressive beyond this stage, the decision is often made to commence dialysis on biochemical grounds alone. Although uraemic symptoms are the most common reason for initiating treatment, other problems may precipitate the need for action. If the patient is becoming malnourished, then this may be an indication to start treatment, since it is difficult to correct malnutrition in a uraemic patient. Recurrent fluid overload (particularly pulmonary oedema, which is not responsive to maximal dosage of diuretic) may also be an indication to start dialysis before it is required on uraemic grounds, particularly in patients with cardiac disease. Rarely hyperkalaemia may be the predominant factor making initiation of dialysis necessary. Normally treatment is initially by dialysis with transplantation at a later stage. In some patients with a suitable living donor, transplantation may be the initial treatment, but this is uncommon.

Treatments Available

Haemodialysis. (See Figure 5.2). This consists of the circulation of blood through an artificial kidney, where diffusion of waste metabolites and electrolytes across a semi-permeable membrane into dialysis fluid occurs. The membrane is highly permeable to small molecules, for example, urea, creatinine, uric acid, but the clearance of larger molecular-weight substances is much lower, for instance, vitamin B_{12}. The membrane is impermeable to proteins and red blood cells. The dialysis fluid is composed of a solution of essential electrolytes and is designed to compensate for electrolyte disturbance. Thus sodium and potassium concentrations enable removal during dialysis, and acetate in the dialysis fluid transfers to blood where it is converted to bicarbonate to correct the acidosis. Similarly, the calcium concentration in dialysis fluid is higher than that in blood so net transfer to the patient occurs during dialysis, compensating for malabsorption of calcium and preventing hypocalcaemia. Water (as well as sodium) is removed during dialysis by applying either a positive pressure in the blood compartment

Figure 5.2: A patient on haemodialysis

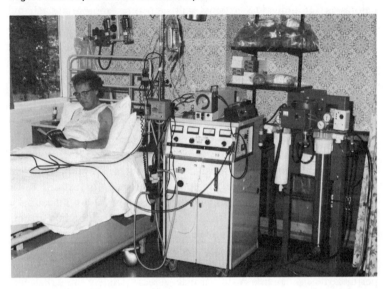

of the artificial kidney, or a negative pressure in the dialysis fluid compartment. This process is termed 'ultrafiltration' and may be performed at the same time as dialysis, or separately. The rate of water removal is determined by the total pressure across the membrane. The dialysis machine delivers dialysis fluid (a mixture of concentrated dialysis fluid and tap-water) at a rate of 500 ml/minute to the artificial kidney and also acts as a safety monitor. It monitors the chemical composition and temperature of the fluid, as well as the presence of blood in the dialysis fluid (resulting from rupture of the membrane), and pressure on both sides of the membrane. Deviation of these parameters outside pre-set limits results in audible alarms and cessation of flow of the dialysis fluid and blood. Most machines now also incorporate an air detector; the detection of air in the blood lines results in the clamping of the blood returned to the patient. These fail-safe devices mean that the risk to the patient from malfunction of equipment is now rare. There are many varieties of machine, but all basically perform the same task. Blood is pumped by a blood pump at a rate of 200 ml/minute from the patient through PVC tubing to the artificial kidney and back to the patient. Heparinisation is required during dialysis to prevent clotting in the extracorporeal circuit. The water for the dialysis fluid is also treated to remove calcium (use of hard water can lead to hypercalcaemia) and aluminium. Water softeners remove calcium, but deionisers or reverse osmosis units are required to remove aluminium.

There are many types of artificial kidney, most of which are now disposable. The main variation is in the surface area of the membrane (thus in efficiency) and in design, but most have a membrane surface area of 1 m². Artificial kidneys also vary in their ability to remove fluid, by variation in the type of membrane. The need to remove fluid during dialysis depends on the amount accumulated between treatments and will vary with residual renal function and compliance of the patient with fluid restriction.

Haemodialysis requires access to the arterial and venous circulation to achieve an adequate blood flow and to perform repeated extracorporeal circulation. This can be achieved by an external silastic arterio-venous shunt (termed a Scribner shunt), which can be placed in the arm or ankle. This has a limited life-span due to clotting or infection, and is reserved for emergency access, since it can be used immediately after insertion. The best means of repeated long-term access is a sub-cutaneous arterio-venous fistula called a Cimino fistula. This is usually performed in the forearm, but can also be created in the upper arm. This results in arteriolisation of the veins which become prominent and allow repeated cannulation with needles. This has a long life-span with a low incidence of clotting and infection, but it takes at least two months to mature and so needs to be created some time before treatment is required. In approximately 25 per cent of patients the venous system may be underdeveloped and a satisfactory fistula may not be possible. In these patients, use of vein grafts and synthetic grafts may be necessary. In addition, these alternatives may become necessary in other patients after some years of treatment, if the primary procedure fails. Current expertise in vascular access means that this is rarely, if ever, a limiting factor in treatment. Care with an external shunt is required in case it comes apart, with resulting haemorrhage, but the risk of damage to the other types of fistulae is minimal. Because of coagulation disturbance associated with uraemia, anti-coagulation is not normally required with these forms of vascular access.

The aim of haemodialysis should be to provide sufficient treatment to prevent uraemic complications and enable adequate rehabilitation. In general, this means maintaining the blood urea around 30 mmol/l (180 mg/dl) and creatinine 1200 μmol/l (13.5 mg/dl), before dialysis, with the patient feeling well between dialyses and free of severe post-dialysis lethargy. The hours of treatment prescribed vary, depending on the views of the nephrologist, but in general range from 9 to 18 hours weekly, with most patients receiving 12-15 hours weekly. The reduction in uraemic toxins with dialysis, as well as electrolyte shifts, may result in the disequilibrium syndrome which consists of lethargy (like a hangover) and, if more severe, nausea, vomiting and convulsions. This is most likely to occur with rapid changes in blood chemistry, particularly when dialysis is first commenced and, if it is persistent, usually indicates excessively rapid dialysis. These symptoms often persist for 24 hours before resolving. To avoid this problem, dialysis is gradually introduced to the new patient, with the hours of treatment being increased slowly until the necessary amount is achieved. For similar reasons, patients usually feel better with treatment three times a week rather than twice weekly treatments, and in addition general health improves because of improved control of uraemia. In general, the hours of treatment are related to body weight and residual renal function. Some patients cannot cope psychologically with treatment three times a week and for them twice weekly treatment results in a happier patient, despite the fact that physical well-being may be less than ideal. As with any treatment, haemodialysis has adverse effects and excessive dialysis can do as much harm as too little dialysis.

Haemodialysis may be associated with circulatory disturbance resulting in hypotension, particularly when large amounts of fluid require to be removed simultaneously. For these reasons, patients are encouraged not to gain in excess of 1.5 kg in weight between treatments. Patients with vascular instability are particularly prone to this problem, for example, elderly patients, patients with cardiovascular disease and patients with diabetes mellitus. For these reasons, such patients are less suited to haemodialysis and are better treated by continuous ambulatory peritoneal dialysis (CAPD).

Haemodialysis does not compensate entirely for failure of renal function, so some restrictions are required. Patients are allowed up to 70 g protein daily with sodium being restricted to a strict no-added-salt level (100 mmol daily) and potassium restricted to 70 mmol daily (this means a restricted intake of high potassium-containing foods, for example, tomatoes, potatoes, chocolate, bananas and most fruits). Fluid intake is restricted to 500 ml plus the urine output, and includes fluid in food. Since fluid restriction may be difficult to comply with, one allows up to 1.5 kg gain between dialyses. Water-soluble vitamins are lost during dialysis and blood loss means the patient is prone to iron deficiency. All patients therefore normally receive supplements of vitamin B complex, folic acid, ascorbic acid and iron. Hyperphosphataemia is not usually controlled by dialysis alone and most patients require phosphate-binding agents before meals. Undoubtedly, patients who comply with the moderate restrictions in diet and fluid are the healthiest patients. Explanation of the reasons for the restrictions often helps compliance.

Haemodialysis is usually initiated in hospital. Once the patient is stabilised, continued treatment may be performed either in hospital or at home. The place of dialysis tends to vary with culture and social circumstance. Rehabilitation is, however, improved by the need not to travel and by an attitude of non-dependence. For these reasons, as well as the risk of hepatitis with large numbers of patients in hospital units, the emphasis has been on home dialysis in the United Kingdom.

Successful self-dialysis requires an appropriate house, a patient who is well on dialysis, psychologically stable and able to accept responsibility for treatment. The patient requires good support at home with a helper to assist with dialysis, and to be available in the event of problems. Thus, selection for self-dialysis is important, if it is to be successful, and experience indicates that patients in the age-range 30–60, with a stable marriage, are the best candidates. Where housing is a problem, as in a large city, minimal-care dialysis units have been created where patients perform treatment with minimal nursing supervision. Such units have been operated successfully in a number of cities in the United Kingdom.

Peritoneal Dialysis. To perform peritoneal dialysis, a catheter is inserted through the anterior abdominal wall below the umbilicus in the midline into the peritoneal cavity, the tip of the catheter being placed in the pelvic cavity. By passing dialysis fluid in and out of the peritoneal cavity through the catheter, the peritoneal membrane acts as a semipermeable membrane allowing dialysis to occur in a similar manner to haemodialysis. Peritoneal dialysis is less efficient than haemodialysis in controlling uraemia – 24 hours of peritoneal dialysis will achieve the same as 6 hours of haemodialysis. By contrast, hyperkalaemia and fluid overload can be rapidly controlled by peritoneal dialysis. A theoretical advantage of this form of dialysis is that large molecular weight substances are cleared more rapidly than with haemodialysis. The dialysis fluid is similar to that used for haemodialysis with the exception that it has a high glucose concentration. Ultrafiltration is achieved by the osmotic effect of glucose and the rate altered by varying the glucose concentration. The gradual correction of uraemia has the advantage that this reduces the risk of disequilibrium. For this reason, peritoneal dialysis is a useful treatment in patients who present with acute severe uraemia.

The major problem with peritoneal dialysis is peritonitis. The development of a silastic permanent indwelling catheter which could be exteriorised through a skin tunnel reduced the risk of infection as well as enabling long-term peritoneal dialysis. Intermittent peritoneal dialysis for chronic renal failure has not, however, been widely practised. This involves three periods of dialysis weekly, usually overnight. Machines to control the procedure mean that patients can perform treatment themselves. Despite good results in a few centres, patients in general are not as well rehabilitated due to inadequate control of uraemia as well as poor nutrition, which may partly result from protein losses from the peritoneal cavity.

The use of peritoneal dialysis as a method of treatment for chronic renal failure has been recently revived with the development of the technique of CAPD (Figure 5.3) (Gokal *et al.,* 1980; Popovich *et al.,* 1978). As in intermittent peritoneal dialysis, a permanent indwelling catheter is placed in the peritoneal cavity. Dialysis fluid is infused into the cavity and left for four hours before being drained and fresh fluid infused. In total, four exchanges are performed daily and involve an aseptic technique for making connections, to reduce the incidence of infection. The volume of each cycle is 2 litres, but they may be less if required, for example, in children. Normally the cycles are carried out continuously seven days a week. Despite reduced efficiency, the continuous nature of dialysis means that sufficient waste metabolites, electrolytes and fluid are removed to control uraemia as effectively as in haemodialysis. Because dialysis is continuous, symptoms due to disequilibration do not occur. Circulatory disturbance is also avoided and this is a potential advantage in the very young, the very old and those with cardiovascular disease. It is also particularly suited to diabetic patients, since glucose can be controlled by adding insulin to the dialysis fluid and heparinisation is not required, minimising the risk of vitreous haemorrhage. Patients in whom vascular access is difficult may also be better treated by CAPD. Because dialysis is continuous, the diet can be more liberal than in haemodialysis. However, the procedure may reduce appetite and, since protein is lost in the dialysis fluid, a protein intake of at least 70 g daily must be encouraged. Excessive weight gain, mainly as adipose tissue, may be a problem in some patients as a result of the calories from glucose in the dialysis fluid, and calorie restriction may be required. Because fluid removal is continuous, a more liberal fluid intake of 1500–2000 ml daily may be allowed, the positive balance being negated by varying the glucose concentration in the dialysis fluid. The main complication of this technique, as with any

Figure 5.3: A patient treated by CAPD, illustrating the indwelling catheter that exteriorises from the anterior abdominal wall and the tubing that connects to the bag of dialysis fluid

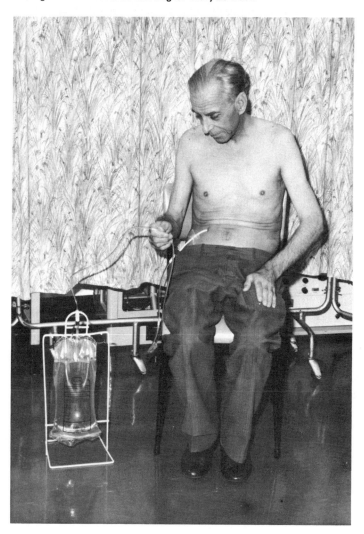

form of peritoneal dialysis, is peritonitis. Despite the use of strict aseptic technique, in most centres a patient can expect to have an episode of peritonitis every 6-12 months. Peritonitis is usually mild, the most common organism being *Staphylococcus albus*. It responds to intraperitoneal antibiotics, but if severe the catheter may have to be temporarily removed with treatment by haemodialysis for two or three weeks before restarting.

In patients with a history of previous abdominal surgery, particularly with intraperitoneal sepsis, this technique may not be successful because of adhesions preventing free infusion and drainage of dialysis fluid, or because thickening of the peritoneal membrane impairs the dialysis process. There is also a risk of herniae, possibly related to increased intra-abdominal pressure and the possibility of an obstructive hernia should be considered in a patient presenting with abdominal pain and apparent peritonitis (Chan *et al.*, 1981). Back pain due to altered posture can occur and occasionally may be a limiting factor in treatment. Similarly, reflux oesophagitis is an important symptom, which usually responds to cimetidine.

CAPD as a method of treatment is still in its infancy. Although in the short term it has been successful, its long-term effectiveness remains to be seen. In some centres, recurrent peritonitis has resulted in the need to transfer to haemodialysis 20–30 per cent of patients initiated on CAPD, but this is not a universal experience. This may partly reflect the use of CAPD as a means of treating patients in the absence of sufficient haemodialysis facilities. As with any form of self-treatment, it is unlikely to be successful unless the patient is motivated to accept responsibility. Peritoneal dialysis is not aesthetically suited to all patients, particularly to the young, since increased abdominal girth may limit the type of clothes which may be worn, and the presence of a catheter may be likened to a fistula. Selection of patients for this treatment is therefore likely to be important, if it is to succeed. Where there are restricted hospital dialysis facilities, CAPD has been used successfully as a means of self-treatment when there is no help at home for haemodialysis. Some patients prefer this form of treatment, since they find it aesthetically more acceptable than haemodialysis and benefit from the fewer haemodynamic changes. The technique of peritoneal dialysis does not interfere with the performance of renal transplantation.

Renal Transplantation. Renal transplantation can be performed using a cadaver kidney or a kidney from a live related donor. Normally the donor and recipient should be ABO blood-group identical, although compatability may be acceptable. Survival of the transplanted kidney is influenced by matching for leucocyte-associated (HLA) antigens. This antigenic system is determined by the major histocompatibility complex on the sixth pair of chromosomes in man. Three loci A, B and C determine the presence of six antigens, of which the A and B antigens are the most important, and are responsible for antibody-mediated humoral rejection. Matching for this system alone does not, however, prevent rejection, there being a 10 per cent difference in graft survival between an O match and a complete match (Van Rood *et al.*, 1979). The HLA-D locus, close to the HLA-B locus, determines cell-mediated immunity and matching for this antigenic system has an important influence on graft survival. Until recently, matching for these HLA antigens could only be assessed indirectly by performing a mixed lymphocyte reaction (MLR) between donor and recipient, a weak reaction indicating compatibility and a strong reaction mismatching. Although this is used with live donor transplants as a guide to whether to proceed with transplantation, there is insufficient time to perform this test before cadaver transplants. More recently, identification of the two HLA-D related antigens has become possible, enabling matching for this system with cadaver transplants. Preliminary results indicate that there is a 26 per cent higher graft survival after six months in transplants matched for both antigens, compared to kidneys with a complete mismatch (Ting and Morris, 1980). Perhaps the most important development, however, has been the observation that prior blood transfusion enhances graft survival (Opelz, Gravier and Teresaki, 1981). Routine transfusion of blood prior to transplantation now takes place in most centres and has been associated with an increase of up to 40 per cent in graft survival.

The best results in transplantation are obtained with an identical twin, there being almost a 100 per cent graft survival. Parents or siblings, if healthy, may also act as donors and are being increasingly looked at in view of the shortage of cadaver kidneys. Although this may raise ethical issues, it may also reduce stress in the family if the patient is successfully transplanted. Most transplants are, however, cadaver. Since the kidneys have to be removed as soon as possible after death, most donors are road traffic accident victims on ventilators. Recent controversies about criteria of death in such cases have affected the co-operation of the public and medical profession, and must be an important factor preventing an increase in the rate of cadaver transplantation in the United Kingdom. Unfortunately, the rate of transplantation has not kept up with the growth in the dialysis population, so that there is a long waiting list for transplantation − in 1980 there were 3786 transplants performed in Europe with 14 084 new patients commencing dialysis therapy in the same year. In most countries there is a central register of patients which is used to try and find the best tissue match for each kidney which becomes available.

The transplanted kidney may be placed in either iliac fossa, the renal artery and vein being anastamosed to the iliac vessels. In general, the recipient's own kidneys are not removed unless they are severely infected or responsible for renin-dependent severe hypertension. The risk of rejection, which may manifest as pyrexia with swelling and tenderness of the graft, as well as deterioration of renal function, is greatest in the first two months, so that the patient is closely monitored over this period. The kidney, however, may not function immediately because of transient ischaemic damage, and this may last between one and three weeks. Continued dialysis is therefore often required for the first few weeks following transplantation. Rejection is prevented by immunosuppression with prednisolone and azathiaprine, with the dosage of steroids being temporarily increased in the event of an acute rejection. There used to be a high morbidity and mortality in the post-transplant period, particularly from infection, but a reduction in the dosage of steroid used has reduced this risk. In addition, if it is evident that rejection is continuing after three or four weeks, then the kidney is removed, rather than persevere with immunosuppression with the risk of killing the patient. In the event of a transplant failing, further transplants are possible but the chances are less good. For these reasons, in second and subsequent transplants matching is of great importance and patients may have to wait some time for a subsequent transplant.

There are few absolute contra-indications to transplantations. Severe atheroma may make this technically impossible. A malfunctioning bladder used to be, but now kidneys can be transplanted into an ileal conduit. This allows children with spina bifida, for instance, to be transplanted. Age is a relative rather than an absolute contra-indication, the mortality being higher in patients over the age of 50. Obviously the general health of the patient at the time of transplant is important since, if this is poor, they are more at risk of complications such as infection. Patients should be well motivated, since this is an anxious period. Following a failed transplant, patients are often debilitated and demoralised and require a good deal of support when dialysis is re-introduced.

Complications in Patients Treated by Dialysis and Transplantation

Haemodialysis and CAPD. Although dialysis does not completely correct uraemia, the appetite should normalise without nausea or vomiting. Similarly, tiredness and lethargy should improve, often strikingly, but can be influenced by the patient's psychological reaction to treatment. Nevertheless, energy does not return to normal, but this need not be a major limiting factor except with heavy physical exercise. Pruritus should also improve, but in some cases can be troublesome at night and require symptomatic treatment. When pericarditis is present at the onset, this should resolve with treatment, but there is a risk of cardiac tamponade with heparinisation which may necessitate surgical drainage of the pericardial cavity. By contrast, if peripheral neuropathy is established, then this resolves only slowly with adequate treatment. In patients successfully established on treatment, pericarditis can recur in association with viral or bacterial infections or surgical procedures, and usually resolves with treatment of the underlying cause and continuing dialysis. The fluid and electrolyte status in dialysis patients is precariously balanced. The weight is stabilised at a level where there is no deficit, no fluid overload and blood pressure is satisfactory. This is achieved by ultrafiltration on dialysis. Maintenance of this state depends on the patient complying with diet and fluid restrictions as well as removing surplus fluid on dialysis treatment. Failure of the patient to comply with fluid restriction or to remove excess weight on dialysis may result in fluid overload and pulmonary oedema. This is more likely to occur with haemodialysis, where the treatment is intermittent, particularly when there is also cardiac disease. Since with CAPD fluid is removed continuously and fluid restriction may be less, fluid overload is less likely to occur. Change in fluid status may also occur in these patients because of changes in nutrition. Thus, improved well-being and appetite with dialysis may result in weight gain. By contrast, decrease in appetite, perhaps associated with an intercurrent infection, may result in loss of flesh. If in these situations the weight is not appropriately adjusted, then symptoms of fluid depletion or overload may arise. Thus, in any patient on dialysis the baseline weight needs to be regularly reviewed and altered appropriately. Acidosis is adequately corrected by dialysis therapy and sodium bicarbonate supplements are not required.

With CAPD, hyperkalaemia is rarely, if ever, a problem. Indeed, in some patients hypokalaemia may necessitate small amounts of potassium supplements. In haemodialysis, life-threatening hyperkalaemia may still arise, either associated with infection or dietary non-compliance. Avoidance of an excess of high potassium foods is an absolute necessity in haemodialysis patients and failure to adhere to this rule can result in tragic death.

Response of anaemia to haemodialysis in unpredictable. Although in some patients with polycystic kidney disease and glomerulonephritis the haemoglobin may normalise, in the majority of patients moderate anaemia persists and is a major factor, limiting exercise tolerance. The mean haemoglobin in haemodialysis patients is 7-8 g/dl and symptomatic anaemia (< 5 g/dl) requiring blood transfusion is uncommon. Anaemia is, however, likely to become symptomatic in patients who require bilateral nephrectomy. Since this interferes with rehabilitation, such patients should have a high priority for transplantation. Initial results with CAPD indicate that anaemia is significantly less than with haemodialysis and this may be an important advantage of this therapy, particularly in patients with cardiovascular disease.

In 90 per cent of patients on dialysis therapy hypertension is adequately controlled by a reduction in weight until there is no evidence of fluid overload, and by sodium and fluid restriction, thus avoiding the need for antihypertensive drugs. In a small proportion of patients, particularly those with vascular disease, this may result in postural hypotension and these patients may be better treated with a small dose of an antihypertensive drug. Only in some 5 per cent of patients is hypertension severe despite these measures, and this is usually associated with high plasma renin activity. Until recently, these patients have been best managed by bilateral nephrectomy, which results in normalisation of the blood pressure. However, the recent availability of captopril may enable medical management of these patients.

Hypocalcaemia is uncommon in dialysis patients since the high dialysate calcium compensates for malabsorption of calcium. Hyperphosphataemia continues to be a problem, due to inadequate removal by the dialysis, and restriction of dietary phosphate with oral phosphate-binding agents continues to be required. With CAPD the plasma phosphate is better controlled and these patients require lower doses of phosphate-binding agents than haemodialysis patients.

The incidence of disabling bone disease increases with increasing duration of dialysis. This may be either osteomalacia or secondary hyperparathyroidism. Osteomalacia due to vitamin D and calcium deficiency is uncommon, provided the dietary intake of vitamin D and calcium is adequate. If this arises, it will respond to treatment with alfacalcidol or calcitriol. When osteomalacia does develop, it is most likely to be the result of aluminium toxicity (see below). Secondary hyperparathyroidism increases in prevalence with increasing duration of dialysis, and is most likely to be severe in those with the longest duration of renal disease. If it is detected at an early stage, it may respond to vitamin D metabolites, but eventually many patients require parathyroidectomy. Vascular and metastatic calcification may still arise and these are best prevented by avoiding hypercalcaemia and hyperphosphataemia.

In recent years a new syndrome of 'dialysis dementia' has been reported in haemodialysis patients. This occurs after a variable period of treatment and initially manifests as speech disturbance, memory disturbance, seizures and myoclonic jerks. Initially these symptoms are most apparent immediately following a dialysis session. The syndrome progresses to severe dementia and death, and is an important cause of death in some units. Following this observation, it became apparent that the condition had a striking geographical variation which related to the use of water with a high aluminium content for dialysis (Parkinson *et al.*, 1979; Registration Committee of European Dialysis and Transplant Association, 1980). In some areas, water treatment with aluminium sulphate is required to precipitate debris and colour, and there may be significant amounts of aluminium in the main water supply. Use of such water results in transfer of aluminium to the patient, with accumulation in tissues. It has subsequently been recognised that this syndrome may be associated with severe osteomalacia, resistant to vitamin D, and exacerbation of anaemia (Parkinson, Ward and Kerr, 1981). Although there is no proof, it seems fairly certain that this syndrome is a result of aluminium toxicity and should be able to be prevented by water treatment to remove aluminium. Treatment of the established condition is difficult and improvement does not necessarily occur following transplantation.

Transplantation. Following successful renal transplantation and a return to near normal renal function, the uraemic syndrome resolves and the electrolyte balance is restored to normal. Both because of correction of the uraemic state and normalisation of erythropoietin production, the haemoglobin returns to normal. The overall effect on the patient is dramatic, the most important being a striking improvement in energy and morale. The liberalisation of diet and fluid restriction, as well as freedom from the restrictions imposed by frequent dialysis sessions, should not be underestimated as important factors improving the well-being of patients.

By contrast, sodium and water retention is a common problem following renal transplantation, particularly in the early stages, as a consequence both of low-grade rejection, hypertension and treatment with steroids, and requires diuretic therapy. Similarly, hypertension, sometimes severe, is also common as a result both of the rejection and the steroid therapy. A successful renal transplant is associated with resolution of hyperphosphataemia and malabsorption of calcium. However, if secondary hyperparathyroidism is severe, this may not resolve and may require parathyroidectomy. The most important bone disease, however, is avascular necrosis, particularly of the femoral heads. This results in pain and immobility and may require operative correction. Although there is no proof, it is likely that this is a consequence of steroid therapy and the incidence has fallen dramatically following the introduction of a low-steroid regime for the treatment of rejection.

The most important complications following transplantation result from corticosteroids and immunosuppression, used to maintain function of the graft. The complications of steroid therapy are no different from those following the use of steroids in other conditions, and include diabetes, weight gain with Cushingoid appearance, fluid retention, acne, muscle wasting and susceptibility to infection. In addition, the use of high doses of steroid may result in avascular necrosis and stress ulcers of the gastrointestinal tract with gastrointestinal bleeding. The susceptibility to infection is added to by azathiaprine and, in addition, warts can not only become troublesome, but occasionally disabling. For this reason, when warts are present, an attempt should be made to treat these prior to transplantation. There is also an increased incidence of malignancy, particularly lymphomas, in transplanted patients (Curtis, 1982). The potentially lethal complications of immunosuppression, particularly atypical infections and gastrointestinal bleeding, have their highest incidence in the first month following transplantation, when large doses of steroids are given to combat rejection. The incidence and mortality of such complications have been strikingly reduced by using lower doses of steroids, without any apparent effect on graft survival (Morris *et al.*, 1982).

Complications Common to All Forms of Treatment

Infection. Patients treated by dialysis or transplantation have an increased susceptibility to infection as well as an increased incidence of atypical infection. Not surprisingly, infection, together with vascular disease, is the commonest cause of death in these patients. For these reasons, prompt detection, investigation and treatment of infection is paramount, with an emphasis on early referral to hospital. In addition to the direct effects of infection, this may also result in worsening of uraemia, and electrolyte disturbance, particularly hyperkalaemia, which may also require treatment.

Hyperlipidaemia and Premature Vascular Disease. Hyperlipidaemia is a common finding in patients treated by dialysis and transplantation, but there is as yet no satisfactory treatment. There is, in addition, an excess mortality from cardiovascular and cerebrovascular disease in these patients; these are the major causes of death. Although it has been suggested that this results from atheroma induced by hyperlipidaemia, there is no proof (Editorial, *Lancet*, 1981). By contrast, there are many other factors which may result in cardiovascular disease in these patients, particularly hypertension, fluid retention, anaemia and arterio-venous fistulae.

Sexual Disturbance. Reduction in libido and impotence are common, occurring in as much as 50 per cent of patients treated by dialysis, with a similar incidence following transplantation. In addition, there is a variable reduction in fertility due to impaired spermatogenesis in the male and ovarian dysfunction in the female. Menstruation may return following dialysis or transplantation and menstrual irregularity is a common problem, often responding to treatment with progestogens.

Although pregnancies are uncommon in women on dialysis, most women of child-bearing age should be capable of conceiving following transplantation. In addition, it is not uncommon for males to father children while receiving dialysis treatment. Since pregnancies do occur and could have disastrous consequences if undesired, such patients should be given clear contraceptive advice; the assumption should not be made that the risk of pregnancy is so small that contraceptive advice is not necessary.

Problems with reduced libido and impotence in these patients are as likely to have a psychological cause as an organic cause. It is not uncommon for an organic cause to be the initiating factor, with sub-sequent psychological reaction then causing persistence of the problem. Drugs may occasionally be an important contributory factor. The spouse as well as the patient may be subject to these problems, either as a reaction to the illness or as a reaction to physical changes in the patient. If the problem is persistent, simple discussion may reveal the cause. If there is a psychological basis, the reason may be simple, for example, fear of damaging the shunt or transplanted kidney, fear of pregnancy. In others it may be more complex and require expert sexual counselling, which should be available in most areas. Few patients come forward with these problems in the United Kingdom, and it seems likely that many patients simply accept these problems as part of the illness.

Psychological Disturbance. Awareness of the patient's reaction to illness is nowhere more important than with chronic renal failure. Acceptance of the illness may mean the difference between survival and death, between rehabilitation and not. The reaction of the patient will also have a marked effect on the ability of the family to come to terms with the illness. Consideration of the patient's and family's ability to cope with the illness is of importance when making decisions about long-term management, particularly self-dialysis, which is unlikely to be a success when the patient and family have not accepted the illness.

Psychological disturbance is, not surprisingly, common, and in the majority can be regarded as a normal reaction to severe stress. Awareness of this and discussion of the problem is often all that is required to support the patient and family through a period of crisis. Experience indicates that morbidity from such reactions can be minimised by discussing fully all aspects of the illness at all stages, explaining what is to happen and recognising the differing needs of patients when making decisions about management. This can be done by all members of staff, but social workers have a critical role to play and a psychiatrist is also of great value in advising about the handling of more difficult reactions. The prescription of anxiolytic or antidepressant drugs is rarely needed in such patients and should not be a substitute for full discussion. One must also encourage a positive attitude in the patient and create independence by encouraging active involvement in treatment. By assessing patients before treatment, one can often detect those who will have most difficulty in adapting. Reaction to illness can often be predicted from the pre-morbid personality and family relationship. Patients and staff should be encouraged to understand that many such reactions are normal, for example, fear of blood, fear of the machine, fear of needles and fear of dying.

Problems are most common when dialysis is instituted. When health begins to deteriorate and the need for dialysis becomes apparent, reactions vary from depression, anxiety, withdrawal, regression to denial. With the institution of treatment, improvement in well-being leads to a 'honeymoon' phase, with often elation. This is then followed by a period of realisation, when symptoms may again arise. The majority of patients eventually come to terms with the illness, but do need continuing support. Although severe anxiety and depressive illnesses requiring drug therapy can occur, such patients can thereafter often go on to be successfully rehabilitated. By contrast, persisting denial or aggressive behaviour have a less good prognosis. Awareness of reactions of the patient in this phase is important when deciding about self-treatment, and all patients should have a period of assessment, if possible on hospital dialysis, before making decisions about self-treatment by haemodialysis or CAPD.

Problems may also arise after a successful period of self-dialysis. This may lead to difficulties within the family and one may need to recognise that treatment will have to be altered and priority for transplantation changed. Patients may become aggressive if they have to wait a long time for transplantation, and explanation of the reasons may help them to accept this. Experience indicates that support groups for spouses of patients help them to cope with continuing treatment.

Following transplantation, patients continue to need support because of anxiety about rejection. Following a failed transplant, depression is likely, associated with physical debility.

Ability to Drive

Fitness to drive is often forgotten, but is of obvious importance. In general terms, guidance on the ability to drive must be based on the general fitness of the patient and the presence of any particular problem which may make driving dangerous, for example, a tendency to epilepsy or to postural hypotension. In particular, patients treated by haemodialysis should be advised against driving immediately after a dialysis treatment, until stabilised on treatment. Once established on treatment, the majority of patients should be fit to drive. Similarly for transplanted patients, most should be able to drive. Doctors should accept responsibility for giving positive advice about the ability to drive.

Who to Treat

With the treatments now available, most patients are suitable for treatment. In the early days, selection was important so that patients did not suffer unnecessarily. Gradual relaxation of criteria for acceptance has followed as the treatments have been refined and the beneficial effects for various groups of patients have become apparent. Thus, for the majority of patients now, the decision should be not who to treat but how to treat. Unfortunately, treatment is expensive and hospital dialysis beds and kidneys for transplantation limited, so that in some countries, including Great Britain, patients who should benefit have been deprived of treatment. The advent of CAPD has improved, but not solved, this situation. One must bear in mind, however, when considering suitability for treatment that, like a drug, it has adverse effects which may outweigh the advantages and as a result place a considerable additional burden on the patient and family without any real benefit. In making a decision about treatment, one must ask if one is going to provide a worthwhile prolongation of life, whether or not one improves the quality of life. The factors limiting suitability for treatment are most commonly physical, but occasionally emotional instability may be such that treatment would simply result in unnecessary suffering. There is a commercial interest in the use of dialysis facilities and this must not influence the decision of doctors to treat the patient, not the disease.

Age by itself is not an absolute contra-indication to treatment. Between the ages of 5 and 60 all patients should be treated, in the absence of other limiting factors. In a patient above the age of 60 in whom the sole problem is renal failure, each individual must be carefully assessed, with the biological age of the patient being an important consideration. Many such patients will have vascular disease, even if not clinically apparent, and this may limit the treatment options. In addition, because of insufficient availability of kidneys, transplantation may not be feasible and one may be embarking on long-term dialysis. These factors must be carefully considered before making a decision. For some such patients, the benefit is clear; for others, the ability to cope with either dialysis or CAPD may be limited and treatment may simply place great stress on a family with little benefit. In some older patients, particularly when the disease is slowly progressive, uraemic lethargy may not be a great problem because of disability related to age. In these circumstances, treatment may simply add a burden with no reward. Such patients may have a better quality of life with conservative management, even if survival is for a shorter period.

The other important factor influencing selection is co-existent disease. Here one is referring to diabetes mellitus, ischaemic heart disease, cerebrovascular disease and, less commonly, connective tissue disorders, including systemic lupus erythematosus. These also are not absolute, but relative contra-indications to treatment and each patient must be assessed in relation to the total problem and quality of life. In such patients, haemodialysis is difficult and associated with a high morbidity and mortality. However, CAPD has provided a more appropriate treatment which may provide a worthwhile prolongation of life. The problem of selection in this group is best illustrated by examples; thus, a diabetic patient with extensive vascular disease and amputations, or with disabling autonomic neuropathy, is unlikely to receive benefit from treatment. By contrast, a diabetic without disabling complications or a diabetic with severely impaired eyesight, but who is highly motivated with good support at home, should almost certainly merit treatment. Particularly in these patients, severity of disease, motivation of the patient and support at home would be important factors determining the success of treatment.

How to Treat

In making a decision about how patients should be treated, one has to consider what is the best medical treatment for the patient, what types of treatment the patient and family can adapt to and the available resources for treatment. Cost, of necessity, comes into the equation, although in an ideal world this should not stop the most appropriate treatment being given. Hospital dialysis is the most expensive and transplantation the cheapest, while home haemodialysis and CAPD are comparable in cost. Since transplantation is the cheapest and, unlike dialysis, replaces all functions of the failed kidney, this would be the ideal therapy. However, there is considerable morbidity with transplantation for some patients but, more important, insufficient kidneys are available to treat all patients as they develop end-stage renal disease. Thus, patients who are suitable for transplantation have a waiting period on dialysis. Because of the inadequate supply of kidneys, one also has to consider priorities for transplantation. For the majority of patients treatment will be by dialysis and transplantation, while in a minority transplantation will not be desirable.

The morbidity and mortality of transplantation is greater in older patients, and survival for this group is better on dialysis. In addition, older patients accept dialysis more readily than younger patients, who tend to be frustrated by the restrictions. Thus, young patients should take priority over older patients for transplantation. Other factors may also influence the degree of priority for transplantation – patients who have difficulty adapting to dialysis treatment, patients who are unwell or who have difficulty with vascular access. In addition, when home dialysis is a treatment option, then – particularly with older patients – those who are unable to do self-treatment and will occupy limited hospital dialysis beds will take priority over patients who are able to perform self-dialysis successfully.

Decisions have also to be taken about the type of dialysis therapy to be used. Reference has been made earlier to the types of dialysis therapy as well as patient suitability. The treatment options will vary with the facilities available. In the United Kingdom, this is likely to include hospital dialysis, home dialysis and CAPD. As indicated earlier,

Figure 5.4: Integration of dialysis and transplant facilities in Edinburgh

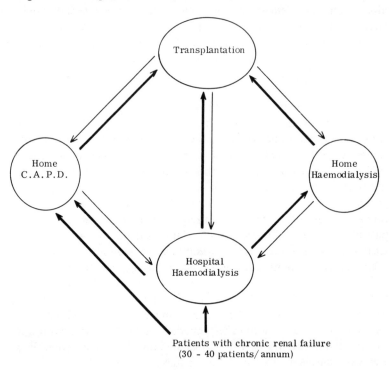

Patients with chronic renal failure
(30 - 40 patients/annum)

Note: The arrows indicate the direction of patient movement between the various treatments.

selection for self-treatment is imperative, if this is to be successful. Each patient and family needs to be carefully assessed to find the most appropriate dialysis treatment, taking all factors into account. For some patients the decision will be easy, for others detailed discussion is needed. Experience indicates that patients are more likely to accept a decision if they feel involved; for example, explanation that the transplantation rate is limited will help patients to accept the need for self-treatment. Similarly, seeing a patient who has successfully performed home dialysis or CAPD often helps patients to make a decision.

For the majority of patients, a period of assessment and stabilisation on hospital dialysis is important before making a decision about self-treatment. This is important to give them time to come to terms with the need for dialysis and enables an assessment of their ability in coping with treatment.

Decisions about dialysis treatment must be reviewed at intervals. The most appropriate treatment at the start may become less satisfactory later, for example, changes in family circumstances, shunt difficulties, recurrent peritonitis on CAPD, failed transplant. Patients should not be allowed to have unrealistic objectives: transplants do fail, and if a patient is allowed to see this as the only objective this will have a disastrous psychological effect.

In reality, the treatment options are likely to change with time. Figure 5.4 shows how the various options in Edinburgh link together to form an integrated service. Use of all these resources enables a continued intake of new patients. The treatment provided is not necessarily ideal, but is the best that can be offered, taking into account the needs of the patient and the facilities available. Thus, young patients go on to hospital dialysis and are transplanted, older patients perform home dialysis with a lower priority for transplantation, and other patients, particularly those with diabetes and cardiovascular disease, are treated by CAPD. However, as the arrows indicate, treatment alters with time as the situation changes.

Results of Treatment: Survival and Rehabilitation

The advances in dialysis and transplantation in Europe have been aided by the collection of statistical information from all centres in Europe by the European Dialysis and Transplant Association (Combined Reports, annually). This audit of treatment has helped to encourage improvement in results, to justify the cost of treatment and has been of value in the management of individual patients by giving an indication of the best form of therapy for the various groups of patient.

As Figure 5.5 illustrates, the survival rate with dialysis and transplantation over five years is comparable to that following a myocardial infarct, and distinctly better than with some forms of cancer. Table 5.6 illustrates survival rates in various age-groups for dialysis and transplantation. These indicate that a considerable prolongation of life can be expected for most patients on treatment. Since mortality with transplantation is higher in older patients compared to dialysis, such patients may be better treated by long-term dialysis, provided they can accept the restrictions.

As well as prolonging life, a treatment must provide a reasonable quality of life if it is to be worth while. Quality of life is difficult to assess, but an indication can be given by looking at the degree of rehabilitation. Table 5.7 indicates that considerable full rehabilitation is achieved with dialysis and transplantation. Although the less good

Figure 5.5: Cumulative survival by dialysis and transplantation compared with some other diseases

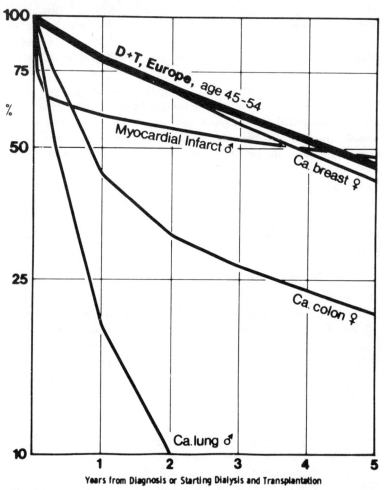

Source: *Proceedings of the European Dialysis and Transplant Association* (1978) vol. 15, p. 22.

rehabilitation with hospital dialysis may partly reflect the need to travel to treatment, it may also result from such patients being physically less well and not able to perform self-treatment or to be transplanted. However, in the present economic climate, rehabilitation may become a less satisfactory method of assessing quality of life. Particularly in older patients, who may sensibly decide to retire early, a good quality of life may be achieved without necessarily working.

Table 5.6: Percentage patient survival according to age-group and mode of therapy, in Europe, 1976-8

Patient survive using:	Age (years)	Sample size	1 year	2 years	3 years
Hospital haemodialysis	15–34	6 305	90.8 ± 0.5	84.4 ± 0.7	80.0 ± 1.1
	35–44	5 271	88.4 ± 0.5	79.5 ± 0.8	72.5 ± 1.3
	45–54	6 989	88.3 ± 0.5	78.5 ± 0.7	71.4 ± 1.1
	55–64	5 452	73.4 ± 0.6	73.4 ± 0.8	63.7 ± 1.3
	65 +	2 982	78.3 ± 0.9	61.2 ± 1.2	51.3 ± 1.7
	All*	27 738	87.1 ± 0.2	76.7 ± 0.4	69.1 ± 0.6
Home haemodialysis	15–34	1 235	97.5 ± 0.5	94.6 ± 0.9	93.3 ± 1.3
	35–44	1 072	95.8 ± 0.7	92.1 ± 1.1	90.8 ± 1.4
	45–54	1 209	94.9 ± 0.7	89.7 ± 1.1	86.5 ± 1.7
	55–64	596	94.0 ± 1.1	86.9 ± 1.9	78.3 ± 3.5
	65 +	103	91.8 ± 3.2	81.0 ± 5.4	†
	All*	4 301	95.8 ± 0.3	91.3 ± 0.6	88.4 ± 0.9
1st Live donor graft	15–34	474	92.3 ± 1.3	87.9 ± 1.8	85.3 ± 2.5
	35–44	145	93.4 ± 2.1	90.6 ± 2.9	†
	45–54	53	91.3 ± 4.2	†	†
	55–64	16	†	†	†
	65+	3	†	†	†
	All*	797	92.3 ± 1.0	88.8 ± 1.3	86.4 ± 1.9
1st Cadaver graft	15–34	2 364	89.4 ± 0.7	85.6 ± 0.8	82.6 ± 1.2
	35–44	1 577	84.2 ± 1.0	76.8 ± 1.3	71.9 ± 1.7
	45–54	1 244	75.1 ± 1.3	66.9 ± 1.6	64.5 ± 1.8
	55–64	406	65.8 ± 2.5	58.4 ± 2.9	49.6 ± 4.1
	65+	42	†	†	†
	All*	5 883	83.3 ± 0.5	77.4 ± 0.6	73.4 ± 0.8

Notes: * Includes patients aged 0–15 years.

† Numbers of patients at risk equals less than 30.

Source: *Proceedings of the European Dialysis and Transplant Association* (1979) vol. 16, p. 36.

Table 5.7: Rehabilitation achieved in patients treated by dialysis in Europe in 1979

	Able to work			Unable to work		
	Working	Not yet working				
					Requires equiva-lent to	
	Full-time (1)	Part-time (2)	No work available (3)	Earning capacity $<$pen-sion/ benefit (4)	Living at home (5)	hospital care (6)	Total patients (7)
Male patients whose potential occupation was full-time employment							
Hospital dialysis	36.7	19.8	14.1	14.5	14.5	1.9	5 600
Home dialysis	63.9	12.3	8.8	9.5	5.2	0.3	3 025
LD transplant	79.1	7.2	3.8	5.7	3.4	0.8	526
CAD transplant	63.0	12.6	7.5	9.2	7.2	0.5	2 215
All modes of therapy	48.0	16.6	11.6	12.3	10.1	1.3	14 366
Female patients whose potential occupation was full-time employment							
Hospital dialysis	39.1	31.1	8.5	7.8	11.7	1.8	2 772
Home dialysis	66.4	19.4	4.1	3.6	5.7	0.7	557
LD transplant	77.7	9.6	2.5	5.7	0.7	0	157
CAD transplant	63.9	20.7	4.7	3.9	5.9	0.8	743
All modes of therapy	48.5	26.9	7.1	6.5	9.6	1.4	4 229
Female patients whose potential occupation was full-time housework							
Hospital dialysis	36.4	34.0	3.7	3.9	19.6	2.5	4 816
Home dialysis	64.0	25.6	1.7	1.2	4.8	0.7	703
LD transplant	84.8	5.1	0	3.8	5.1	1.3	79
CAD transplant	70.1	17.3	2.1	1.9	7.3	1.2	723
All modes of therapy	43.9	30.8	3.3	3.4	16.6	2.1	6 321

Note: The figures shown are the percentage of the total patients in each category of rehabilitation.
Source: *Proceedings of the European Dialysis and Transplant Association* (1979) vol. 16, p. 45.

References

Chan, M.K., Balloid, R.A., Tanner, A., Raftery, M., Sweny, P., Fernando, O.N. and Moorhead, J.F. (1981) 'Abdominal hernias in patients receiving continuous ambulatory peritoneal dialysis', *British Medical Journal*, 283, 826

Combined reports on regular dialysis and transplantation in Europe, in *Proceedings of the European Dialysis and Transplant Association*, Pitman Medical, Tunbridge Wells (published annually)

Curtis, J.R. (1982) 'Cancer and patients with end-stage renal failure', *British Medical Journal*, 284, 69–70

Editorial (1981) 'Adult polycystic disease of the kidneys', *British Medical Journal*, 282, 1097–8

Editorial (1981) 'Uraemia, lipoproteins and atherosclerosis', *Lancet*, ii, 1151

Editorial (1982) 'Prescribing in renal impairment', *British National Formulary*, 3, 10–14

Gokal, R., McHugh, M., Fryer, R., Ward, M.K. and Kerr, D.N.S. (1980) 'Continuous ambulatory peritoneal dialysis: one year's experience in a UK dialysis unit', *British Medical Journal*, 281, 474–7

Jacobs, C., Broyer, M., Brunner, F.P., Brynger, H., Donckerwolcke, R.A., Kramer, P., Selwood, N.H., Wing, A.J. and Blake, P.H. (1981) 'Combined report on regular dialysis and transplantation in Europe', *Proceedings of the European Dialysis and Transplant Association, 18*

Knapp, M.S. (1982) 'Renal failure – dilemmas and developments', *British Medical Journal*, 284, 847–50

Morris, P.J., Chan, L., French, M.E. and Ting, A. (1982) 'Low dose oral prednisolone in renal transplantation', *Lancet*, i, 525–7

Office of Health Economics (1978) *Renal Failure – a Priority in Health?*, White Crescent Press, Luton

Opelz, G., Gravier, B. and Teresaki, P.I. (1981) 'Induction of high kidney graft survival rate by multiple transfusion', *Lancet*, i, 1223–5

Parkinson, I.S., Ward, M.K. and Kerr, D.N.S. (1981) 'Dialysis encephalopathy, bone disease and anaemia: the aluminium intoxication syndrome during regular haemodialysis', *Journal of Clinical Pathology*, 34, 1285–94

Parkinson, I.S. Feest, T.G., Ward, M.K., Fawcett, R.W.P. and Kerr, D.N.S. (1979) 'Fracturing dialysis osteodystrophy and dialysis encephalopathy: an epidemiological survey', *Lancet*, i, 406–8

Pendreigh, D.M., Heasman, M.A., Howitt, L.F., Kennedy, A.C., Macdougall, A.I., MacLeod, M., Robson, J.S. and Stewart, W.K. (1972) 'Survey of chronic renal failure in Scotland', *Lancet*, i, 304–7

Popovich, R.P., Moncrieff, J.W., Nolph, K.D., Ghods, A.J., Twardowski, Z.T. and Pyle, W.K. (1978) 'Continuous ambulatory peritoneal dialysis', *Annals of Internal Medicine*, 449–56

Registration Committee of European Dialysis and Transplant Association (1980) 'Dialysis dementia in Europe', *Lancet*, ii, 190–2

Ting, A. and Morris, P.J. (1980) 'Powerful effect of HL-DR matching on survival of cadaver renal allografts', *Lancet*, ii, 282–5

Van Rood, J.J., Persijn, G.G., Lansbergen, Q., Cohen, B., van Leeuwen, A. and Bradley, B.A. (1979) 'How can HLA matching improve kidney graft survival?', *Proceedings of the European Dialysis Transplant Association*, 16, 297–303

Waterfall, W.K. (1981) 'Dialysis and transplant', *British Medical Journal*, 282, 1097–8

Recommended Further Reading

Anderton, J.L., Parsons, F.M. and Jones, D.E. (eds) (1978) *Living with Renal Failure*, MTP Press, Lancaster

Atkins, R.C., Thomson, N.M. and Farrell, P.C. (eds) (1981) *Peritoneal Dialysis*, Churchill Livingstone, Edinburgh

Black, D. and Jones, N.F. (eds) (1979) *Renal Disease*, 4th edn, Blackwell Scientific Publications, Oxford

Brenner, B.M. and Rector, F.C. (eds) (1981) *The Kidney*, 2nd edn, W.B. Saunders, Philadelphia

Davison, A.M. (ed.) (1978) *Dialysis Review*, Pitman Medical, Tunbridge Wells

Earley, L.E. and Gottschalk, C.W. (eds) (1979) *Strauss and Welt's Diseases of the Kidney*, Little, Brown, Boston

6 PALLIATIVE CARE IN RESPIRATORY DISEASES

David Flenley

Chronic respiratory disease, which cannot be cured, but may be considerably alleviated by treatment, forms a major burden on the economic, social and personal life of many patients in western societies. This chapter will concentrate on chronic bronchitis and emphysema, the major source of this burden, but will also consider briefly chronic bronchiectasis, cystic fibrosis and bronchial asthma. Other major diseases of the respiratory system, including pneumonia, which is usually too short-lived to constitute a chronic problem, will not be considered. The specific problems of lung cancer, the commonest of all malignant disease in men, and second only to cancer of the breast in women, will be considered elsewhere.

Chronic Bronchitis and Emphysema

Incidence and Epidemiology

Chronic bronchitis and emphysema is by far the commonest disease causing 30 million working days to be lost in British industry each year, as a result of respiratory disease, a major burden therefore on the British economy (Royal College of Physicians, 1981). England and Wales have the highest incidence of chronic bronchitis in the world, with Scotland close behind. A major risk factor, epidemiologically, is undoubtedly cigarette smoking, but life in an industrial area, low social class, recurrent childhood respiratory illnesses and parents who smoke are also recognised factors.

Definition

Chronic bronchitis is defined as chronic cough or spit, occurring for three months of each year for three consecutive years. Emphysema is defined pathologically: as dilatation of the distal air spaces of the lungs, with destruction of their walls. In clinical practice the two conditions are nearly always associated to a greater or lesser degree, but the extent of chronic bronchitis, or the extent of emphysema, cannot be estimated with accuracy in any individual patient during life (Thurlbeck, 1976). It is thus recommended that the term chronic bronchitis and emphysema be used to describe the clinical condition, recognising that the exact pathological changes can only be ascertained accurately at post-mortem.

Pathogenesis

The way in which smoke from cigarettes damages the lungs is now becoming clearer. In chronic bronchitis the mucous glands lining the airways are hypertrophied, so that excess mucous is produced, in response to the chronic irritation of inhaled cigarette smoke. We do not yet know which constituents amongst the 2000 different chemical substances in cigarette smoke are responsible for this. The irritation also causes airways to constrict, so producing a major feature of the disease, progressive breathlessness. Cigarette smoke also causes destruction of the lung tissue, producing the 'holes in the lungs' characteristic of emphysema, from damage to cells which protect the lungs in health. These alveolar macrophages lurk deep within the air spaces, but are irritated by cigarette smoke to release chemical factors which attract inflammatory cells (the polymorphonuclear leucocytes) from the bloodstream into the lungs. These polymorphonuclear leucocytes then release proteolytic enzymes (similar to biological washing powders) when exposed to cigarette smoke. The proteolytic enzymes literally dissolve the nearby parts of the lungs. In health, any attack from proteolytic enzymes is antagonised by anti-proteolytic substances within the lung-lining fluids. However, cigarette smoke is now known to oxidise these anti-proteolytic proteins, so inhibiting their action. The net result is an increased release of proteolytic enzymes, with reduction in the body's defences against their action, leading to local destruction of the lungs, or emphysema (Snider, 1981). As with lung cancer, the only effective prevention is abolition of cigarette smoking. But we still do not know why only about half of those who smoke develop emphysema, and why the others do not.

Clinical Presentation and Course

As the definition implies, a recurrent winter cough, usually with the production of mucous sputum, is the characteristic of chronic bronchitis. Eventually, after some years of continued cigarette smoking, the patient begins to have purulent sputum each winter, episodically associated with an increase of breathlessness, often causing two or three weeks off work, and consultation with the general practitioner. These episodes of chest infection gradually increase in frequency and severity, the patient will then begin to be breathless (and possibly wheezy) on even modest exertion, even when he does not have an exacerbation of chest infection. Breathlessness progresses, until eventually after many years the patient becomes breathless even when at rest, or undressing, washing and moving about the house. By this time he will have two or three bouts, each lasting a couple of weeks or so, in bed each winter with a chest infection, and has probably had to retire early because of disabling breathlessness. None the less many such patients continue to smoke!

By this time two distinct clinical patterns of the disease are beginning to emerge in different patients, although in many features of both may co-exist. The 'pink and puffing' patient is very breathless, with hyper-inflation of his chest, as shown by indrawing of intercostal spaces. How-ever, he still has relatively normal levels of oxygen and carbon dioxide in his arterial blood, and does not develop heart failure (cor pul-monale), nor does he have an increase in circulating haemoglobin (secondary polycythaemia).

In contrast, the 'blue and bloated' patient has hyperinflation of the chest, but may complain less of breathlessness, despite a similar degree of obstruction to air flow. Cough is also prominent (as with the 'pink and puffing'), but he has central cyanosis (blueness) and often ankle oedema unless treated with diuretics (hence the bloated). The 'blue and bloated' patient has right heart failure (cor pulmonale) with secondary polycythaemia. Such patients have a very grave outlook (Figure 6.1); only about 30 per cent survive for five years (Warren *et al.*, 1980). Recently 'blue bloaters' have been found to have markedly abnormal sleep, with recurrent severe transient oxygen lack recurring many times each night (Figure 6.2) (Douglas *et al.*, 1979). These hypoxaemic episodes, which are associated with transient increase in pulmonary arterial pressure, occur particularly in the rapid eye movement phase of sleep (REM).

Treatment of Chronic Bronchitis and Emphysema

First, the patient must *stop smoking* for life. Repetition of this advice, given without humour by both the hospital doctor and general prac-titioner, is probably the best way of achieving this (Russell *et al.*, 1979). The patient should know of the serious nature of his disease, and that persistent cigarette smoking is the major cause. Anti-smoking clinics, although laudable in their aims, in practice have contributed little to effective prevention of cigarette smoking. Nicotine chewing gum may be helpful in some patients attending anti-smoking clinics (Fee and Stewart, 1982), but in hospitalised patients suffering from

Figure 6.1: Survival of patients with chronic bronchitis and emphysema following first admission to hospital with an acute exacerbation of respiratory failure, compared with survival in a Scottish population of similar age and sex

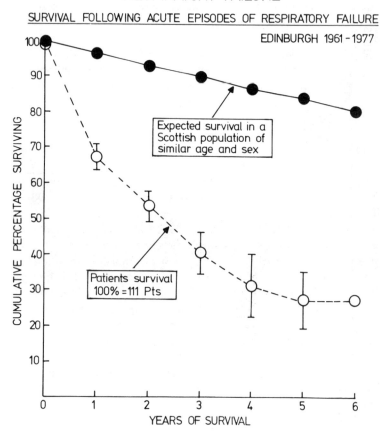

Note: These patients were not treated with long-term oxygen therapy.

cigarette-related diseases a controlled trial has shown no significant success with nicotine chewing gum in obtaining smoking cessation at six months (British Thoracic Association, 1982), as compared to a placebo chewing gum.

Second, drugs can relieve breathlessness by *dilating the airways*. Thus β_2-sympathomimetics (either salbutamol, terbutaline or fenoterol),

Figure 6.2: Ear oxygen saturation (below) and EEG sleep stage (above) in a 'blue and bloated' chronic bronchitic throughout a normal night's sleep, when breathing air

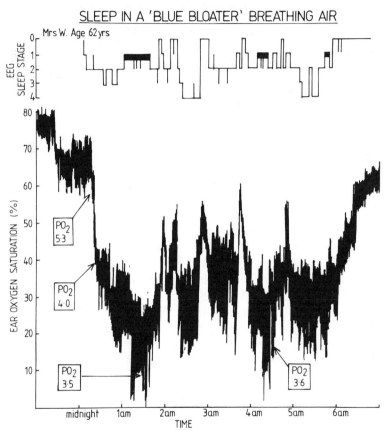

Notes: 0 = wakefulness

4 = deep sleep

■ = rapid eye movement during sleep

Note the severe recurrent hypoxaemia.

given by metered-dose aerosol, can usefully be combined with ipratropium bromide (Douglas *et al.*, 1977). Two puffs of each drug are taken, one after the other, three or four times a day. The patient must be shown how to use a metered-dose inhaler. After a full expiration to empty the lungs as far as possible, the inhaler is placed between his lips and the canister depressed during a slow inspiration. The patient should then hold his breath at the end of the inspiration for as long as possible, and then exhale slowly. Oral bronchodilators, such as salbutamol or terbutaline delayed-release preparations, or delayed-release theophyllines, have not yet been shown by controlled trials to be of particular value in such patients, although they are in widespread use. Rarely oral corticosteroids may be of benefit, but the dose should never exceed 10 mg of prednisolone per day on a long-term basis. Prednisolone should only be used if the peak expiratory flow (or forced expiratory volume − FEV_1) is shown to increase.

Third, episodes of *infection*, as shown by purulent sputum, require prompt antibiotic treatment, although controversy persists as to the value of this in patients with relatively good respiratory function (Bates, 1982). The usual organisms are *Haemophilus influenzae* and *Streptococcus pneumoniae*; both are susceptible to ampicillin, as 500 mg four times a day for ten days, or amoxycillin 250 mg four times daily, both taken by mouth. An alternative is cotrimoxazole, two tablets twice daily for ten days. These drugs are as effective as the much more expensive cephalosporins in treatment of infection with these common organisms (Nev, 1982). Antibiotics given for a short course to treat an exacerbation of purulent sputum are preferable to continuous long-term antibiotics in most patients. Routine culture of sputum from patients with purulent exacerbations of chronic bronchitis and emphysema is not recommended in general practice, as it is most unusual for organisms other than *H. influenzae* or *Str. pneumoniae* to be isolated in patients who have not previously been treated with antibiotics (Valentine *et al.*, 1980).

Infection with influenza virus (either A or B) can be very dangerous in these patients who have severely compromised respiratory function. Death from complicating staphylococcal pneumonia is well recognised to be a risk in such patients during an influenza epidemic. Thus prophylaxis against influenzal infection is recommended to be given by influenza vaccine, each October or November, by intramuscular injection. Immunity only lasts for one season, and the vaccine should contain the strains of influenza virus thought to be prevalent for the forthcoming winter (Flenley, 1979). Immunisation against fourteen of the most prevalent strains of *Str. pneumoniae* is now available, using an inactivated vaccine, but the efficacy of this has not yet been proven in patients with chronic bronchitis and emphysema. However, this vaccine has been shown to prevent pneumonia from *Str. pneumoniae* infection in other closed communities who are particularly at risk.

Pneumococcal vaccine can be combined with influenza vaccination given at the same time, provided that the two vaccines are given at a different site (Schwartz, 1982).

Exercise training can improve breathlessness on exercise, by training both the muscles of respiration (for the ventilation increases on exercise) and the other skeletal muscles (Grimby and Skoogh, 1980). This can be simply achieved by practising stair climbing or outdoor walking. However, patients with chronic bronchitis should stay indoors in foggy weather.

Cor pulmonale, or right heart failure in the 'blue and bloated' bronchitic, is an indication for diuretics, but the role of digoxin in these patients is much more controversial. If powerful diuretics (e.g. frusemide 40-120 mg/day) are used to control oedema, potassium supplements (Slow-K 1.2 g up to three times a day) are also desirable.

Physiotherapy with percussion and breathing exercises has been traditional, but its value has never been convincingly demonstrated by controlled clinical trials. Claims that an imposed breathing pattern with slow deep breathing, both at rest and during exercise, can improve exercise tolerance and reduce CO_2 retention in these patients have yet to be confirmed (Gimenez *et al.*, 1976). None the less, physiotherapy to assist in coughing and raising secretions during an acute exacerbation, particularly if coupled with postural drainage if the secretions are predominantly in the lower zones, can be very helpful in these patients.

Respiratory Failure

In health the lungs add oxygen to the arterial blood and remove carbon dioxide. In advanced chronic bronchitis and emphysema these functions fail. Oxygenation is affected at first, when central cyanosis reveals inadequate oxygenation of the arterial blood. This is Type I respiratory failure, whereas in the more advanced disease, characteristically seen in the 'blue and bloated' patient, or in an exacerbation of chronic bronchitis with chest infection, the patient cannot also remove sufficient carbon dioxide. As a result, the tension of carbon dioxide (PCO_2) in his arterial blood rises. In Type II respiratory failure, hypoxaemia is combined with a high PCO_2, a combination which can be especially dangerous during an acute exacerbation. These patients should be treated in hospital. They will have severe central cyanosis, purulent sputum, breathlessness and often drowsiness. Their survival depends upon controlling the chest infection, bronchodilatation and *controlled oxygen therapy*.

In the controlled oxygen therapy regime, oxygen is given at a flow rate of 1-2 l/min by nasal prongs, continuously, so as to give enough oxygen to the body cells, but without removing totally any drive to breathing from oxygen lack. This would, of course, result in an excessive rise in PCO_2, and death from respiratory acidosis. The treatment is controlled by repeated measurements of arterial blood gas tensions, and if success cannot be obtained by this simple measure alone, respiratory stimulants may be needed and eventually mechanical ventilation. However, most such exacerbations can be managed by controlled oxygen therapy alone (Warren *et al.*, 1980).

Respiratory stimulant drugs (e.g. doxapram) can be useful to avoid mechanical ventilation, if controlled oxygen therapy alone is not working. The respiratory stimulant doxapram is given by continous intravenous infusion, the dose rate being controlled by repeated blood gas measurement. Doxapram causes tremor, tachycardia, perineal burning and agitation, so that it is rarely possible to use it for more than 24-72 hours. However, this may buy enough time to allow the factor precipitating the acute exacerbation to be controlled (this is often the chest infection, but may also be a fractured rib, spontaneous pneumothorax, pulmonary oedema, etc.).

Admission to Hospital

Many acute exacerbations of chronic bronchitis and emphysema, with purulent sputum, can be managed at home, using the treatment outlined above. However, if the patient has severe central cyanosis, with the signs of acute exacerbation of CO_2 retention (flapping tremor of the outstretched hands, rapid bounding pulse and distended forearm veins), controlled oxygen therapy may be required, and this means admission to hospital. Again, if the sputum has not cleared from purulence within two or three days on the antibiotic regimens outlined, or if the patient has signs of pneumonic consolidation, hospital admission is usually desirable. If the patient cannot cough effectively to clear secretions, the exacerbation of infection may precipitate more severe respiratory failure, making hospital admission desirable. Localised chest pain, which may indicate pleurisy associated with pneumonia, spontaneous pneumothorax or a fractured rib, are also often indications for hospital admission in an established case of chronic bronchitis and emphysema. Clouding of consciousness, which can be due to hypoxia combined with CO_2 retention and respiratory acidosis, also requires hospital admission. Of course, if adequate nursing care cannot be provided by the patient's relatives at home, this may also be an indication for admission.

Sedatives

It must be emphasised that these patients are very susceptible to the respiratory depressant effect of any sedatives, hypnotics or tranquillisers. There is no safe hypnotic for the patient with CO_2 retention, which is usual in the 'blue and bloated' pattern of patients with chronic bronchitis and emphysema. Nitrazepam, diazepam and other benzodiazepines and, of course, barbiturates can all be very dangerous in such patients, and should not be administered without careful monitoring of arterial blood gas tensions, which means hospital admission.

Long-term Domiciliary Oxygen Therapy

Two recent controlled trials have shown that the length of life, and its quality, can be improved in many of these patients who are given oxygen over a long term at home (Nocturnal Oxygen Therapy Trial Group, 1980; MRC Working Party 1981) (Figure 6.3). A flow rate of 2 l/minute or more is given for at least 15 hours in the 24-hour day. This treatment, given both by day and night, improves the delivery of oxygen to the body cells, but does not affect the underlying lung disease. None the less, the treatment can improve the quality of sleep, mental ability and prevent further rise in pulmonary hypertension, which would lead eventually to failure of the right heart. Long-term oxygen can also correct secondary polycythaemia, provided that the patient stops smoking (Calverley *et al.*, 1982).

The treatment is expensive, being given by either oxygen cylinders in the patient's home (where 15 of the F size (48 ft^3) cylinders are required each week to provide 15 hours of treatment per day at 2 l/minute), or much more economically by the oxygen concentrator. This device is the size of a domestic refrigerator, and uses an electrical compressor to remove nitrogen from the air, so giving up to 95 per cent oxygen. Unfortunately, this equipment is not yet available on the NHS drug tariff. The cost of providing long-term oxygen by the oxygen concentrator is probably less than £1000 per patient per year, as compared to £3000–£4000 per patient per year for similar treatment with oxygen from cylinders, the only method currently available on the NHS.

Clearly the cost and inconvenience of such long-term treatment indicate that it should only be given to those patients most likely to benefit. The results of the controlled trials only apply to patients with proven hypoxaemia (arterial PO_2 below 60 mmHg, 8.0 kPa)

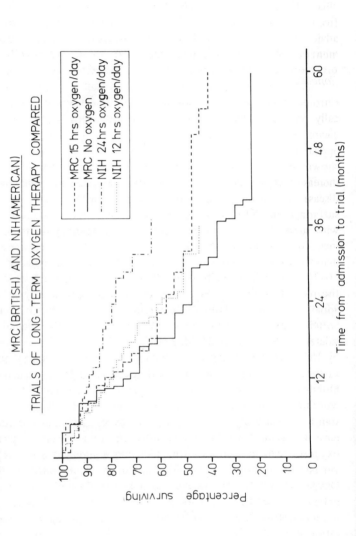

Figure 6.3: Five-year cumulative survival in patients with chronic bronchitis and emphysema with arterial hypoxaemia (PO$_2$ 50 mmHg) treated with long-term oxygen, of varying durations (see insert) compared with those receiving no oxygen (results combined from MRC and NIH controlled trials)

and this treatment is only recommended after full investigation, so as to establish the severity of hypoxaemia, and the extent of chronic bronchitis and emphysema. Any patient receiving long-term domiciliary oxygen should also have stopped smoking for life, for death from flash fires has occurred in patients who have not followed this advice. Smoking also prevents the physiological benefits of the treatment being reached (Calverley *et al.*, 1982).

Conclusion

Chronic bronchitis and emphysema remains a major burden economically on the health of our society. As with lung cancer, abolition of cigarette smoking would improve this position, but as a society we appear peculiarly reluctant to adopt the one measure which has been shown to be effective in achieving this desirable end, namely, a severe increase in cigarette tax. As we appear capable of preventing the disease, we must as a society accept the consequences, and treat those suffering from it. This will involve the general practitioner principally, with support from hospitals, social services including home helps and meals on wheels, etc. and the evolution of an effective home oxygen delivery service. Chronic bronchitis and emphysema progresses for some 10-20 years before finally killing its victim, and for much of this time the patient becomes progressively disabled, although this may not be apparent to those observing him casually, as he does not have the crutches, sticks or obvious appliances to distinguish those usually considered as 'the disabled'. None the less, mobility is seriously limited by his exercise breathlessness. Thus aids to improve mobility are indicated, although they have not yet been of much success in these patients. Mobility allowance, providing the patient with transport to work without having to expose himself to the cigarette fumes on public transport, can help to keep a patient in work when otherwise he would have to retire. Portable oxygen, possibly best given by the liquid oxygen system currently only available on an experimental basis, may yet be proved to have a role in keeping some of these patients at work. Oxygen on exercise can reduce the need for ventilation, make the patient less breathless and thus improve his mobility. The decision to use a wheelchair for such a patient is never easy, but may be the most rational solution to a reasonable life-style. However, more work is needed to indicate when this step should be taken, and experience with the aids to mobility used in those disabled by orthopaedic or joint conditions could with advantage be deployed for the patient with chronic bronchitis and emphysema.

Bronchial Asthma

In some patients, particularly children and post-menopausal women, bronchial asthma may be so severe as to justify palliative care for its management. Such palliative treatment aims to alleviate increasing severity of airflow limitation, while recognising that restoration of normal airway calibre may not be possible in these severely affected chronic long-standing asthmatics. The principles of management are to reduce the burden of known antigens which may be triggering the asthmatic attack; in these types of patients with exacerbations of a continuous level of persistent airways obstruction, a combination of drug therapy is used to try and dilate the airways. It is now recognised that the common house-mite asthma is largely due to high concentrations of the antigen in the house-mite faecal pellets, and these may be concentrated in carpets, mattresses and soft cuddly toys (for example, the British teddy bear). Sensible measures to sterilise these sources of house-mite antigen seem reasonable (Tovey *et al.*, 1981).

Drug therapy starts with regular β_2-agonists (salbutamol or terbutaline), by metered-dose inhalers, given in the adult as two puffs of the inhaler up to four times daily. Alternatively wet nebulisation of these drugs may be more effective in the severe asthmatic. This can be given as terbutaline 5 mg by a compressor-driven nebuliser up to four times daily, and in asthmatics over the age of 40 years this may be usefully combined with ipratropium bromide 0.4–2.0 ml of a 0.025 per cent solution (100–500 μg of ipratropium by a wet nebuliser driven by compressor) up to four times daily. These again are adult doses. If nocturnal wheeze or exercise-induced asthma is prominent, sodium cromoglycate, given by two spincaps four times a day, can be added. All of these, though less with the wet nebulisers, require some co-ordination from the patient, and a simpler regime may be to use a terbutaline metered-dose inhaler with the 'spacer', to improve distribution of aerosol in those who cannot co-ordinate properly with an ordinary metered-dose aerosol inhaler. Beclamethasone, again given by metered-dose inhaler, as two puffs four times daily in the adult, is also very valuable, and is probably, combined with β_2-agonists, the first-line treatment of severe asthma. Oral slow-release preparations such as aminophylline or theophylline can also be helpful, but as the toxic-therapeutic ratio of theophylline is very narrow, monitoring of drug levels in the plasma can be very valuable, aiming for a concentration between 10–20 μg/ml for maximal effect, without serious side-effects of theophyllines. In addition to the well-known gastrointestinal side-effects and tachycardia, these can include serious cardiac irregu-larities, and epileptic fits at higher levels which may be attained in-advertently if drug levels are not monitored.

If this regime combining aerosol medication with oral theophyllines does not keep the peak flow rate above 150-200 l/min in the adult (this should be monitored by the patient using a Mini-Wright peak flow meter), long-term continuous steroid therapy should be considered. Contra-indications or need for great caution using this treatment include known peptic ulceration, diabetes mellitus, pre-existing obesity, hypertension and psychosis. The aim should be to use a long-term dosage no higher than 10 mg prednisolone daily, although it may need to be increased to 30 mg over short periods (for a few days), reducing thereafter rapidly to 10 mg over the course of one week, in patients whose asthma is otherwise intractable. However, such steroid side-effects will occur if a dose above 10 mg in the day is kept up con-tinuously for longer than one week or so. These patients should be advised to self-medicate themselves with steroids to relieve an acute attack of asthma, using up to 30 mg reducing thereafter by one 5 mg tablet daily within a week, if they cannot obtain medical attention. This regime, of proven efficacy, in treating the acute exacerbation of chronic asthma, must carry the risk that over-usage of the regimen can cause steroid side-effects. Patients receiving long-term steroids for chronic asthma should be seen regularly to check body weight, blood pressure, urine for sugar, an enquiry as to back pain (osteoporosis) and examination for other steroid side-effects.

In children, oral steroids can inhibit pubertal growth spurts, but depot tetracosactrin (0.5-1.0 mg twice weekly at most for adults, and 0.25-0.5 mg every 2-8 days for children of school age) by intra-muscular injection can relieve symptoms of asthma, without impeding growth. Such treatment requires careful supervision, and in children the charting of height and weight on appropriate growth charts is essential when using this regime. Severe asthmatics can die in an acute attack, and an emergency asthma admission register, whereby such known patients can be admitted directly to hospitals skilled in their emergency treatment by self-referral, can be shown to reduce the death rate in such very severely affected patients.

Bronchiectasis

Bronchiectasis, which means persistent dilatation of the bronchi, has declined in frequency in developed countries where antibiotics have been widely employed for treatment of respiratory infections. However, there are still some patients who persistently produce large volumes of offensive sputum over many years due to bronchiectasis, and thus require long-term continued palliative care. In those relatively uncommon patients where bronchiectasis is associated with a localised abnormality of the respiratory tract, with the disease confined to one lobe of the lungs, surgical resection may be curative. However, it is more usual that the disease involves more than one lobe, so preventing surgical resection, and in such patients the mainstay of therapy is postural drainage with antibiotics to control infection.

Postural drainage uses gravity with assisted coughing and chest wall percussion to drain secretions from the infected lower lobes, which must therefore be placed uppermost. As the basal segments are most usually involved, this means that the foot of the bed should be raised, for at least 15 minutes twice daily, or for longer if secretions are profuse. In some patients the bronchi can only be kept clear if the patient sleeps with the affected lobe elevated. The patients themselves and their relatives should be taught the technique, by a trained physiotherapist who can teach the relatives to carry out percussion over the affected lobe after a period of postural drainage, to assist the patient with coughing to clear secretions.

Antibiotics

The common bacterial pathogens, as in chronic bronchitis and emphysema, are *Haemophilius influenzae* and *Str. pneumoniae*, and these can thus be adequately controlled with ampicillin 250 mg four times a day, or even 500 mg four times a day. Tetracycline 500 mg four times a day is also of value in this context, and it has been found useful to alternate courses of ampicillin lasting 10–14 days, with cotrimoxazole, for a similar period, followed by tetracycline again for a similar period. This provides a cyclical regimen of anti-infective agents, the three drugs being used sequentially in this fashion, aiming to control infection rather than attempting to eradicate it.

In those patients whose bronchiectasis is a result of *agammaglobulinaemia*, replacement therapy with 25–50 mg/kg body weight of immune serum globulin given every week by intramuscular injection is needed, for life. Further doses of fresh plasma may be helpful during exacerbations of infection which break through this regimen in these patients (Hill, 1981).

Allergic broncho-pulmonary aspergillosis can also be complicated by bronchiectasis, but such patients are usually also subject to severe bronchospasm, and high doses of steroids may then be necessary to control this symptom and also to clear radiological infiltrates associated with the aspergillosis. This may require doses of 30 mg prednisolone per day, which of course will lead to steroid side-effects unless the dosage can be reduced rapidly. When such high doses are used potassium supplements should be given, and the patient regularly examined for evidence of side-effects (moon face; obesity of the trunk; purple striae of the skin of the abdomen, buttocks and shoulders; hypertension; osteoporosis; induction of diabetes mellitus; psychosis; hypokalaemic alkalosis and susceptibility to infection). These side-effects are all uncommon, if the dose of steroids does not exceed 10 mg of prednisolone per day in the adult over a prolonged period.

The prognosis of bronchiectasis is good, if the treatment outlined above is used. The treatment will usually need to be lifelong, but in most cases this can probably ensure that the patient's life is indeed long.

Cystic Fibrosis

This is the commonest Mendelian genetic disorder in Caucasians, occurring in about 1 in 2000 births in Europe and North America, but the disease is very rare in Asians and Africans. Improved management of these patients during childhood has now meant that increasing numbers are surviving to adult life, but the respiratory problems are the major hazard to life (Mitchell-Heggs *et al.*, 1976). There is little doubt that these patients are best managed by co-operation between the general practitioner and a special management centre, with skilled physiotherapists, experienced consultant physicians and sympathetic nursing and social workers who can provide continued advice to help these patients through the many social, economic and work problems which they encounter living in the community.

The major aim of medical management in such adult cystic fibrotic patients is to control respiratory infection, relieve bronchospasm and, in the later stage, attempt to control the terminal cor pulmonale and hypoxaemia which usually herald death between 20 and 30 years of age in these patients. As with bronchiectasis, the hallmark of control of respiratory infection is postural drainage and antibiotics. However, an important new manoeuvre has now been proved to be of value to these patients, that of draining secretions themselves using the 'huff' technique. During expiration from mid-lung volume and low-lung volume, the patient carries out huffs, combind with sharp adduction of the upper arms, then followed by a few minutes of relaxed diaphragmatic breathing, and then coughing. This can raise as much sputum as can physiotherapists who assist in postural drainage. The ability to clear the chest themselves using these 'huffing' techniques greatly increases the patient's independence.

Some patients find that five or ten minutes of inhaling a saline aerosol, with or without a bronchodilator (for example, terbutaline respiratory solution 5 mg/ml) from a compressor-driven nebuliser, can liquefy secretions and thus make the raising of sputum more effective (di Sant'Agnese and Davis, 1979).

Antibiotics can be used continuously, depending upon the pathogen currently infecting the patient. Staphylococcal infection, common particularly in children and young adolescents, can usually be controlled by flucloxacillin or clindamycin, given in high doses early in an infective episode. In later life *H. influenzae* and *Str. pneumoniae* again become dominant pathogens, and respond to amoxycillin, ampicillin and cotrimoxazole as for bronchiectasis and chronic bronchitis.

Pseudomonas aeruginosa is a major threat to these patients in later adult life. The development of a mucoid strain of this organism in the sputum often indicates a grave prognosis. Parenteral treatment with intramuscular gentamicin, combined with intravenous carbenicillin has been the traditional treatment, but unfortunately in many of these patients the mucoid strains of *Pseudomonas* is resistant to these antibiotics. A careful controlled trial from Brompton Hospital has recently shown that gentamicin and carbenicillin given by aerosol using a compressor-driven inhaler, three or four times a day over many months, can prevent progression of respiratory impairment in such adult cystic fibrotic patients (Hodson *et al.*, 1981). However, this complicated therapy is best controlled by a specialised centre with experience of the technique. The new cephalosporin, ceftazidime, appears to be promising, at least in the laboratory studies against mucoid strains of *Pseudomonas* (Ceftazidime Symposium, 1981), although this expensive antibiotic cannot yet be recommended on the basis of proven controlled clinical trials in such patients.

References

Bates, T. (1982) 'The role of infection during exacerbation of chronic bronchitis', *Annals of Internal Medicine*, 97, 130–1

British Thoracic Association (1982) 'Smoking withdrawal study', *Annals of Internal Medicine*, London, pp. 130–1

Calverley, P.M.A., Leggett, R.J., McElderry, L. and Flenley, D.C. (1982) 'Cigarette smoking and secondary polycythaemia in hypoxic cor pulmonale', *American Review of Respiratory Disease*, 125, 511–16

Ceftazidime Symposium (1981) *Journal of Antimicrobial Chemotherapy*, 8, suppl. B

Di Sant'Agnese, P.A. and Davis, P.B. (1979) 'Cystic fibrosis in adults. 75 cases and a review of 232 cases in the literature', *American Journal of Medicine*, 66, 121–32

Douglas, N.J., Sudlow, M.F. and Flenley, D.C. (1977) 'Bronchodilatation with ipratropium bromide in severe chronic bronchitis', *Thorax, 32*, 645

Douglas, N.J., Calverley, P.M.A., Leggett, R.J.E., Brash, H.M., Flenley, D.C. and Brezinova, V. (1979) 'Transient hypoxaemia during sleep in chronic bronchitis and emphysema', *Lancet*, i, 1–4

Fee, W.M. and Stewart, M.J. (1982) 'Controlled trial of nicotine chewing gum in a smoking withdrawal clinic', *Practitioner*, 226, 148–61

Flenley, D.C. (1979) 'Vaccination against influenza', *Health Bulletin*, September

Gimenez, M., Uffholtz, H. and Panafiel, C.M. (1976) 'Physiotherapy and directed breathing: methodology', *Bulletin Européen de Physiopathologie Respiratoire*, 12, 140

Grimby, G. and Skoogh, B.E. (1980) 'Rehabilitation of the respiratory patient', in D.C. Flenley (ed.), *Recent Advances in Respiratory Medicine* II, Churchill Livingstone, Edinburgh

Hill, H.R. (1981) 'Infections complicating congenital immuno deficiency syndromes', in R.H. Rereben and L.S. Young (eds), *Clinical Approach to Infection in the Compromised Host*, Pleenham Medical, New York and London

Hodson, M.E., Penketh, A.R.L. and Batten, J.C. (1981) 'Aerosol carbenicillin and gentamicin treatment of pseudomonas aeruginosa infection in patients with cystic fibrosis', *Lancet*, ii, 11–37

MRC Working Party (1981) 'Long-term domiciliary oxygen therapy in chronic hypoxic cor pulmonale complicating chronic bronchitis and emphysema: a clinical trial', *Lancet*, i, 681–5

Mitchell-Heggs, P., Mearns, M. and Batten, J.C. (1976) 'Cystic fibrosis in adolescents and adults', *Quarterly Journal of Medicine*, 45, 479–504

Neu, H.C. (1982) 'Clinical uses of cephalosporins', *Lancet*, ii, 252–5

Nocturnal Oxygen Therapy Trial Group (1980) 'Continuous or nocturnal oxygen therapy in hypoxemic chronic obstructive lung disease: a clinical trial', *Annals of Internal Medicine*, 93, 391–8

Royal College of Physicians (1981) 'Disabling chest disease, prevention and care. Report of the Royal College of Physicians by the College Committee on Thoracic Medicine', *Journal of the Royal College of Physicians of London*, 15, 3

Russell, M.A.H., Wilson, C., Taylor, G. and Baker, C.D. (1979) 'Effect of general practitioners' advice against smoking', *British Medical Journal*, 2, 231–5

Schwartz, J.S. (1982) 'Pneumococcal vaccine: clinical efficacy and effectiveness', *Annals of Internal Medicine*, 96, 208

Snider, G.L. (1981) 'The pathogenesis of emphysema; twenty years of progress',

American Review of Respiratory Disease, 124, 321–4

Thurlbeck, W.M. (1976) *Chronic Airflow Obstruction in Lung Disease. Major Problems in Pathology* V, W.B. Saunders, London

Tovey, E.R., Chapman, M.D., Wills, C.W. and Platts-Mills, T.A.E. (1981) 'The distribution of dust mite allergen in the houses of patients with asthma', *American Review of Respiratory Disease*, 124, 630–5

Valentine, U., McHardy, J.M., Inglis, J.M., Calder, M.A. and Crofton, J.W. (1980) 'A study of infective and other factors in exacerbations of chronic bronchitis', *British Journal of Diseases of the Chest*, 74, 228–38

Warren, P.M., Flenley, D.C., Millar, J.S. and Avery, A. (1980) 'Respiratory failure revisited: acute exacerbations of chronic bronchitis between 1961–1968 and 1970–1976', *Lancet*, i, 467–71

Further Reading

Crofton, J.C. and Douglas, A.C. (1981) *Respiratory Diseases*, 3rd edn, Blackwell Scientific Publications, Oxford

Flenley, D.C. (1980) *Recent Advances in Respiratory Medicine* II, Churchill Livingstone, Edinburgh

Flenley, D.C. (1981) *Respiratory Medicine*, Ballière Tindall, London

7 PALLIATIVE CARE IN CARDIOVASCULAR DISEASES

Michael Matthews

To sudden death, described by the ancients as 'life's greatest blessing', diseases of the heart, often previously unrecognised, make a splendid and quite disproportionate contribution. If there is not to be this happy exit from life, there can be discussion as to whether neoplasia or chronic organ failure provides the less forbidding road. All chronic organ failures have their own trials; in chronic heart failure, except terminally, the rationing system imposed by the restricted cardiac output arranges that the brain continues to receive an adequate blood supply and to remain clear. As a result, the problem is usually a very demanding one and also only too apparent to the patient. The acceptance of the humiliating physical restrictions, the loss of well-being and of mobility, the reconciliation to the inevitable restrictions imposed on others, even if willingly and lovingly accepted, all require a formidable adaptation. But the medical attendant with a bright eye, listening ear and well-stored mind can provide effective palliation, and because chronic heart failure is usually such a slow process, this of course implies that it is the general practitioner who must usually provide it.

Perhaps the doctor's most precious contribution is time; time to listen, time to look and, a much appreciated courtesy, time to conceal that he has not much of it. Perhaps none of the advice which follows is as important as to underline the necessity of conveying to the patient that his need is understood, and to give him the feeling that he is being cherished in what may prove to be a prolonged trial.

Palliation is derived from the latin verb *palliare*, to cloak; it implies the hiding or concealing of symptoms, and at its best the alleviation of symptoms or mitigation of suffering, but, of course, by definition, no cure. We must assume, then, that we are dealing with the patient who is not one of those who can be cured. How inappropriate it would be, however, to be using palliation in a patient with gross heart failure due, for example, to beri beri — in this country almost peculiar to those who seriously abuse alcohol or to zealot diet faddists — when a few injections of vitamin B_1 could produce a prompt and total cure. Even in the elderly, division of a hitherto unrecognised persistent ductus

171

arteriosus can produce a prompt cure of heart failure. Of course these are exquisite rarities, and it is only a relatively small proportion of patients with heart failure who are amenable to cure e.g. the grossly anaemic, the hyperthyroid, and the patient with a correctable left-to-right intracardiac shunt or a systemic ateriovenous aneurysm, for example. For the most part the practice of cardiology *is* palliative, whether surgical or medical. Operations for valvotomy, coronary arterial bypass grafting and cardiac valve replacement are all palliative rather than curative. In all such cases, continuing observation of the patient is required, and active further steps may be needed in order to provide further help where appropriate.

What, then, are ways of ameliorating the cardinal symptoms of heart disease? Rather than to reiterate what is available in the standard textbooks of medical practice, those practical measures will be described which are often overlooked in the management of the symptoms of heart disease, especially with those patients for whom surgical treatment has been properly rejected, often on the grounds of old age. We are concerned, then, disproportionately with the elderly patient for whom surgery is inappropriate, and whose lot can be capable of improvement by suitable attention to detail. The cardinal symptoms of heart disease result from fluid retention, e.g. with dyspnoea, oedema, ascites, etc., from cardiac ischaemia or from rhythm disturbances; for these, palliation is achieved first and foremost by precise and careful medical management.

General Considerations

There are potentially reversible adverse factors in many patients with the symptoms of chronic heart disease, and their importance is often underestimated. They are common and by no means, of course, peculiar to those with heart disease.

Obesity

The patient who is 10 kg overweight, if asked to carry a similar amount in a rucksack all day, would readily come to recognise the difficulty of the acute added burden, though he is unaware of the effects of the more long-standing one. It would be inappropriate here to try to deal fully with a difficult problem which requires patient and persistent medical supports, and which all too often defies the doctor's best efforts. In men success often depends on the degree of concern and skill in the spouse in her role as cook. Patients can be encouraged in the view that appropriate calories can become reliable friends. The eyes can be trained to look on sugar, flour and potato as enemies, and to recognise that a whole orange will give some comfort to the stomach used to being stretched. Weight reduction with a weight chart displayed in the bathroom at home and, if possible, a family competitor may help to put the responsibility also upon others. This is by no means to underrate the ill effects on calorie balance of the enforced inactivity of cardiac failure, or the comfort of good food when other interests wane. However, patients often have little idea of how the calorie requirement reduces with age, and especially with inactivity, or the extent to which the stomach-stretching process is a matter of habit. Sometimes it is useful to remind patients that they usually taste the first few mouthfuls; the disposal of the rest of the meal is more akin to the action of the vacuum cleaner. Slowing the eating process avoids being the first to finish when helpings are smaller. As in so many other aspects of patient care, it is communication between doctor and patient which counts most, and the realisation by the doctor that the problem is a difficult one. The 'brown fat' story − still hotly debated − with its news that some patients are not adequately provided with these useful furnaces for the destruction of surplus dietary fat, has done something to stifle pejorative medical comments. The need for weight reduction of heart disease is no different from what is so urgently required in the management of an osteoarthritic hip, emphysema or a stroke, so that the physican can expect plenty of practice in this respect.

Anaemia

No patient with angina or heart failure can be assumed not to be anaemic until the blood has been examined. The occasional patient is entirely relieved of angina by attention to bleeding haemorrhoids, for example. Ruling out anaemia should invariably precede long-term anti-anginal therapy or treatment for heart failure; if possible, of course, a revealed anaemia should be corrected. If cardiac failure or angina becomes worse, anaemia must be considered as a cause of the deterioration.

Exercise

There is evidence that exercise encourages coronary and leg collateral vessel development, and the walking range of patients with intermittent claudication or angina pectoris can be improved in this way. In the early stages of heart failure, modest exercise is acceptable. Sensible patients can tell how much they can do. In general, there is much to be said for encouraging patients to listen to what their body is saying to them. Children have few problems in this respect, they are either in bed or up and about; but adults have theories, and their spouses and their medical attendants often have more.

In our present context we are dealing mainly with those patients who have reached the stage when all exercise may have become a challenge, the patient who is breathless in a chair or in bed and who may have real difficulty in crossing the room. He knows that he cannot do more, and advice needs only to reinforce what the patient's body is clearly telling him. At this stage of dyspnoea exercise is not only difficult or impossible, but often leads to further deterioration. When the cardiac output is much reduced, the rationing system already mentioned preserves the cerebral and myocardial blood flow by differential adjustment of arteriolar resistance. When with exercises, the limbs require more blood, the kidneys may be further deprived, and more water retention result, and there are important changes in renal tubular function which further exacerbate the condition. The patient who is nearing the end of the cardiac-failure road nearly always loses water weight when relieved from struggling with the daily chores by confinement to bed, at home if circumstances permit, or in hospital if they do not. The value of rest in these severely incapacitated patients in order to restore the fluid balance cannot be overestimated. Such patients when admitted to hospital lose weight even without change in the diuretic treatment; then proper assessment of day-to-day progress is not possible without regular reliable weighing, for measuring fluid balance is usually unreliable.

Fluid Retention

Checking on Sodium Intake. It is surprising how infrequently there is an enquiry into the patient's salt-eating habits. These habits vary widely, as can be readily observed with fellow eaters in public places. There is a section of the population who pour salt on food without a prior taste, as if testifying that it will inevitably be inedible unless grossly saline – a practice which the discriminating cook, of course, finds reprehensible. The permanently freckled hand of the former tea planter from Sri Lanka, when he develops heart failure, will have to be trained not to be putting the amount of salt on food which a tropical environment required. The grossly hypertensive man who had been in three teaching hospitals and still brushed his teeth with sodium chloride, the lady who scoured London for salt-free bread while her husband, the patient, used 'fruit salt' (50 per cent sodium bicarbonate) every night for his bowels, are examples which come to mind of the ways in which excessive sodium intake may be overlooked. Anyone on diuretic therapy with significant water retention should not add salt to his food, and the salt in cooking should be reduced as much as possible. These patients should also avoid bacon, kippers and other excessively salty foods.

The salt-free diet has been described as not prolonging life, but making it seem longer, and it is not this which is being discussed. Rather, we are dealing with the need to keep sodium intake to a reasonable minimum. Patients' taste for salt, just like their taste for sugar, can be made to change; many a patient with chronic heart failure comes to develop a distaste for salt. When fluid retention is difficult to control, enquiry of some patients may reveal that they have a taste for a familiar beef extract, about which a Cambridge professor used to say that it was '50 per cent an extract of the inedible portions of the beef carcase, and 50 per cent salt which keeps it from putrefaction which it so richly deserves.' A patient unexpectedly re-admitted to hospital with pulmonary oedema during the night said that he had thought that his hostess's soup was very salty, but that he had been too polite not to finish it. Such is the price which can be paid when the fluid balance is critical. Some may find 'salt substitutes' palatable.

Fluid Restriction. Many patients with heart failure are subjected to restriction of fluid intake which they find irksome, and which is usually quite unnecessary. Most patients should take whatever fluid they feel that they need, avoiding of course those containing excessive sodium. The only exception to this general rule is the patient with dilutional hyponatraemia, that is, the patient with gross water retention whose serum sodium is low. In such patients both total body water and total body sodium are increased. The situation can be improved by continuing sodium restriction and restricting water intake to 600–800 ml/day, until the sodium has risen to about 135 mmol/l (Avery, 1980). Many continue diuretic therapy despite the development of dilutional hyponatraemia. Knowledge of the blood urea and electrolyte levels in patients with severe heart failure on diuretic therapy is necessary from time to time at least. Enforced inactivity leads to increased tissue breakdown, and this contributes to uraemia (Domenet and Evans, 1969), which may be made worse by inappropriate restriction of fluid intake and can contribute significantly to the patient's loss of well-being. Occasionally, hyponatraemia and uraemia also result from the over-enthusiastic use of diuretics in patients who no longer have oedema; all that is required then is to reduce or terminate the diuretic therapy.

Assessment of Heart Failure and Control of Diuretic Therapy. The ideal diuretic therapy is one which, in combination with a reasonable restriction of dietary sodium, maintains the patient free of cardiac failure without significant side-effects. The most sensitive indicators of efficient management are the weight control, the repeated examination of jugular venous pressure, freedom from attacks of nocturnal breathlessness and absence of oedema. The test of hepato-jugular reflux is not reliable in specifying that there is heart failure (Matthews and Hampson, 1958) because of unpredictable accompanying changes in the intrathoracic pressure and because in normal subjects there is an elevation of jugular venous pressure, albeit transient, with compression of the abdomen. It is, however, a useful manoeuvre in helping to identify the upper level of distention in the jugular veins when this is in doubt. The oedema may be predominantly sacral or at the back of the thighs and therefore readily overlooked in patients confined to bed. The basal crepitations so dear to the physician's heart are too common an accompaniment of the ageing process to be reliable; even post-tussive crepitations are often present with radiologically clear lungs. Only if crepitations are present over a fairly large area bilaterally, are fine and are persistent after vigorous coughs, can they be regarded as a fairly reliable indicator of left heart failure. (It is, important, however, not to be misled by the extensive crepitations of fibrosing alveolitis; in these patients evidence of heart disease is usually lacking.)

In the early stages of the management of heart failure, the cheapest diuretic with potassium supplement is usually appropriate. There are now 23 diuretics presented in about 60 different products (Ramsay, 1982). Except for the more resistant cases, thiazides are usually the appropriate diuretics, given once daily; they usually cause no problems, although gout and diabetes may be precipitated. The least expensive of them is bendrofluazide, and this should therefore be the drug of choice. There is disagreement about the requirement for potassium supplementation, but occasional examples of the ill effects of induced hypokalaemia tend, disproportionately perhaps, to influence most physicians in favour of simultaneous potassium supplementation. Potassium supplementation is usually provided in the form of the proprietory preparation Slow-K. This can cause grave harm to the oesophagus if allowed to lie there and should be given with a drink or with food to prevent this. There is a particular risk to post-operative patients if an adequate drink is omitted. The elderly, those liable to episodes of arrhythmias or those also taking corticosteroids or digoxin are particularly vulnerable to hypokalaemia, and then potassium-sparing diuretics may be particularly appropriate, e.g. spironolactone, amiloride or triamterine.

When severe heart failure requires loop diuretics such as frusemide, bumetanide or ethacrynic acid, these promote a diuresis lasting up to six hours or so. The cheapest is frusemide BP, and in severe chronic cardiac failure as much as 500 mg or even more frusemide per day may be required. Spironolactone 100 mg orally once a day is often useful together with the frusemide in such cases. This combination, together with restriction of exercise and moderate restriction of salt, should prove effective as a rule. In the severely disabled patient whose water retention increases despite such measures, a period of more complete physical rest between a bed and a chair may result in the required water loss, particularly if aminophyllin is given slowly intravenously followed by intravenous frusemide.

Spironolactone, just like potassium chloride and digitalis preparations, is notorious for its effect in reducing the appetite, and may cause gynaecomastia. Anxiety as a result of this may require explanation, but gynaecomastia is on the whole an acceptable price to pay for useful improvement in maintaining fluid balance. Many patients find a high diuretic dose more acceptable than extreme restriction of dietary sodium.

The patient with severe congestive heart failure does not suffer only from breathlessness and oedema; the dropsy of former days is no longer seen with effective use of diuretics. The cost of freedom from waterlogging may be heavy in terms of loss of appetite and electrolyte disturbance. Congestion of the liver and stomach, and the use of diuretics and digitalis may all depress the appetite; the patient may be helped if the particular cause of the anorexia in his or her case can be identified. There is a need for special skills in cooking, particularly when the salt is to be restricted; a more than usually generous use of herbs and lemon juice, for example, may be very helpful for the patient with a cultivated palate. Some patients find salt substitutes acceptable. Discussion between the patient and the patient's wife with a dietician may prove particularly worth while.

In the occasional patient in whom death seems to be imminent despite these measures, the use of a regime regarded as appropriate in terminal cancer may prove to be the best form of management. The increased rest and the reduction in anxiety may prove extremely effective palliation. Sometimes the use of opiates may result in a surprising degree of remission in the cardiac failure, and the opiates themselves may prove to be required only temporarily. The regular use of opiates in what appears to be pre-terminal heart failure can bring about an ease of mind and acceptance of disability in an impressive way. For some reason there is reluctance to learn that there is a phase in heart failure which requires the methods generally and successfully used in pre-terminal illness of other kinds.

The Management of Acute Pulmonary Oedema

Pulmonary oedema leads to a breathlessness even more alarming, often, than that of the asthmatic attack, and every reasonable step should be taken not only to relieve the attack, but to prevent a recurrence. In the acute attack, by far the most important measure is the injection of an adequate amount of morphine or diamorphine, preferably intravenously and accompanied by cyclizine. The current fashion of giving a diuretic without an opiate is to be strongly deprecated. The good effect of the intravenous opiate is almost immediate; the breathlessness becomes less, anxiety is allayed, the catecholamine level is reduced, and there is an effect of peripheral venous dilatation which leads to an advantageous peripheral sequestration of the blood. The occasional patient who has severe emphysema − and he should be identifiable as being usually breathless and with an over-inflated chest − is the only common exception to this general rule. An intravenous fast-acting loop diuretic such a frusemide, bumetanide or ethacrynic acid is a necessary accompaniment.

The prevention of further attacks is along the lines of the management of chronic cardiac failure already described, and except when the pulmonary oedema has been the result of an acute myocardial infarction, diuretic therapy is then likely to be a life sentence. It is, of course, far more important to prevent recurrences of pulmonary oedema than it is to keep the ankles shapely.

Digitalis

The role of digitalis in patients with atrial fibrillation with a rapid ventricular rate is not in doubt, but there is dispute about its use in the management of patients with cardiac failure in sinus rhythm (Smith and Haber, 1975; Editorial, *British Medical Journal*, 1979). On the one hand, it has been amply demonstrated since the early days of cardiac catheterisation that by the use of digitalis in patients with heart failure the cardiac output is usually augmented (Harvey *et al.*, 1949). On the other hand, numerous clinical trials (for example, Dall, 1970; Hull and Mackintosh, 1977) have suggested that most patients in sinus rhythm with heart failure fail to show deterioration when digitalis is withdrawn. However, 16 per cent of 341 patients collectively reported in these and several other trials showed evidence of deterioration when digitalis was discontinued (Griffiths *et al.*, 1982). A recent study on M-mode echocardiograms and systolic time intervals showed that there were significant inotropic, and therefore presumably beneficial, effects from the long-term administration of digitalis (ibid.). Very numerous variables in cardiac failure and its management suggest that invasive studies or carefully controlled echocardiographic studies, most of which show benefit for such patients with long-term digitalis therapy, should guide our decisions, rather than clinical trials.

It is necessary to use well-formulated digoxin preparations, because otherwise there may be a bio-availability problem; with high bio-availability preparations such as Lanoxin (BW) maximal plasma concentrations are reached in 25-60 minutes. Much of the drug is eliminated in the urine, so that toxic levels of digoxin in the blood may be a feature if there is co-existing renal failure. It is necessary then, to re-emphasise the relative intolerance of the elderly to digoxin, probably mainly due to reduced renal function, but also when there is reduced lean body mass; in such patients 0.0625 mg of digoxin twice daily may prove adequate and not toxic. Occasionally the stomach is intolerant of digoxin even though the level in the blood is within the therapeutic range. In such rare cases another preparation of digitalis, such as digitoxin, may be better tolerated. Digitoxin, however, has the disadvantage that it has a much longer half-life, so that if toxic symptoms develop they take longer to resolve. The special risks of hypokalaemia in elderly patients should perhaps be reiterated.

Peripheral Vasodilators

Patients with severe cardiac failure unresponsive to digitalis, diuretics, bed rest and sodium restriction may have benefit from the use of vasodilator drugs. Of these isosorbide nitrate (40 mg four times daily), hydralazine (25-100 mg per day in divided doses), and prazosin (4 mg twice a day) have been widely used. Captopril (25-100 mg three times daily) is also proving very effective (Cowley *et al.*, 1982). These drugs tend to reduce both the pre-load of the heart as a result of venodilatation and the afterload as a result of reduction in peripheral resistance.

Measurable reduction occurs in the left ventricular diastolic pressure, and hence pulmonary venous pressure, result which of course tends to reduce pulmonary oedema. The good effect of peripheral vasodilators in terms of increased cardiac output is readily demonstrable in the cardiac laboratory (e.g. Rouleau *et al.*, 1982). There is a growing tendency to use vasodilators early in the management of cardiac failure, rather than to restrict their use to those patients in whom conventional methods have failed.

Chronic Cor Pulmonale

Cardiac failure, when it results from respiratory failure, is usually precipitated by an acute intercurrent respiratory infection. Cardinal palliation is therefore the treatment of the respiratory failure, usually with antibiotics, physiotherapy and, if indicated, bronchodilators and oxygen by controlled oxygen therapy or other suitable equipment. Success in these respects will be likely to improve the cardiac failure, which will usually require diuretic therapy also. Under experimental circumstances digitalis has also been demonstrated to be useful (Harvey *et al.*, 1951) and should therefore probably also be employed.

The Management of Angina Pectoris

All treatment for angina pectoris is palliative, although least so in patients whose angina can be relieved by the replacement of a stenotic aortic valve or by the surgical bypass of single or multiple localised coronary arterial obstructions.

The assessment of the value of medical therapy for angina pectoris is fraught with difficulty, as many studies have shown that a significant proportion of patients improve with the demonstration of medical interest and concern (e.g. Cole, Kaye and Griffiths, 1958) and in addition trials using lactose as placebo almost invariably show benefit in 20-30 per cent of patients (Evans and Hoyle, 1933). How good then to be selling a remedy for angina, unless it is not even as good as placebo!

The managment depends on whether the patient is experiencing only effort angina, or whether he is having, either alone or in addition, episodes of cardiac pain at rest, that is, Printzmetal angina. For both, the use of the general methods already described (pp. 173-4) is essential. In the management of exercise angina, when it is disabling, and particularly in the younger patient, assessment for surgery is becoming mandatory; the benefits of successful surgery are considerable and, from the symptomatic point of view, temporarily at least curative. When such an option is available, medical palliation is therefore inappropriate.

It is essential that the mechanism which produces the pain is clearly described to the patient, and it is often helpful to say that the way to get angina if you have such a liability is to walk uphill against the wind with a full stomach on a cold morning. In this way he can see how to avoid the pain, if possible. He should also know that in about 30 per cent of cases with time the angina disappears, though he need not know that the disappearance may be only temporary. It is helpful for him to know that there is a natural process of coronary bypass; it is surprisingly little realised that innumerable intercoronary anastamoses develop in the ageing heart. No step in the management of angina pectoris is more important than the exercise of communication skills.

Glyceryl trinitrate has now been in use for more than a century and, this being so, it is vastly surprising that it is so often used wrongly. It is almost without value for the *treatment* of stable exercise-induced angina, for this is generally relieved promptly by rest even before the glyceryl trinitrate can take effect in the two to three minutes required. For a bad attack, however, it may be invaluable, especially if the (fresh) pill is crunched and the pieces held in the mouth. By far the most important use of glyceryl trinitrate is to use it *prophylactically*, for example, two minutes before setting out on the journey which experience indicates will be likely to cause pain; the protection may last for 20 minutes or so. The patient with angina should form the habit of slipping in his glyceryl trinitrate tablet much as the patient with osteoarthritis picks up his walking stick. The side-effects of glyceryl trinitrate are few, and it is worth stressing that the headache experienced by some with the first pill tends to become less as more are used. Patients expect that they are 'habit forming' — implying that they will lose effect, which they will not. They fear using too many, and can be reassured that even two per hour would cause no harm. Glyceryl trinitrate is an excellent, reliable friend to the patient with angina pectoris, but one who needs an effective introduction by the physician. It is still the best and safest treatment available. Glyceryl trinitrate may also be administered by inunction.

Beyond this there are now innumerable forms of treatment. There is dispute about the value of long-acting nitrates, but they are unlikely to be as ineffective as they are often held to be; glyceryl trinitrate itself was introduced by Murrell (1879) to be used three times a day, and it survived this triumphantly. The next line of treatment is the use of the β-receptor blocking drugs; of these, propranolol is one of the cheapest and has the great merit that it has been more used than any other, so that the potential ill effects are best understood. This is by no means unimportant, for it took ten years for the dangerous side-effects of practolol to be discovered. It has the disadvantage that there is great variation between patients in their susceptibility to the drug, because of the different handling of propranolol by the liver. The dose has therefore to be tailored to need. Unless significant slowing of the heart is achieved, the dose is probably inadequate and should be increased until this has occurred. 80 mg four times a day or even more may be required; one sees many patients maintained on very small doses of propranolol (for example, 10 mg twice a day), who can expect to enjoy the placebo effect, but not the therapeutic one.

Of the other β-receptor blockers available, atenolol and metoprolol are among the most widely used. Being more cardioselective, they are less liable to cause asthma. β-Blockers function by reducing cardiac work from bradycardia and reduction of arterial pressure; many may eliminate angina. This is, however, often done at the cost of disturbed sleep, dreams and even hallucinations, cold limbs, tiredness, anorexia, bronchoconstriction, impotence, etc. One has therefore to be alert to the possibility that the side-effects may be more disabling than the angina.

Of the other treatments, nifedipine (10–20 mg three times daily) appears at the present time to be the most valuable, either alone or in combination with β-blockers. It is also the drug of choice in capricious or Printzmetal angina. Some patients have dramatic improvement from perhexiline (100 mg three times daily), but it has the disadvantage of producing a peripheral neuropathy and disturbance of 'liver function' tests; both are reversible.

The Surgical Treatment of Angina

Coronary artery bypass grafting (CABG) is now the single most common surgical operation in the United States; the United Kingdom is well down the ranking order in this respect as compared with many other EEC countries. It is extremely effective in relieving pain in well-chosen cases and there is growing evidence too from the European trial (among others) that the operation may also improve life expectancy. Coronary angiography is now a very safe procedure and is still essential in making a proper assessment of the coronary arterial disease. It is, of course, only appropriate as an investigation if the patient has said that, should the arteriogram indicate that he is suitable for surgery, he would be prepared to undergo such an operation. Ideal patients are those with localised obstruction in one to four coronary arteries which are capable of bypass with the patient's leg veins. The vein is sewn to the aorta and to the coronary artery beyond the block. This operation requires patience and care, but in good hands carries a mortality of less than 1 per cent. There are naturally some potential complications of thoracotomy and in some cases there may be an intra-operative infarct.

Myocardial Infarction

It seems inappropriate to deal with the vast topic of the management of acute myocardial infarction under the heading of palliative care. However, for the older patient for whom hospitalisation and continuous monitoring may be considered unsuitable, it is necessary to consider some of the crucial points in the management at home.

Home management requires adequate domestic circumstances, and therefore usually means that the patient left at home will be male. Bed rest is useful when the patient feels he needs it, but should be kept to a reasonable minimum. The essential consideration is adequate analgesia, and during the first three days or so the medical practitioner or practice nurse should between them aim to visit the patient twice a day, mainly so as to ensure adequate analgesia, with either diamorphine or morphine and cyclizine. The patient usually suffers from the disease only for a few days; from then on he suffers from medical restrictions which should therefore not be too forbidding or arbitrary, and he should be guided by the severity of complications rather than by the diagnostic label. Control or arrhythmias may be difficult or impossible at home; alleviation of cardiac failure along the usual lines should not however present significant problems.

Arrhythmias

In the later stages of heart disease atrial fibrillation is one of the commonest developments and one which is often overlooked by those who do not feel the pulse for long enough and conclude erroneously

Figure 7.1: Patient's chart of attacks of supra-ventricular tachycardia

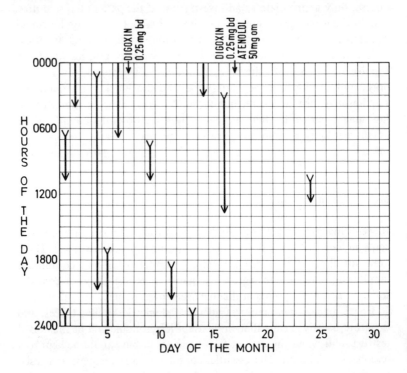

that there are extra-systoles. When recognised, and if the ventricular rate is rapid, this can usually be effectively and readily managed by the use of digitalis preparations. When atrial fibrillation develops unexpectedly in a previously fit elderly patient, the possibility that it may be due to hyperthyroidism should not be overlooked. The troublesome and eminently treatable arrhythmias are the bradycardias, which include sino-atrial disease and complete heart block, and the tachycardias, particularly recurrent ventricular tachycardia.

Bradycardias

Sino-atrial disease is now recognised to be common as the cause of both periods of bradycardia and attacks of tachycardia. It does not usually shorten life (Shaw *et al.*, 1979), but may impair its quality considerably by causing Stokes-Adams attacks or attacks of supraventricular tachycardia. Such patients require cardiological assessment, and if the attacks are sufficiently troublesome, a pacemaker is usually required which not only provides protection from undue bradycardia but also permits the use of digoxin, which might otherwise induce dangerous brady-cardia.

Recurrent supraventricular tachycardia should be manageable with digoxin, a β-blocker, the combination of these two or with one of the newer anti-arrhythmic agents. It is usually a matter of trial and error to work out the method of management. It may be helpful if the patient keeps a chart of attacks such as that shown in the diagram (Figure 7.1). This will allow the physician to see quickly how frequent and how long the attacks are and how effective his treatment is proving to be.

The management of ventricular arrhythmias needs expert assessment and there is nowadays a bewildering array of anti-arrhythmic agents, each with its particular advantage and disadvantage.

Cardiac Transplantation

This is so far available to a minuscule proportion of patients under the age of 40 with cardiac failure so severe that life is intolerable despite maximal diuretic therapy. At the present time it is available to so few that it is inappropriate to consider this at length here.

The Sick Room and Cardiac Failure

The physician's eye should include the ability to see whether the patient looks cherished in the terms of the social milieu. The patient with chronic heart failure requires a comfortable chair which really provides support, as well as a back rest in bed; pillows alone will not provide the sort of comfort which the breathless require at night. Is there water within reach? Is the urinal in a socially acceptable housing to hand? Flowers are often a good indication of cherishment. Are radio and television available? And now that loneliness has become one of the commonest disorders in society, what steps are being taken to fill the extra social gap imposed by inactivity? Chronic heart failure is a good test of friendship. Circumstances which allow the patient to give something of himself fill a need which the invaluable radio and tele-vision cannot. As in the prisoner of war camp, the patient with intel-lectual interests and/or a meaningful faith can often cope better. The reader, the writer of letters, the knitter and the stamp collector all can maintain their interest and find enjoyment in a very restricted life. The former athlete without other interests suffers most; the golfer deprived of golf has a serious disorder of his own, which can be lessened by supporting visits from those still able to play.

In the restricted life of the patient with severe heart failure, social isolation seems for some to be made more bearable by what seems to them to be the friendly presence of a glowing cigarette tip. It is easy enough for the physician to pontificate on the well-established ill effects of the habit, and its power to hasten degenerative arterial disease. Indeed, in the context of chronic cor pulmonale, ischaemic heart disease and intermittent claudication in particular, the medical adviser is failing in his duty if he does not point out the almost inevitable ill effects of continuing to smoke. But in doing so, he can hardly be giving 'palliative' advice – for the patient often knows that it is he who requires 'palliation' of his lonely and often unhappy lot with the cigarettes which have long been a 'friend'. The physician may have to accept that when some patients say that life is not worth living without tobacco, they really mean it – though for many a patient the environment of the illness may make smoking quite inappropriate if the needs of neighbouring patients are to be met. Each patient has to be assessed on his own merits.

References

Avery, F.S. (1980) *Principles and Practice of Clinical Pharmacology and Thera-peutics*, 2nd edn, Churchill Livingstone, Edinburgh, p. 620
Cole, S.L., Kaye, H., Griffiths, G.C. (1958) 'Assay of antianginal agents; the rapport period', *Journal of the American Medical Association*, 168, 275
Cowley, A.J., Rowley, J.M., Stainer, K.L. and Hampton, J.R. (1982) 'Captopril therapy for heart failure', *Lancet*, ii, 730
Dall, J.L.C. (1970) 'Maintenance digoxin in elderly patients', *British Medical Journal*, i, 1103-4
Domenet, J.G. and Evans, D.W. (1969) 'Uraemia in congestive heart failure', *Quarterly Journal of Medicine*, 61, 117
Editorial (1979) 'Digoxin in sinus rhythm', *British Medical Journal*, i, 1103-4
Evans, W. and Hoyle, C. (1933) 'The comparative value of drugs used in the continuous management of angina pectoris', *Quarterly Journal of Medicine*, 26, 311
Griffiths, B.E., Penny, W.J., Lewis, M.J. and Henderson, A.H. (1982) 'Main-tenance of the inotropic effects of digoxin in longterm treatment', *British Medical Journal*, ii, 1819-22
Harvey, R.M., Ferrer, M.I., Cathcart, T., Richards, D.W. and Cournand, A. (1949) 'Some effects of digoxin upon heart and circulation in man; digoxin in left ventricular failure', *American Journal of Medicine*, 7, 439-53
Harvey, R.M., Ferrer, M.I., Richards, D.W. and Cournand, A. (1951) 'Influence

of chronic pulmonary disease on the heart and circulation', *American Journal of Medicine*, 10, 719

Hull, S.M. and Mackintosh, A. (1977) 'Discontinuation of maintenance digoxin therapy in general practice', *Lancet*, ii, 1054–5

Matthews, M.B. and Hampson, J. (1958) 'Hepato-jugular reflux', *Lancet*, i, 873–6

Murrell, W. (1879) 'Nitroglycerin as a remedy for angina pectoris', *Lancet*, i, 80, 113, 151, 225

Ramsay, L.E. (1982) 'Choosing a diuretic', *Prescriber's Journal*, 22, 49

Rouleau, J.L., Chatterjee, K., Benge, W., Parmley, W.M. and Hiramatsu, B. (1982) 'Alterations in left ventricular function and coronary haemodynamics with captopril, hydralazine and prazosin in chronic ischaemic heart failure', *Circulation*, 65, 671

Shaw, D.B., Bolwell, A.G., Gowers, J. and Holman, R.R. (1979) 'Prognosis in sino-atrial disorder (sick sinus syndrome)', *British Heart Journal*, 42, 233

Smith, T.W. and Haber, E. (1973) 'Digitalis', *New England Journal of Medicine*, 289, 945, 1010, 1063, 1125

Recommended Reading

English, T.A.H. (1982) 'What price excellence?', *Journal of Medical Ethics*, 8, 144–6

Ewy, G.A., Kapadia, G.G., Yao, L., Lullin, M. and Marcus, F.I. (1969) 'Digoxin metabolism in the elderly', *Circulation*, 39, 449

Greenblat, D.J. and Koch-Weser, J. (1976) 'Drug therapy: intramuscular and injection of drugs. The digoxin dilemma', *Clinical Pharmacokinetics*, 1, 36

8 PALLIATIVE CARE IN NEUROLOGICAL DISORDERS

Ernest Jellinek

Most fatal neurological diseases terminate in coma, which is usually peaceful, albeit often quite noisy; our role at that stage is relatively easy, confined to essential nursing duties and support for the family. The real problems arise in the pre-terminal stages of the illness. The two most major neurological crippling disorders that are occasional killers are cerebrovascular disease and multiple sclerosis, and the latter should be supplemented by a group of paraplegias from other causes. Parkinson's disease is a possible killer, although it often does not do so, as the late stages tend to coincide with the later years of life, with all their other medical and social problems. The invariable fatalities in neurology occur in patients with Alzheimer's disease, in cerebral tumours, and lastly, and fortunately much less commonly, in motor neuron disease.

The palliation of advanced muscular dystrophy usually falls into the territory of the paediatrician. Rarities such as the encephalitides and system degenerations are not discussed specifically, although the principles of management of some of the above conditions, of course, also apply.

Cerebrovascular Disease

The patient who is more or less bed-bound in the last year of his life, as a result of cerebrovascular disease, is likely to have suffered a number of strokes, rather than just one. Some patients have reached this stage as a result of innumerable little strokes spread over many years, some after only two fairly major cerebrovascular accidents. Disease of one cerebral hemisphere, even of great severity with hemiplegia and aphasia, is unlikely to shorten survival, but bilateral cerebral hemisphere troubles or severe trouble in the brain-stem are invariably associated with a profound disturbance of mood and higher mental function. Great lability of mood is the rule, with uncontrollable outbursts of rage, frustration or, more rarely, laughter. Many patients do not lose insight and become appropriately and deeply depressed. Endless patience

188

may be a counsel of perfection when there is no rotation of attendants. Sometimes there is a case for sedation, especially with phenothiazines, but quite often this is ineffective and produces disagreeable side-effects (mental and motor retardation and Parkinsonism). Chlormethiazole and diazepoxides are more effective in some patients, and hypnotics are indicated when insomnia aggravates the mental agitation. Again, various medicaments may need to be tried.

The intellectual impairment may be difficult to assess in the presence of an obvious medical disturbance and perhaps a disturbance of speech. Sometimes members of the family have a better intuitive knowledge of the degree of intellectual preservation: this should help in avoiding the mistakes of either pitching too high or too low, that is, to frustrate the patient with impossible intellectual challenges or to treat him unnecessarily like a child.

The problems of disordered speech in cerebrovascular disease can be great, and any combination of motor or receptive disorders, and of dysarthria, will be encountered. Inexperienced persons may often fail to appreciate that a patient with an almost total expressive loss of speech may still understand almost normally, and there are many instances in the literature of recovered aphasiacs who were maddened by attendants and family talking across them as if they did not understand. Inability to express oneself is, of course, incredibly frustrating, and empathetic attendants are the greatest boon. In a few cases, the patients derive comfort from the efforts of a speech therapist; moreover, the speech therapist may be able to advise on possible alternative methods of communication.

Bilateral cerebral hemisphere disease or disease in the brain-stem produces spastic dysarthria, and also quite often appreciable difficulty in swallowing, with a tendency to choke, and poor coughing. Experienced nurses are, of course, familiar with the benefit of certain postures of the head in these patients in feeding, and the advantages of semi-liquid or liquid diet in some. Where these difficulties are extreme, naso-gastric tube feeding may become mandatory to avoid distressing dehydration. Parenteral nutrition is hardly ever justified in really advanced cerebrovascular disease. Major throat and swallowing problems, of course, provoke chest complications. These can be retarded or prevented for a while by suitable posturing, and by chest physiotherapy and suction.

Although physiotherapy has probably not very much to offer in the restoration of true active mobility in these advanced cases, passive movement and good posturing will prevent painful complications, especially of the shoulder joint, where there may be some subluxation. Ideally, there should be passive movements of all paralysed limbs as often as possible to prevent painful subluxation and contractures which will also hinder essential nursing procedures. These are naturally mainly concerned with attention to bowel and bladder. Incontinence is almost the rule in advanced cerebrovascular disease, and may still cause great distress to the patient, and certainly also to the family. At some stage an indwelling catheter becomes necessary.

Particular problems may arise in patients with damage to one or other parietal lobe of the brain, when there is lack of feeling on the contralateral side of the body, and also loss of half of the field of vision to that side, which may lead to injuries to the limbs on that side, and sometimes also to the patient falling out of bed, unless that side is blocked by a rail or placed against the wall.

The end usually results from chest complications or further strokes, which bring about coma, with or without convulsions.

Multiple Sclerosis (Paraplegia)

The majority of patients with multiple sclerosis never become seriously disabled. Even those who do become severely disabled do not usually progress in their disability, and last a normal life-span in a wheelchair. A very small proportion of cases in all age-groups suffer from progressive disease which may kill, directly or indirectly. The former outcome is really most uncommon, and happens when there is extensive demyelination in either the brain-stem or the upper spinal cord, leading to bulbar palsy and respiratory failure. When this happens very early in the disease, and there is no strong evidence of extensive neurological damage elsewhere (for example, in the visual system), there may be a temptation to place the patient in an intensive care unit. Although this is sometimes justified by results, it is more often followed by only very limited recovery: most neurologists would probably let nature take its course under these circumstances. When multiple sclerosis does lead to premature death, it does so more often indirectly as a result of complications of immobility and disturbed sphincter control, that is, by infections and renal failure.

The scatter of lesions in the white matter of the central nervous system (brain and spinal cord) in this disease is a random process, and multiple lesions are therefore most likely to affect the longest tracts most seriously, that is, the motor and sensory connections to and from the lower limbs and bladder. Accordingly, most patients with really advanced disease are liable to be paraplegic and incontinent. There are some other patients in whom the brunt of the disease has fallen on the cerebellar connections in the cerebellum itself or in the brain-stem, whereby patients are crippled by ataxia. As in advanced cerebro-vascular disease, there tends to be an affection of mood and higher mental functions in advanced cases of multiple sclerosis. The classical state of euphoria is by no means the rule. When it does occur, it can be particularly annoying to the attendants who have to do everything for a totally unrealistic patient. Appropriate and indeed pathological depression occurs quite commonly, and does seem to respond to some extent to anti-depressant medication. Advanced-disease patients usually have a fairly severe disorder of vision as well, that is, either lack of vision through optic neuritis, or disturbed vision from disordered eye movements with diplopia, which can be corrected by occluding an eye, or more rarely a distressing jumping about of vision with nystagmus (oscillopsia). Quite often reading becomes impossible and watching television likewise, Radio, record players and talking books then come into their own.

The really advanced case of multiple sclerosis will usually have become bed-bound after a period of wheelchair existence, when the patient may or may not have developed pressure sores. These should not occur where attendants are properly instructed in repeated changes of posture. However, this is clearly not always possible in a domestic situation at night time, and sores supervene regrettably often even in properly staffed hospitals. Posturing and skin care by the nurses is probably more important in the prevention of bed sores than the provision of special beds and pneumatic mattresses (ripple beds, Simpson air beds, etc.), which do, however, reduce the need for frequent turning. Once pressure sores have occurred in these advanced cases, they must be attended to within reason (that is, removal of necrotic tissue, meticulous cleansing with Eusol solutions, etc., and changing of dressings, if necessary several times a day). Further pressure in the same area should be avoided as far as possible: all this, of course, is made much more difficult by great spasticity of the limbs, and flexor or extensor spasms, or any intercurrent infection. Local antibiotics have probably no place, but systemic antibiotics may be indicated, especially when the sores are badly infected and lead to septicaemia.

Disturbed bladder control is almost the rule in advanced cases of multiple sclerosis. Usually the bladder starts off by being irritable and urgent, and gradually becomes more and more spastic and uncontrollable. A flaccid bladder with retention and overflow incontinence is much less common in this disease. All this is aggravated by infection, which may be treatable. The irritability of the bladder can usually be reduced by belladonna derivatives and analogues, for example, propantheline bromide.

Incontinence is almost always complicated sooner or later by a bladder infection and this, in turn, will lead to retrograde pyelonephritis and often to stone formation. A good fluid intake should reduce these risks, but this, of course, adds to the volume of incontinence. Appropriate antibiotic therapy should be given following bacteriological examination and tests for sensitivities of the organisms. Sooner or later catheterisation becomes the lesser evil, especially when there is also trouble with the skin. Modern silastic catheters do not need to be changed very often (under good conditions as rarely as once every two months), but catheters in the bladder do contribute to stone formation, and a further reduction in bladder size.

Bowel control is usually less troublesome than bladder control in these patients, and a well-timed evacuation can often be achieved by an oral laxative alone, or in combination with suppositories or (disposable) enemas, where the patient is in a position to retain these. Some patients and their nurses prefer moderate constipation and manual evacuation of the rectum.

Chest complications are frequently the terminal event in advanced cases of multiple sclerosis, especially those weakened by chronic urinary infections and pressure sores.

The palliative care of paraplegias from other causes than multiple sclerosis depends to some extent on the underlying condition (trauma, tumour or vascular disease of the spinal cord). The complications from pressure sores and bladder trouble are the same as in multiple sclerosis, and the end is often caused by irreparable renal damage or sepsis from the infected pressure sores.

Catheters are often particularly unsatisfactory in the female bladder on account of 'bypassing', and there may be an indication for diversionary urinary surgery in patients who are not too near the end.

Occasionally flexor spasticity is so disturbing or painful in patients with either multiple sclerosis or paraplegia that destructive procedures are called for, that is, if there is no response to such drugs as baclofen or dantrolene in full dosage. The introduction of either of these alone or in combination must be very gradual, for example, increasing baclofen by only 10 mg at weekly intervals. The easiest procedure for the expert is probably the injection of intrathecal phenol dissolved either in myodil or glycerol. Phenol in myodil can be injected in a strength of 5-10 per cent; phenol in glycerol is much more potent, and should not be used in a strength beyond 2 per cent or 5 per cent. 1 cm^3 of such a solution is injected into the spinal theca with the patient lying on his side and near the nerve roots of the muscles one is trying to weaken, for example, the upper lumbar roots for spasticity around the hip, and the lower lumbar and first sacral roots for spasticity lower down. These injections may be repeated if the effect wears off after a few weeks, as it often does. The main disadvantage is the weakening of any remaining bladder control and the aggravation of sensory loss in the skin, which could predispose to skin damage or aggravation of existing sores. On rare occasions, the surgeon may wish to carry out rhizotomies or destructive injections of alcohol, etc. into the spinal cord to bring relief for a limited period of time. Stereotactic spino-thalmic tractotomy is an option which the present author has never had to adopt in these diseases. There is a limited place for tenotomies.

Pain other than that caused by spasticity is most unusual in multiple sclerosis or spinal cord disease. In the former condition, one occasionally gets trigeminal and other neuralgias that are transient and should respond to full doage of carbamazepine, alone or in combination with analgesics. On rare occasions, symptomatic herpes (Zoster or simplex) may complicate spinal cord disease.

Parkinson's Disease

The management of Parkinsonism from all its causes was transformed by the introduction of laevo-dopa in the late 1960s. Although drug-induced Parkinsonism need not be considered in this context and post-encephalitic Parkinsonism is more or less extinct, Parkinson's disease itself continues to be an increasing problem as the population ages. Although it varies in its rate of progression, there is probably a steady deterioration in almost all patients, which is masked to a varying extent by treatment, but becomes apparent if for any reason anti-Parkinsonian treatment needs to be discontinued. Unfortunately, in the majority of cases the control of the disease becomes increasingly difficult after five to ten years from the onset of medication with laevo-dopa and its combination with carbidopa and benserazide. Over the years, in each individual patient there tends to be a diminishing tolerance of laevo-dopa, and increasing difficulty in getting the right concentration in the central nervous system without fluctuations from too little to too much, that is, a fluctuation from under-treatment to over-treatment. Under-treatment is liable to manifest as sudden akinesia, over-treatment as dyskinesia with sometimes quite wild involuntary movements, of which patients paradoxically seem to complain very little, although it is a most upsetting sight for their families, and indeed for their nursing and medical attendants. In the late stages, the doctor is under increasing pressure to over-treat, as this seems less intolerable to the sufferer. When akinetic, the patient may find it quite impossible to move himself (for example, to turn over in bed), and immobility in certain postures causes discomfort and indeed pain, and may lead secondarily to pressure damage to the skin. Sensation and sphincter control remain intact in the majority of patients, as does the intellect, although there are a small minority in whom dementia is associated with Parkinson's disease. Although the crises described in Parkinson's disease in the older texts, with deviation of the eyes and laryngeal spasms, are seen rarely nowadays (they occurred mostly in patients with post-encephalitic Parkinsonism), there is, of course, increasing difficulty with nutrition and sometimes also with breathing and coughing in the advanced disease.

When the patients do manage to get to their feet, there is grave danger of falls and fractures at this stage. The immobility also leads to increasing risk of chest infections. Some of these are probably brought about by the aspiration of food and drink, and of saliva.

The problem of drug control may be lessened by switching from one laevo-dopa preparation to another, by repeated intake of small doses of laevo-dopa every two hours when awake, or by the increase of anti-cholinergic drugs, even though these may add to the confusional state and cause bladder problems, and by brief courses of amantadine. All anti-Parkinsonian drugs are liable to cause confusion and unpleasant hallucinations and the anti-cholinergic drugs in addition aggravate constipation and affect the pupils, which may make it difficult to focus and to read. The anti-cholinergic drugs may need to be given parenterally for laryngeal and oculogyric crises.

The late stages of the disease, when drug control fails for at least part of the time, become increasingly distressing to patients with an intact intellect, and psychotropic medication may be indicated. Phenothiazines tend to aggravate Parkinsonism, but tricyclic antidepressants are tolerated, and there is also a place for the judicious use of amphetamine. When intractable rigidity causes muscle aches and pains, analgesics in generous dosage should be given. Rather surprisingly, it is less common to get joint problems and contractures in Parkinson's disease than in the hemiplegias of vascular disease or in multiple sclerosis.

Although other authors suggest that there is invariably an increasing deterioration in Parkinson's diease with the passage of time, the present author has found a number of patients who seem to have levelled out after mounting difficulties eight or even ten years after the initiation of laevo-dopa therapy.

Alzheimer's Disease (Cerebral Atrophy)

The majority of patients with pre-senile dementia present with an increasing memory problem, especially for recent events. Medical advice is usually sought when this leads to professional and social embarrassment. An increasingly purposeless existence continues over the next few years, and serious problems usually arise between five and ten years after the onset, although in some patients the downward course is much more rapid. At this stage, members of the family suffer far more than the patient, who is usually lacking in insight and becomes more child-like and clinging. Lack of personal cleanliness and incontinence usually occur fairly late, and most families at this stage need support and indeed a break from continuing care, with attendance at a day hospital in the first instance. With increasing restlessness, sedation and admission to hospital eventually become necessary.

In the earlier stages, patients often become depressed and may require appropriate medication, but no such treatment is of any use or indeed indicated in the later stages. Needless to say, the family needs more and more support and understanding in coping with a situation of prolonged and drawn-out cortical failure in a person who is otherwise physically quite fit. In the later stages, physical incapacity is added to the mental failure, and patients begin to totter and fall and break limbs; they eventually become bed-bound and malnourished, and usually succumb to chest troubles.

Where families opt for domestic care until the very end, there may be a period when quite heavy sedation is required – at a stage when the patient is liable to wander or interfere with the cooking or heating and cause fire risks. Only a minority of families can tolerate the situation at home, or be capable of supporting it, without suffering damage.

Brain Tumour

Cerebral tumours are, of course, more rapidly fatal than cerebral atrophy, and it is therefore more often possible to keep a patient in his home environment once a diagnosis has been made. On occasion, benign cerebral tumours like some astrocytomas or meningiomas that are not removable for technical reasons (for example, when they envelop a major blood vessel) drag on, and the illness can then be extremely prolonged. Most cerebral tumours, however, are either metastatic from somatic malignancies, or malignant astrocytomas. In either of the latter group, the duration of illness is often less than one year. In the more benign group of astrocytomas and the inoperable meningiomas, the patients and their families must be prepared for years of increasing incapacity.

Symptoms from cerebral tumours are either irritative (epileptic attacks), or increasing defects of cerebral function (intellect, speech, motor power or vision), or they are due to an increase in intracranial pressure. The last may cause pain and severe headache, although this is decidedly unusual. Complaints of pain in cerebral tumour patients tend to occur early in the illness and are usually controlled by a fairly mild analgesic regime. Where the intracranial pressure continues to be elevated, there is usually a general blunting and lessening of awareness of everything, including pain.

With the exception of a few rare metastatic tumours, cerebral tumours are not amenable to chemotherapy or hormone therapy, although radiotherapy is used fairly often both for some metastatic tumours and for some malignant gliomas. This will, in turn, produce its own symptoms and complications, for example, lasting loss of hair and sometimes a period of more brain swelling.

Although nothing can be done to alleviate lack of cerebral function, as in patients with cerebrovascular disease, attention must be paid to the control of epilepsy when fits occur. Symptomatic epilepsy of this nature is often rather intractable, and the physician may have to accept defeat and not push drugs to a toxic level in the vain hope of controlling fits. Patients themselves are usually not disturbed by their fits, although they may have a transient increase in their cerebral deficits afterwards. Families, of course, are greatly upset, and in need of explanation. There is probably nothing much to be said for one anticonvulsant versus another in this setting: the present author prefers to use phenytoin and carbamazepine, or a combination of drugs. Inadequate dosage may be indicated by serum anticonvulsant levels; the usual dosage is about 300 mg of phenytoin daily, and carbamazepine 200–400 mg eight-hourly.

The most potent therapeutic option in cerebral tumours is the use of dexamethasone, which is designed to reduce cerebral oedema around the tumour. The more malignant the tumour, the more effective the treatment is in the first instance. It will relieve the symptoms of raised intracranial pressure and lessen cerebral deficits such as dysphasia and hemiplegia. The initial treatment, if there is acute swelling, is an injection of dexamethasone 4 mg eight-hourly, to be followed by an oral dose of about 4 mg eight-hourly, reducing to 2 mg eight-hourly. Dosages of this level are apt to produce Cushing's syndrome, and in the long run may produce muscle weakness (steroid myopathy). Patients develop an appetite, bloating of the face and neck and abdomen, sometimes mild diabetes and hypertension, and later osteoporosis and vertebral collapse. All this, of course, is acceptable in the medium run, if good alleviation of the symptoms is produced, but as the tumour progresses a time will be reached when it becomes wrong to persevere with steroid therapy. A sudden withdrawal of steroids will often lead to a very rapid clinical deterioration, which may be in the best interest of the patient and his family when the cerebral deficits have become intolerable.

At this stage it may become necessary to introduce generous analgesics with diamorphine, but this is not usually necessary at the terminal stage of cerebral tumours, as the swelling leads to increasing stupor and coma.

Motor Neuron Disease

This rare but hideous disease afflicts roughly one person per 100 000 of the population per annum. Epidemiological studies have shown no particular groups at risk, except for some Pacific islanders. The disease is relentlessly progressive and lasts from a few months to up to ten years; the majority last about two years. The disease causes progressive paralysis, with or without spasticity, and may start in the upper part of the spinal cord with wasting in the upper limbs and spasticity of the legs, or, less commonly, in the bulbar muscles (progressive bulbar palsy), or, rarely, in the lumbar enlargement of the spinal cord with an ascending paralysis. Each manifestation causes its own peculiar problems.

When the disease starts in the cervical spinal cord, patients become less and less able to manipulate, and then less able to walk and stand. Breathing and swallowing are affected late, that is, at a stage when they have become chair-bound or bed-bound. The patients with a bulbar presentation usually succumb from asphyxia long before their limbs become paralysed, and are crippled by increasing difficulties with swallowing, and choking, and by dysarthria. The management of either form of the disease poses a crescendo of problems to all concerned.

Although this is the most predictable of all neurological diseases in its inevitable downhill course, few patients can be expected to have the moral fibre to take the prognosis, and most neurologists will give a guarded prognosis, indicating that there may well be deterioration for some time, without extinguishing all hope of future recovery. Failure to indicate likely future deterioration leads, of course, to a total lack of confidence as the downward course becomes only too obvious, and leads to a search for quack treatments, etc. One tends to be much more explicit to the family, who may in turn be less able to take it than the patient. As things get worse, the patient and his family are liable to be showered with well-meaning, but ill-informed advice. In most cases, the author tends to transmit his grave misgivings both to the patient and even more to the family, while going through the motions of a number of placebo treatments.

As the disease progresses and paralysis of the limbs sets in, the patient may experience a good deal of discomfort, especially when in bed; sometimes splinting of the limbs helps.

In the bulbar variety of the disease, or in the later stages of what was originally the spinal form of the disease, swallowing problems make it mandatory to pass a nasogastric tube. This makes it possible to maintain reasonable hydration, and to administer whatever drugs are necessary to alleviate apprehension and pain. The author has no hesitation in using diamorphine at this stage for these two purposes.

Intellectual functions, sensations and sphincter control remain intact throughout this distressing illness: this means, at least, an absence of pressure sores of the skin. The author considers it quite inappropriate to treat chest complications in this disease, either by bronchoscopy and aspiration, or by antibiotics.

Most certainly in this disease, and to a lesser extent also in the other conditions mentioned above, Sir William Osler's statement about pneumonia in *The Principles and Practice of Medicine*, written almost a century ago, apply: 'pneumonia may well be called the friend of the aged. Taken off by it in an acute, short, not often painful illness, the old man escapes those "cold degradations of decay" so distressing to himself and to his friends.'

Further Reading

* Texts designed for lay readers.

Cerebrovascular Disease

Marshall, J. (1976) *Management of Cerebrovascular Disease,* 3rd edn, Blackwell Scientific Publications, Oxford
*Rose, F.C. and Capildeo, R. (1981) *Stroke. The Facts,* Oxford University Press, Oxford

Multiple Sclerosis and Paraplegia

Hallpike, J.F., Adams, C.W.M. and Tourtellotte, W.W. (eds), (1983) *Multiple Sclerosis: Pathology, Diagnosis and Management*, Chapman and Hall, London
*Matthews, B. (1980) *Multiple Sclerosis. The Facts,* Oxford University Press, Oxford
Guttmann, Sir Ludwig (1976) *Spinal Cord Injuries,* Blackwell, Oxford

Parkinson's Disease

Marsden, C.D. and Fahn, S. (1981) *Movement Disorders,* Butterworth Scientific Publications, London
*Stern, G.M. and Lees, A.J. (1982) *Parkinson's Disease. The Facts,* Oxford University Press, Oxford

Alzheimer's Disease

Miller, N. and Cohen, G. (1981) *Clinical Aspects of Alzheimer's Disease and Senile Dementia,* Raven Press, New York

Cerebral Tumours

Thomas, D.G.T. and Graham, D.J. (eds) (1980) *Brain Tumours,* Butterworths Scientific Publications, London

Motor Neuron Disease

Norris, Forbes and Kurland, Leonard (eds) (1968) *Motor Neuron Disease: Research on Amytrophic Lateral Sclerosis and Related Disorders,* Grune and Stratton, New York
Rose, F.C. (ed.) (1977) *Motor Neuron Disease*, Grune and Stratton, New York
Rowland, L.P. (ed.) (1982) *Human Motor Neuron Disease*, Raven Press, New York

9 PALLIATIVE CARE OF THE CANCER PATIENT

John Smyth

Introduction

The majority of malignant diseases do not declare themselves until they have reached a relatively advanced stage. Unfortunately this means that with currently available treatment, it is only possible to attempt to cure the disease in a minority of patients. Strictly speaking, therefore, most cancer therapy is carried out with 'palliative' intent. The term 'palliation', however, encompasses a variety of different approaches to management which depend on the type of cancer, the age and general condition of the patient, coexisting or previous medical problems, and the patient's own attitude to his or her disease. Obviously an entirely different approach is required for the young woman who presents with inoperable breast cancer for whom, although the disease is incurable, the prognosis may be measured in years, compared with the elderly patient who presents with metastatic carcinoma of the colon, for whom life expectancy is only a few months.

It is not possible in the scope of one chapter to give a comprehensive account of the palliative management for all forms of cancer, and emphasis will be placed on conditions where life expectancy is relatively short. The general principles of palliative management will be outlined before considering the management of some specific organ dysfunctions as a consequence of malignant disease. The psychological problems faced by patients and their relatives will be discussed, and problems relating to therapy described.

The cornerstone of palliative management is to relieve suffering. This requires a detailed elucidation of symptoms and provision of the most efficacious treatment that is compatible with the minimum disruption to the patient's way of life. For patients with cancer, this is often a difficult balance to achieve. The symptoms of cancer include psychological disturbances, generalised symptoms such as malaise and cachexia, and symptoms related to the failure of specific organ systems. Any or all of these factors may be relevant to the planning of specific palliative management for the individual patient. For most patients, the knowledge that they have been diagnosed as having a malignant

200

disease inevitably causes considerable anxiety. The word 'cancer' is still interpreted by many patients as implying a death sentence, and a distressing and harrowing death at that. The first and most important aspect in planning palliative care for a patient with cancer is to establish a relationship where the doctor acknowledges the patient's anxieties and starts to initiate the process of attempting to reassure the patient that many aspects of his or her situation can be improved, even if the disease cannot be eradicated.

Non-specific symptoms such as anorexia, lethargy and malaise are common sequelae of malignant diseases; a second, important principle of palliative care is to recognise that very often the best and the only way to improve these generalised symptoms is to take active measures to treat the underlying disease. It is not infrequently thought that the kindest thing to do is to adopt a policy of 'least intervention', but as with the problems relating to a specific organ dysfunction, discussed later, one should always consider the possibility of actively treating the disease as being the best way to relieve distressing symptoms, even if for only a relatively short period of time.

When planning active treatment, consideration must be given to the difference between the need for local treatment and the need for generalised systemic treatment. Surgery and radiotherapy offer treatment for localised problems, and chemotherapy forms the mainstay for generalised treatment. Surgery has a relatively minor role in palliative care, but may be useful in such circumstances as the removal of painful subcutaneous metastases or toilet operations for fungating skin masses such as occur in breast carcinoma, for example. In exceptional cases, surgical procedures are used for the control of widespread problems, for example oophorectomy in pre-menopausal women with breast cancer that has metastasised to bone, a procedure which can have a dramatic effect on relieving bone pain.

Radiotherapy is used for palliating many forms of cancer. It is not appropriate here to describe radiotherapeutic procedures in detail, since these are the responsibility of the radiotherapist, but when not used with curative intent radiotherapy is prescribed for the relief of pain, to reduce the size of tumours which may be compromising vital organs, or for cosmetic improvement to unsightly or distressing tumours, for example, of the head and neck or in the breast.

Chemotherapy can be used to palliate a wide variety of problems caused by malignant diseases, but being less familiar to many people there is sometimes a reluctance to consider the use of cytotoxic drugs in the palliative setting. Indeed, particular caution is required in the prescribing of cytotoxic drugs since most of these compounds can cause unpleasant side-effects if not properly administered and monitored. For these reasons the use of cytotoxic drugs will be described in greater detail in this chapter than the use of surgery or radiotherapy.

Gastrointestinal Complications of Malignancy

The gastrointestinal tract is affected by many malignant diseases as a secondary phenomenon, in addition to the symptoms caused by primary carcinomas of the oesophagus, stomach, pancreas and large bowel.

Anorexia (see Chapter 13) is a common accompaniment of advanced malignancies from many sites. Prolonged anorexia leads to cachexia and malnutrition, which can cause secondary phenomena that further debilitate the patient. Anorexia may result from primary carcinoma in the upper gastrointestinal tract, but it is frequently an accompaniment to carcinomas in other sites such as the lung. Irrespective of the cause of anorexia, attention should be given to advising the patient on the most appropriate diet which his or her system will allow. It should never be underestimated how inappropriate the diet is that many patients select for themselves in the absence of professional advice. Careful attention to oral hygiene and the early treatment of oral candida infections can frequently improve patients' ability to tolerate appropriate foods. Dysphagia and early satiety may be caused by oesophageal candida infection, and vigorous treatment with amphoteracin and nystatin can result in a dramatic improvement in patients' ability to increase their nutritional intake. The presence of hepatic metastases frequently results in anorexia and nausea. The treatment of this depends on the site of the primary tumour. Carcinoma of the breast or lung metastasising to the liver may be sensitive to cytotoxic drugs, but unfortunately the commonest cause of hepatic metastases arising from carcinomas in the gastrointestinal tract — carcinoma of the colon — is a disease which is resistant to the action of available cytotoxic drugs and palliative management of the anorexia and nausea associated with this rests with the use of anti-emetics. For some patients prednisolone (20 mg/day) is beneficial for the palliation of symptoms arising from hepatic metastases. The use of steroids can stimulate the appetite, and for some patients will relieve the nausea associated with this form of anorexia. However, caution is required in the use of steroids, particularly in the elderly, in whom confusion or disturbance in sleep pattern may contra-indicate their use.

Biliary tract obstruction can arise from carcinoma in the head of the pancreas or from metastases in the liver secondary to carcinomas in the gastrointestinal tract or elsewhere, particularly in the lung and breast. The site of the primary tumour is of paramount importance in considering the treatment of complications arising from biliary tract obstruction, for the same reasons as those concerning intrahepatic metastases. Obstruction of biliary outflow results in a decrease in the level of bile salts in the intestinal lumen; this leads to malabsorption and diarrhoea, jaundice, and pruritis secondary to bile-salt deposition in the skin. In obstructive jaundice pruritis can be an extremely distressing symptom and frequently requires palliation. Surgical intervention with external drainage of bile through a T-tube may provide relief of the symptoms (see Chapter 3), but in patients for whom this is not technically feasible, the use of cholestyramine should be considered.

Advanced carcinomas of the stomach, pancreas or large bowel may result in intestinal obstruction. The palliation of the abdominal pain, nausea and vomiting associated with this follows standard procedures, but particular consideration should be given to the intestinal obstruction which can arise from advanced carcinoma of the ovary. Over the past few years it has been appreciated that carcinoma of the ovary is responsive to treatment with cytotoxic drugs. The use of cyclophosphamide, chlorambucil, methotrexate, 5-fluorouracil, adriamycin and *cis*-diamminedichloroplatinum – either singly or in various combinations – has been shown to have a profound effect on the palliation of carcinoma of the ovary and can be considered even in advanced cases presenting with sub-acute intestinal obstruction.

Particular attention should be paid to the correction of electrolyte abnormalities and the prevention of secondary problems related to the temporary nausea or vomiting which can result from the use of some of these compounds. The appropriate use of cytotoxic drugs for advanced carcinoma of the ovary can temporarily relieve intestinal obstruction and its associated symptoms. Recurrent ascites is a common problem in advanced carcinoma of the ovary. When this occurs in a patient who has not received previous cytotoxic drugs, then the same considerations as mentioned above pertain and systemic treatment with cytotoxic drugs is the treatment of choice. When recurrent ascites presents in a patient who has failed to respond to cytotoxic drugs, then management consists of repeated paracenteses. As a routine, it is not advisable to instil cytotoxic drugs into the peritoneal space. A number of studies have failed to confirm the therapeutic efficacy of this approach and the installation of drugs such as bleomycin has occasionally resulted in severe toxicity secondary to systemic absorption.

Pulmonary Complications of Malignancy

Dyspnoea is a common problem in the palliative care of many forms of malignant disease. Apart from the symptoms and signs of primary bronchogenic carcinoma, the lungs are a frequent site of metastatic disease from carcinoma of the breast and colon amongst many others. Bronchopneumonia is frequently a terminal event in patients who are severely debilitated by carcinomas of many sites, and dyspnoea can arise from anaemia or cardiac failure consequent upon malignant cachexia, hypoproteinaemia, renal failure, etc.

Carcinoma of the Lung

Carcinoma of the lung usually presents in a form that is incurable by surgery, but where palliation with radiotherapy or chemotherapy is eminently warranted. Distressing symptoms such as persistent cough or haemoptysis can frequently be relieved with the appropriate use of radiotherapy, and in recent years the sensitivity of *small cell anaplastic* carcinoma of the bronchus to cytotoxic drugs has resulted in significant improvement in the control of symptoms and the survival of patients.

In centres specialising in the use of cytotoxic drugs for this disease, median survival in excess of one year is now attainable, and a proportion of patients survive for two years or more. A number of drugs are useful in this situation, including cyclophosphamide, methotrexate, CCNU, adriamycin, procarbazine, the vinca alkaloids and the epipodophyllotoxin VP-16. Combination chemotherapy has been shown to be superior to the use of these drugs individually, but the associated potential increase in the toxicity requires particular care in patients who are often seriously ill at the time of presentation.

Small cell anaplastic carcinoma of the bronchus frequently presents with extrathoracic manifestations including cachexia, hyponatraemia and carcinomatous neuropathies, in addition to symptoms relating to metastatic disease in the liver, adrenal glands or elsewhere. For all these reasons the palliative treatment of choice is systemic chemotherapy.

For lung cancers other than small cell anaplastic carcinoma, cytotoxic drugs have not been found to be of sufficient benefit to warrant their routine use in palliation. The exception to this is for the management of recurrent pleural effusions, where the introduction of bleomycin into the pleural space (after draining the effusion to dryness whenever possible) can frequently result in significant delays in the reaccumulation of pleural fluid. A dose of 60 mg of bleomycin is usually adequate and can be introduced with only minor discomfort to the patient – other than the occasional occurrence of fever over the few hours following administration of bleomycin.

The differential diagnosis of chest-wall pain in malignant disease requires a distinction between rib pain secondary to bone metastases, particularly from carcinomas in the colon, breast or lung, and subpleural deposits or extensions of primary intrapulmonary carcinomas. Radiotherapy can frequently alleviate rib pain with significant short-term benefit to the patient.

For patients presenting with superior vena caval obstruction, management depends on the aetiology of the bronchus or lymphomas, particularly Hodgkin's disease. Treatment consists of the use of steroids (dexamethasone 16 mg daily) to reduce oedema, and radiation therapy to the mediastinum. For some patients with incomplete superior vena caval obstruction, if it is known that this is secondary to Hodgkin's disease, the use of combination chemotherapy may effect as satisfactory a resolution of symptoms as the use of radiotherapy. Similarly, for small cell anaplastic carcinoma of the bronchus the treatment of choice for incomplete superior vena caval obstruction or obstruction of very recent onset is combination chemotherapy rather than radiotherapy, since in addition to providing treatment of the vena caval obstruction, chemotherapy, is also providing palliative treatment for the disease at other sites.

Haematological Complications of Malignancy

Apart from primary carcinomas of the blood-forming organs, many carcinomas cause secondary effects on the haematopoietic system. Thus bleeding may lead to acute or chronic anaemia, metastatic disease in the liver may cause clotting diatheses, and infiltration of the bone marrow may result in anaemia, leukopenia or thrombocytopenia. Malignancies such as renal carcinomas can be associated with polycythaemia or thrombocythaemia. The correction of anaemia is almost always associated with improvement in a patient's well-being and patients should be transfused, even if it is not possible to correct the primary source of blood loss or failure in blood production. Infiltration of the bone marrow by secondary carcinoma from, for example, carcinomas of the breast or lung, presents as anaemia, leukopenia and/or thrombocytopenia. For carcinoma of the breast or for small cell anaplastic lung carcinoma, the use of cytotoxic drugs in this situation can have a significant benefit. This treatment, however, frequently results in temporary worsening of the haematological state with added risk of infection or bleeding during the period immediately following the administration of chemotherapy. The use of appropriate antibiotics and in selected cases the use of leucocyte transfusions and/or platelet transfusions should be considered. Prophylactic platelet transfusions are not warranted and should only be provided when there is evidence of spontaneous haemorrhage such as haematuria or epistaxis or when there is severe, spontaneous bruising. There is sometimes a reluctance on the part of clinicians to use cytotoxic drugs which are known to cause haematological toxicity when the patient presents with bone marrow failure. The decision whether or not to use chemotherapy in this situation clearly rests with an assessment of the overall condition of the patient and his or her prognosis.

Electrolyte Disturbances

Attention to the correction of electrolyte abnormalities is an important part of the palliative care of a number of different situations.

Hyponatraemia

Hyponatraemia is not infrequently a presenting sign in small cell anaplastic carcinoma of the bronchus resulting from tumour production of antidiuretic hormone (ADH). This presents as drowsiness and somnolence and may mimic intracranial metastases; when severe, this can be associated with coma. Treatment of the primary tumour with combination chemotherapy, whilst at the same time instituting severe water depletion (500 ml/24 hours fluid intake), can result in a resolution of symptoms within 24-48 hours. In refractory cases the use of dimethylchlortetracycline to antagonise the effects of ADH in the kidney will further contribute to the correction of hyponatraemia.

Hypercalcaemia

Hypercalcaemia (see Chapter 13) may arise from metastatic cancer in the bone or, more rarely, from ectopic parathyroid hormone production from a squamous carcinoma of the bronchus. Hypercalcaemia affects a number of different organs and can present with a variety of signs and symptoms that are common in patients with malignant disease. It is important to remember the possibility of hypercalcaemia when patients present with otherwise unexplained anorexia, nausea, vomiting, constipation, polyuria or disordered mental state progressing to coma. The treatment of hypercalcaemia is essentially the treatment of the underlying disease, but severe hypercalcaemia can be life-threatening and requires urgent treatment. A high fluid intake with a minimum of 3 l of parenteral fluids per 24 hours together with diuretics is the first approach to its management. Prednisolone can further lower the serum calcium and should be instituted when the serum calcium is greater than 3.0 mmol/l. If fluids and steroids fail to lower the serum calcium, then mithramycin should be used. Oral or parenteral phosphate can be used in addition, but this is associated with profound diarrhoea and is less favourable than the use of the measures indicated above.

Psychological Problems

The most important aspect of providing palliative care for any patient with cancer is to help him or her with the anxiety and depression that so often accompanies advanced malignancy. The extent to which one discusses the aetiology and significance of signs and symptoms will depend on the individual patient, and it is imperative in planning palliative care to establish how much the patient really understands about the nature of his or her disease. Failure to do so can lead to confusion and distrust, two factors which must be avoided at all cost. With changing attitudes amongst both the general public and the health profession, there is a tendency nowadays to be much more open about the nature of malignant diseases and about patients' prognoses. All palliative care is greatly helped if the patient has trust and confidence in those who are caring for him or her. The most important principle is to adopt a sympathetic and *positive* attitude to the relief of distressing symptoms, and to avoid inappropriate optimism where this is not likely to be realised. Although it is in the patient's best interest sometimes to withhold information, one should never impart misleading information suggesting that given problems are unrelated to the underlying malignant disease.

The timing of when to tell patients about their prognoses is a matter for individual judgement. Patients frequently ask about their future at the first encounter, but usually it is best to defer lengthy explanations until a plan of palliative management has been made and the patient is more familiar with medical and nursing staff, and has had time to begin to adjust to the knowledge that he or she has a malignant disease. It should never be underestimated how confusing and alarming this first disclosure of information is, and that in consequence the patient's ability to comprehend and retain detailed knowledge is frequently very poor. Though time-consuming and requiring a significant commitment from medical staff, the most successful counselling is achieved by frequent and sometimes necessarily repetitive explanation of the patient's situation and prognosis. It is essential to allow time for patients to express their anxiety and uncertainties as to the nature of any treatment that is being administered.

In general, psychotropic drugs form a relatively small part in the palliative management of cancer, although mild sedatives such as diazepam and, in selected cases, anti-depressant agents may be useful. Clouding of consciousness should be avoided as much as possible and can indeed be a significant problem in the use of opiate analgesics for severe pain. Patients frequently find that the confusion and disorientation caused by such drugs is distressing and depersonalising, and though of immense value, great care should be taken to titrate the analgesic requirement with a preservation of consciousness and dignity (see Chapter 12).

Problems Related to Therapy

Most forms of therapy for cancer are associated with some secondary side-effects. The consequences of surgery may result in psychological difficulties following, for example, mastectomy or amputation, but these are well appreciated and will not be discussed here. Radiotherapy may acutely give rise to skin discoloration over the treated area or to mucositis, resulting in soreness of the mouth, dysphagia and dyspepsia when the upper intestinal tract is irradiated. Irradiation of the lung can result in the chronic delayed toxicity of dyspnoea, resulting from radiation fibrosis, a condition which is partially relieved by the use of systemic steroids.

However, the treatment which causes most problems in palliation is the use cytotoxic drugs. The relatively poor specificity of these compounds for damaging tumour cells, over and above causing damage to normal host tissues, results in a variety of acute and chronic problems. The acute effects associated with the administration of some cytotoxic drugs include bone marrow depression, resulting in anaemia, leukopenia with an increased risk of infection, or thrombocytopenia with an increased risk of haemorrhage, and effects on the gastro-intestinal tract resulting in nausea and vomiting. The drugs which are most myelotoxic are the alkylating agents such as cyclophosphamide, chlorambucil and busulphan, the nitrosoureas such as CCNU, and the anthracyclines such as Adriamycin. Nausea and vomiting are seen particularly with Adriamycin, cyclopphosphamide, CCNU and *cis*-platinum. *cis*-Platinum universally causes severe nausea and vomiting, but there is considerable patient variation in the degree of emesis engendered by most cytotoxic drugs. Anti-emetic agents such as meto-clopramide or prochlorperazine are partially successful in ameliorating this unpleasant side-effect. Due to the necessity to administer cytotoxic drugs at repeated intervals, agents that cause emesis frequently induce psychogenic nausea and vomiting over a course of treatment.

Alopecia resulting from interruption in the growth of the hair follicle is seen particularly following the administration of Adriamycin and cyclophosphamide. The latter may also cause a degree of bladder irritation, resulting in dysuria and occasionally frank haematuria. These symptoms are minimised by encouraging a high fluid intake, since they are caused by direct irritation of the bladder mucosa by a metabolite of cyclophosphamide.

The vinca alkaloids, vincristine, vinblastine and vindesine can cause a dose-related peripheral sensory and motor neurotoxicity. Initially mild sensory paraesthesia is the presenting sign, but this can progress to areflexia and motor weakness. These symptoms are reversible on cessation of treatment, but may take many months to disappear fully. Peripheral neuropathy is occasionally seen with the long-term administration of *cis*-platinum. Bleomycin as used for some lymphomas and squamous carcinomas of the head and neck, lung and cervix can accumulatively cause pulmonary fibrosis, which may be irreversible.

A toxicity unique to the anthracyclines, Adriamycin and dauno-rubicin, is a form of cardiomyopathy, the incidence of which is considerably increased above a total dose of 450 mg/m^2 of Adriamycin. For this reason it is only in very exceptional circumstances that this total dose should be exceeded.

An understanding of the side-effects of cytotoxic drugs is essential to their safe use. Not all cytotoxic drugs cause side-effects and the degree to which these present a problem to individual patients is variable and depends particularly on the way in which the drugs are used either singly or in combination, on the age of the patient, and on the disease for which the drugs are being used. Provided that they are used carefully and with a full understanding of the individual toxicities of the different drugs, then these compounds can be highly beneficial in the palliative setting. Their injudicious use can of course result not only in failure to achieve relief of symptoms, but can even make these worse. A major problem in the use of cytotoxic drugs for palliation is to know for how long it is appropriate to continue their administration. Simple procedures such as the use of chlorambucil for palliating chronic lymphocytic leukaemia are innocuous and can be continued for months and even years. A more aggressive combination chemotherapy for the palliation of breast cancer, however, poses a different spectrum of problems. The use of drugs such as vincristine, Adriamycin or cyclophosphamide for the palliation of advanced breast cancer can result in a temporary remission of distressing symptoms which are held at bay for the duration of therapy. When treatment is discontinued, the symptoms often recur. Judgement is therefore needed for the individual patient to know whether the continued administration of such drugs is indicated in comparison with the risks and emotional consequences of allowing the symptoms to return. For diseases such as small cell lung carcinoma, where the use of cytotoxic drugs with or without radiotherapy can alter life expectancy from a matter of two or three months to twelve months or more, there are some patients for whom a moderately aggressive approach to treatment is eminently worth while. For ovarian carcinoma, where the disease frequently presents at an advanced stage, it has been found that cytotoxic drugs administered over a period of six to nine months can result in significant disease-free palliation for periods in excess of five years. For such patients the discomfort and problems associated with the treatment period are usually eminently worth while in terms of the disease-free interval that follows the attainment of remission.

The recent increase in the use of cytotoxic drugs provides a rapidly changing pattern of medical practice. Fortunately the results of clinical research over the past few years have shown significant improvements in our ability to palliate many of the distressing symptoms and signs of incurable cancers. There is still much that needs to be improved and many of the treatments are complicated and time-consuming. Nevertheless, the time taken to administer such programmes of treatment affords an opportunity to establish a relationship with the patient, to acknowledge their fears and anxieties and, while trying to relieve some of their suffering, to provide an atmosphere of comfort and re-assurance.

Recommended Further Reading

Calman, K.C., Smyth, J.F. and Tattersall, M.H.N. (1980) *Basic Principles of Cancer Chemotherapy*, Macmillan, London and Basingstoke
Carter, S.K., Bakowski, M.T. and Hellmann, K. (1977) *Chemotherapy of Cancer*, John Wiley, New York, London, Sydney and Toronto
Devita, V.T., Hellman, S. and Rosenberg, S.A. (1982) *Cancer – Principles and Practice of Oncology*, J.B. Lippincott, Philadelphia and Toronto
Saunders, C.M. (1978) *The Management of Terminal Disease*, Edward Arnold, London

10 PALLIATIVE CARE OF THE DYING CHILD

James Farquhar

The child . . . said his mother was dying. The brown eyes expressed
no emotion: it was a fact. You were born, your parents died, you
grew old, you died yourself.

Graham Greene, *The Power and the Glory*

In the churchyard near my home a headstone praises a mother of
thirteen children. She was buried with the last a few days after his
birth. She had already buried four. Within a few paces, others tell the
same story of the nineteenth-century familiarity with child death. In
the short terraced street of my childhood fifty years ago we watched
fascinated as black horses drew away the coffins of young friends.
Others in smaller white coffins had not lived or emerged to become
playmates; in the neighbouring streets of the working class, common
infectious diseases took a heavier toll. Too many children struggled on,
before finally surrendering to rheumatic fever, kidney failure and tuberculosis. The infant hymn 'Jesus loves me' then contained the lines
'He will take me when I die, to His heavenly home on high.' Older
children, instructed about more immediate hazards, repeated 'if I
should die before I wake. I pray the Lord my soul to take.'

Then, as now in poor developing countries, children played happily
undeterred by these common reminders of their mortality; they
accepted death because of its very familiarity. The family was as distressed and as grieved then as now, but friends and neighbours seemed
less shy and more confident about the support which they should
immediately give. My medical unit of the Royal Hospital for Sick
Children in Edinburgh (RHSC) admitted 486 children in 1930 and 89
died (18.3 per cent), whereas in 1980, only 8 of 1465 admissions did so
(0.5 per cent), although it had by then given a proportion of its beds
for children whose progressive neurological degeneration certainly
proves fatal.

It is wrong to imply, as Easson docs (1981), that there are now more
slow deaths than in the past. The physician in western societies no
longer deals with the thousands of children who lived precariously and
died slowly of rheumatic heart disease, chronic nephritis, bronchiectasis

212

and tuberculosis. It is true, however, that cystic fibrosis has emerged starkly from the previous carnage; that neurological handicap and leukaemia are now stressful long-term problems; and that unfamiliarity with dying, death and the comfort of the bereaved create a new problem. This is what now makes education necessary for the professionals and the people. Furthermore, the much wider dispersal of family units in the new society and the greater isolation within crowded urban communities seem sadly to make the provision of comforting and supporting a professional task. The decreasing expertise of professionals and people was stressed by Yudkin (1967), whose succinct and classical paper with its sensitive recommendations remains compulsory reading for all who must handle such sad events.

The Size and Nature of the Problem

The Edinburgh area has a population of about one million people. The registered causes of 205 consecutive child deaths (under the age of 16 years) there in 1980 are broadly classified by age and diagnosis in Tables 10.1–10.7. The implication of each group is then considered.

Death Before 1 Week (Table 10.1)

These accounted for one in three of all the deaths, and almost two of every three of them were associated with pre-term delivery in maternity hospitals. Almost all of the others were caused by malformation.

Table 10.1: Broad classification of cause of death in 1980: Lothian children aged less than one week

Cause	Number
Pre-term birth, associated illness	45
Malformation	24
Birth asphyxia	2
Infection	1

Death Between 1 and 4 weeks (Table 10.2)

These make up a further 10 per cent of the total and most are associated with pre-term and difficult birth or malformation. Sudden infant death syndrome (SIDS) accounts for less than 10 per cent of the groups, but dominates the next one.

Table 10.2: Broad classification of cause of death in 1980: Lothian children aged 1 but less than 4 weeks

Cause	Number
Pre-term birth, associated illness	8
Asphyxia	1
Convulsions, cause unknown	1
Malformation	6
Infection	3
Sudden infant death syndrome	2

Death Between 1 and 12 months (Table 10.3)

SIDS accounts for 32 of the 46 deaths in this group. The Procurator-Fiscal (the public prosecutor in Scotland, after the style of the chief law officers of the crown under the Roman law which applies in Scotland) authorises autopsy in every such case by the head of the paediatric pathology service at the RHSC in association with the forensic pathologist, so that diagnosis is accepted only after exhaustive studies.

SIDS is the most feared, silent and unexpected angel of death in an age-group from which most of the past threat has been removed. Some 2000 babies are estimated to die thus each year in the United Kingdom. Perhaps one in every 500 live births suddenly expires between the ages of 1 week and 2 years, although the figure varies from region to region, depending perhaps upon such factors as social disadvantages and pollution.[1]

Most happen between four weeks and six months. Prior symptoms, if any, seldom exceed those shown by most babies during the peak winter months. Many escape comment. Parents put the baby into the pram or cot, ignorant of impending disaster. A few hours, sometimes a few minutes, later the baby is found dead. The ensuing scenes involve neighbours, ambulance and police services, hospital casualty departments and general practitioners. Shock, guilt and anger are general. The subject is well described in *Medicine, Science and Law* (Symposium on Cot Death, 1980) and separately in other careful studies, for example those from Sheffield and Edinburgh, where the epidemiology seems to show regional differences. The devastating effect on parents is universal. The knowledge that some parents lose more than one baby in this way and the discovery of other parents of babies 'nearly dead' who are restored by mouth-to-mouth breathing (so-called 'near miss' cases) fuels the anxiety of all parents and receives support from some

Table 10.3: Broad classification of cause of death in 1980: Lothian children aged 1 but less than 12 months

Cause	Number
Sudden infant death syndrome	32
Pre-term birth, associated illnesses	1
Malformation	10
Infection	1
Kidney failure	1
Brain haemorrhage	1

scientific studies which suggest intrinsic variations of respiratory control.

Malformation plays an important but smaller part (22 per cent).

Death Between 1 and 3 years (Table 10.4)

Accidents, always unheralded and commonly immediately fatal, appear in association with the child's inquisitive exploration and new mobility. Malformation continues to take its toll throughout childhood and malignancy is first represented. Infection plays a small primary role, but slow problems of metabolism and muscular activity feature.

Table 10.4: Broad classification of cause of death in 1980: Lothian children aged 1 but less than 3 years

Cause	Number
Accident	
Traffic	1
Fall	1
Asphyxia	1
Drowning	1
Malformation	2
Malignancy, solid	1
Infection	1
Progressive paralysing disease	2
Biochemical disease	1

Death Between 3 and 6 years (Table 10.5)

Accident, malformation and malignancy account for more than half of the deaths. A grossly handicapped child succumbs and children with cystic fibrosis die of respiratory infection and failure.

Table 10.5: Broad classification of cause of death in 1980: Lothian children aged 3 but less than 6 years

Cause	Number
Malformation	3
Traffic accident	2
Malignancy, solid	1
Acute infection	3
Inhalation of vomit	1

Death Between 6 and 10 years (Table 10.6)

The same pattern holds of accident, malformation, malignancy and chronic degenerative diseases in the nervous and respiratory systems. Acute infection is a rare cause and might most often take the form of a meningococcal septicaemia in which, as in SIDS, an apparently well child may die within 24 hours or possibly overnight.

Table 10.6: Broad classification of cause of death in 1980: Lothian children aged 6 but less than 10 years

Cause	Number
Malformation	2
Traffic accident	4
Malignancy	
Blood	2
Solid	1
Gross mental handicap and epilepsy	1
Chronic respiratory failure	1
Cystic fibrosis	3
Acute infection	1

Death Between 10 and 16 years (Table 10.7)

With the exception of diabetes which should not now kill properly cared-for children, the same pattern continues.

Accidents are usually swift and without previous anxiety or prolonged fear of dying. The shock to the family is very great.

Malformation terminates life, the quality of which has been worsening. Increasing weakness and discomfort make impending death apparent to all. Sometimes, however, reasonable quality may be abruptly terminated by a need to take definitive surgical action in, for example, a complex structural heart defect.

Malignancy presents problems which are as great in the area of social

Table 10.7: Broad classification of cause of death in 1980: Lothian children aged 10 but less than 16 years

Cause	Number
Accident	
Traffic	7
Fall from a height	2
Drowning	3
Malformation	2
Malignancy	
Blood	3
Solid	6
Muscular dystrophy	1
Brain haemorrhage	1
Degenerative disease of brain	2
Diabetes	1
Cystic fibrosis	2

and spiritual support as they are in the physical. Until the 1950s acute lymphoblastic leukaemia (ALL) usually caused death in 12-16 weeks from first symptoms. Solid tumours were excised and/or irradiated, but most progressed so that only analgesia and sedation were prescribed. Blood and solid malignancies can now involve years of treatment, long returns apparently to normal, sudden relapse, disfigurement, isolation, anguished suspense and for some children, a final failure. The 1980 British paediatric report on childhood malignancy estimates 1200 affected children in the United Kingdom at any time compared with 200 000 adults.

Muscular dystrophy, although rare in this small series, is particularly tragic because of its inheritance so that, more obviously in cystic fibrosis, the child may watch a brother die before him and the parents live with the inevitable sentence of death on loving and loved children. These two diseases represent a large group of individually rare genetic problems.

The Problem in Practice

In an area which has approximately 460 general practitioners, 205 deaths per annum are lightly spread, especially if almost half occur in the first month of life within the neonatal paediatric units of maternity hospitals. Even in these, however, the family doctor has responsibilities to bereaved parents which continue before and through further pregnancies. SIDS affects general practitioners very acutely and most may expect to be involved at some time in the course of their professional life. Accidental death, similar in its unexpected blow to the family, differs in its cause.

Slower and unexpected, sometimes welcome, death always involves the family doctor and his or her partnership with the hospital and community health services, social workers, schoolteachers and clergy.

The Child's Concept of Death

At the age of 5 years I was crying bitterly in bed one night. It was my father's birthday and he seemed to me to have achieved an advanced age. He came to ask me what distressed me. I told him he was old and would soon be dead. He took the news cheerfully and reassured me. I had no personal fear of death, since heaven meant kind grandparents, seaside holidays, endless ice-cream and an eternal Christmas happily compounded. My fear was the dissolution of my present world: parents, home and love. A 6-year-old relative in the next generation rushed in front of a London bus and was snatched from instant extinction. Asked for an explanation by a shocked mother, he said he 'wanted to know what it feels like to be dead', and showed some irritation that this precocious research project had been frustrated.

From the age of group play (well established by 6 years) boys kill: 'Bang! bang! you're dead!' Grief is also shammed. In the market place 2000 years ago, children at pay were heard to chant 'We have piped unto you and ye have not danced; we have mourned unto you, and ye have not lamented' (Matt, 11: 16-17). Such death carries with it the certainty of resurrection: the school bell or call to dinner sees each Lazarus immediately standing forth.

Children's talk about death has been recorded by Raimbault (1981) in a sensitive paper based on fifteen years as a psychoanalyst in a paediatric nephrology unit in the Children's Hospital in Paris with more than 100 children of all ages. No questionnaire was used. The patients were simply allowed to speak freely to a familiar friend. A few quotations illustrate their knowledge, or at least what they had been told. A 6-year-old boy: 'When one is dead, one is dead. That's all. One is in a grave. The grave is a room in the graveyard. One is dead. That's all.' A 7-year-old boy: 'Dead people are no longer on earth. They cannot live anymore. They cannot open their eyes. They cannot move . . . I'm going to know all the hospitals and I am going to die.' A 12-year-old boy: 'If I died, I'd just sleep for ever.' A 14-year-old girl painted a picture about her father's death from the same disease. She saw herself in it: 'The person cannot believe that the other one is dead . . . she loved the dead one . . . she will go home very sad and look for death . . . and will die quite soon.'

In a reviewing monograph Easson (1981) gives 3 to 4 years as the age at which children recognise body changes resulting from disease or treatment. Their much earlier appreciation of others and their assertion of personal wishes pass through the realisation of *me* and *you* to the point, again by 5 or 6 years, of there being states of *not me* and *not you*: a home, a garden, a class from which he or she or a loved one is absent. Between then and 7 years, the child appreciates that being unwell could involve death (unable to open his eyes, to move, to live any more, to be asleep for ever).

Allowance must be made for the experience of the child at this age. The isolated and protected may grasp the significance of death later than those in families where death is known or discussed. The intelligent child will quickly see the link between the death of a pet or a scene on television and himself. Orthodox Christian teaching of the love of God and the assurance of family survival can be given a grotesque and terrifying face by adults who use the threat of supernatural retribution to achieve an inexcusable end. Not all children of this age share the phlegmatic personality of the small Glasgow boy who was threatened with God's fury because he failed to finish a supper of rice and prunes. He was then submitted by chance to an extraordinary storm of thunder and lightning, but was overheard, alone in his bedroom, heaping scorn on the Almighty for making such a fuss over nothing.

Nor at this age should childish reserve and silence exclude appreciation of sharp ears, wary observation, careful thought and anxiety. Parental comment under happier conditions that 'Big Ears is listening' is particularly true when the discussion deals with threat. A child needs neither to hear nor to understand the jargon of doctors and nurses to sense possible danger. Their behaviour and expressions on ward rounds are usually as easy to read as a silent movie.

Increasingly from the age of 8 or 9 through puberty and adolescence the child's education — secular and religious — takes him toward the wide range of views held by adults. It may extend from superficial café talk to silent ponderings of Hamlet's incomparable soliloquy and the words of the community's scripture to the writings of the great philosophers. He is trained by then to sift and weigh these before making his own judgements about God, the meaning of death and how it affects him. Raimbault (1981) concludes: 'as soon as a child can express himself freely on this subject, no further age-dependent progress concerning the concept of death can be observed. Faced with disease and death, the child is led to the same images and conclusions, to the same order of ideas as the adult.'

The child's intelligence, its development, or what is left of it, determine his understanding of death, his anticipation and anxiety. Clearly the pre-term baby, the infant and young toddler experience pain or distress, but have no knowledge of death. Those killed outright or scarcely regaining consciousness after accident do not know. Nor do those severely brain damaged from birth or soon afterward, and the comprehension of the mentally handicapped may be slower and incomplete. They may, however, as in Down's syndrome, learn to experience both anxiety and grief.

A review of the Edinbrugh deaths (Table 10.8) shows that in only 13 per cent of them was the child likely to be aware of impending death. They would be enormously outnumbered by the masses of children who fear death but are without significant disease, and even by those whose illnesses engender such anxiety but will never kill. The unfamiliarity of normally intelligent children with real rather than fantasy death is therefore not surprising: nor is the uncertainty and embarrassment of their doctors, nurses and social workers unless they gain experience in a specialised unit or keep in intimate contact with its teaching practice.

The Child's Reaction to Dying

The children reported by Raimbault (1981) seem strangely composed, but this depends in part on the period available for adjustment. Not all are so philosophical and they are likely to pass through the same stages, modified by their phase of development, as are described by Kubler-Ross (1970) in adults: denial and isolation, anger, bargaining, depression and acceptance. Faced even with a promise of eternal happiness and sunshine, they may agree with an Edinburgh girl who replied: 'I like it fine here.' With time, however, and fatigue, their quiet resignation may humble the adult observer. Many years ago I sat all night beside a well-educated 14-year-old girl dying of cystic fibrosis. To my shame none of the staff had ever mentioned death, and I would be surprised if that excluded the kindly chaplain. 'I shall die tonight,' she whispered, 'I'm sorry to have caused so much trouble.' Within an hour her prediction was true. We had failed her in the valley of the shadow: but I suspect she was not alone.

Table 10.8: Estimated awareness of impending death: Lothian children
by age-groups, 1980

Age-group	Number of deaths	Instant or very rapid death	Significant warning of death	
			Aware	Unaware
0 < 1 week	72	72*	0	0
1 week < 1 month	21	21*	0	0
1 month < 1 year	46	32	0	(14)**
1 year < 3 years	11	5	0	(6)**
3 years < 6 years	10	6	3 possible	1
6 years < 10 years	15	5	7 probable	3
10 years < 16 years	30	14	13	3
Total	205	155	23	27

Notes: * Very little warning; life precarious from the start in the majority.
      ** Certainly the majority was unaware.

The child, the severity of whose illness is apparent to him, must face many problems at different stages. Children of all ages, of all grades of intelligence and from all backgrounds react in varying degree to the symptoms themselves, the visit to the family doctor, the referral to hospital, admission to a foreign environment, possible limitation of visiting hours (unless in a paediatric unit), living with uniformed strangers, investigative attack, strange bedside discussion amongst staff and students, parental reaction to the diagnosis and therapeutic side-effects. Those whose pathology remits and relapses but who worsen over time or who have watched others die have a long time to think about it.

A very young child takes his cue from the parents and family. At this age perfectly normal children have outbursts of temper and breath-holding and may strike or bite parents and family when intense simple desire (a toy, an ice-cream, father's razor) are withheld. It is not then surprising that a sick tired child, possibly in pain, may be more easily provoked. By the age of 6 to 8 years, the fear of dying is much likelier and occasions more anguish and weeping, more withdrawal and perhaps difficulty in sleeping or frightening dreams.

The young adolescent, with greater experience and education, may be distressed by increasing weakness, loss of mobility, exclusion from the virile games of an age-group attaining to manliness and loss of the team society which has been moving away from parental company. The girl's aroused interest in body shape and dress, whether 'pretty' or 'sloppy', is crushed as the disease spoils and distorts her appearance and the dreams of future womanhood turn sour. Increasing dependence on parents and other adults accentuate all these reversals of normal development and often generate resentment of those who seek to care. Enough can have been learned by this age about the community's religious belief, not only to stimulate thought but to provoke anger. Children raised in the philosophies and practices of other cultures may simply await the ultimate with resignation, but in the Christian tradition the delightful simplicity of 'let little children come to me because my heaven is made only of such nice people as they are' can be overlaid with the most terrible threat. Alternatively, it can have been made a Santa Claus religion where goodness, kindness, provision and protection are to be expected for all *good* children. This prepares the way for 'Why me? What have I done?' and the anger of injustice or the false guilt of imagined misbehaviour with all its attendant misery.

In later adolescence behaviour is more adult, conforming recognisably to the Kubler-Ross stages (1970), but modified by age. The patient is not looking down on the sunset in the valley with all the memories of the climb, but from the valley to sunlit mountain tops which she will not reach. A 15-year-old girl reported by Raimbault (1981) said: 'I did not want to be treated because I was ashamed to see myself so fat with the cortisone. I found myself disgusting. Do you know what life means to me? It can be beautiful, but if I lose it, I'll never know it.' There is room for bitterness, but the older adolescent's greater ability to think and discuss helps him or her to express gratitude for the care offered: to accept the comforting and the companionship of parents and relatives.

Parental Reaction

Breaking the news of a child's death or fatal illness was at one time common, but never easy — miliary tuberculosis, tuberculous meningitis, acute lymphoblastic leukaemia. These and others involved announcing the absolute certainty of death within 3–16 weeks and the total absence of effective treatment. A house officer could face this ordeal once or twice a month and the declaration that death had already occurred in acute cases was a weekly and sometimes daily matter. I felt that the news should be given at home; that the hospital doctor should fully brief the family doctor and that the latter, possibly with his hospital colleague, should call and quietly tell the parents among the familiar things of their daily lives. My offer was never accepted, although I was sometimes given the freedom to 'do it yourself'. This did not result from callousness, but from a feeling of inadequacy and inexperience. If that were so 25 years ago, there is much less experience now. There were of course problems like the presence of other children at home and the absence of privacy. Are these necessarily bad? There was a time when a community grieved and rejoiced together. Is the problem not compounded by silence and secrecy? The usual alternative is worse. The parents are called from the child's bedside and often promise 'to be right back'. In too many NHS hospitals the news is broken in a multi-purpose room, the telephones ring, doctors/nurses/students come and go, the surroundings are spartan. The news is broken. Comfort is given by a devoted staff painfully aware of the inappropriate surroundings. The shocked parents stumble out. Often they decide to leave immediately. The child, puzzled and alarmed by their appearance, watches them from a window. Ordinary parents without cars wait for a bus and then perhaps for another. The central station offers transport 10 or 15 miles to home. Fellow passengers eye them curiously. The rest of the family waits. The hospital staff grieves. Too often the nation 'cannot afford' a better environment.

Neonatal deaths (see Tables 10.1 and 10.2) stress the big contribution (45 per cent) made by deaths in the first month of life, Table 10.9 shows that in the mixed urban/rural community represented by the Edinburgh area, at least 39 per cent died in maternity units. (Other babies certainly died in medical and surgical paediatric units after transfer from maternity hospitals.) This should not exclude involvement of the family doctor, nurse and health visitor.

Table 10.9: Place of death of 205 Lothian children

Place	Number
Home or outdoors	54
Royal Hospital for Sick Children	47
Maternity units' newborn nurseries	80
General hospital without paediatric unit	9*
General hospital with paediatric unit	10
Infectious disease hospital	1
Others	4

Note: * Mostly in central head injury unit (traffic accidents).

The baby's death may be sudden and unexpected, as in intrauterine death, with or without difficult labour or in lethal malformation. It may follow a few hours, days or even weeks (in that order of likelihood) after birth, especially in pre-term deliveries. In such cases the mother is likely to have sat beside her baby's incubator in the special care unit and to have anguished with him in his fight for survival.

The anticlimax is profound after months of anticipation and preparation. The reaction is likely to be severe and to endure it in hospital may be intolerable. Other babies are sleeping, crying or suckling. Other mothers are happy and fulfilled. The staff goes about its duty, relatives rejoice over the new arrivals. The parents of the dying or already dead baby, lonely in their grief, see only unfamiliar, rather clinical surroundings and their need of home is intense. Yet they want to know the cause of death, whether they were at all to blame and whether it was preventable. Doubts reassail them from time to time and anxieties recur before and during a subsequent pregnancy.

The experience of parents afflicted by *sudden infant death syndrome* (SIDS) in an English study of three separate areas is mostly predictable, but it is also worrying (Watson, 1978; Watson, Gardner and Carpenter, 1981). The parents were first interviewed as soon as possible after the death and ranged from the most socially deprived to the most affluent. 'Over 70 per cent of the parents mentioned anger, bewilderment, self-blame, guilt and anxiety about a possible recurrence; guilt feelings were particularly apparent where abortion had been considered or the pregnancy unplanned.' Sudden death commonly prompts suspicion and gratuitous inferences about possible murder are always disturbing. The attitude of general practitioners or hospital outpatient departments consulted shortly before the death may induce bitterness. Bereaved parents are in no state to accept the fact that many babies seen during the day with identical mild symptoms have remained well. Inevitably the tone of the original interview decides the parents' feelings. Seldom will they blame a doctor who has been kind and careful.

The second interview, three weeks after the death, naturally showed continued grief, depression and anxiety, but parents were more able to talk and to see things in better perspective. They were still distressed. The events had been repeatedly rediscussed. Doctors were sometimes thought to have been negligent. Watson provides a table (reproduced here as Table 10.10) of helpful support experienced by afflicted parents. More than one source may be included for each family. The role of parents and friends is natural, but reassuring. Health visitors rank highly as the skilled early counsellors. General practitioners and ministers of religion are surprisingly poor and the absence of hospital support, although it will surprise few, should concern many. Limerick's

Table 10.10: Sources of help experienced by parents of SIDS

	Area I	Area II	Area III
Relatives	69 (1)	72 (1)	72 (1)
Friends	44 (2)	32 (4)	40 (2 =)
Health visitors	36 (3)	39 (3)	50 (2 =)
Coroner's officer	21 (4)	17 (6)	18 (6)
General practitioner	18 (5)	41 (2)	31 (4)
Minister of religion	10 (6)	30 (5)	30 (5)
Total	198	231	251

Source: Watson (1981).

study (1981) includes quotations from bereaved parents. There are tributes to ambulance men, police, coroners, health visitors and doctors, but there are complaints too; for example, 'my GP was utterly useless . . . he did not offer any support and he stayed only about 10 minutes'; 'I felt very angry that the health visitor called to visit a young family next door regularly, yet never called to see us once, despite coming before our baby's death'; 'it was very hurtful when the paediatrician asked if he'd been a wanted baby'. These may tell us as much about the parents as about the professionals, but it may be the parents, difficult as the interviews may be, who need the professionals most. It is interesting that Lady Limerick quotes no comments about clergymen or funeral undertakers, although both can help or worsen the mourning experience. These findings are likely to vary with the community studied, quite apart from social class, in different parts even of the British Isles. Changes in family circumstances following such cot deaths are said to be common and range from mothers returning to work (where employment is available) to attempted suicide, neglect of or assault on other children and parental separation. As in all of life's acute stresses, the outcome depends on the prior ability of the parents and of their marriage.

The effects of *long-continued stress* also depend on personal and marital stability. Studies of child diabetics and their families in my own clinic have shown that this stress alone causes symptoms in half the mothers and that marriages which were already under strain threatened to break unless supported. The news that their child had a fatal illness may be disbelieved. The doctor's therapeutic approach may be rejected as the disease deteriorates or the side-effects of drugs begin to bite. The less educated the parents, the likelier are they to doubt. Their concern is natural. No matter how great the confidence of the doctor in his diagnosis and programme, they need reassurance, if necessary from medical colleagues, if they are to be protected from quacks and charlatans.

The threat of death, as in malignant disease undergoing long-term treatment, the devotion to nursing a child who is weak, mutilated and in pain, and the loss of relaxation and friendship out of the home: these may cause depression and despair in the parent as well as in the child. If employed, the father's work may suffer, the mother's household responsibilities may be ignored and family meals may deteriorate. The care of the dying (even if poorly organised) may replace the care of the living. As it drags on, the existence may become a living death and the parents may go through the normal process of grieving and mourning while the patient is still alive. This is common and is part of the preparation for separation. On the other hand, it can be an ennobling and enriching experience. My wife's slow downhill progress with cancer was perhaps the richest part of our 27 years together. As the end approached, each day became fuller, more to be savoured and enjoyed. 'It will not be today', we would say as we sipped our tea, spoke of the day's experiences and found infinite pleasure in each minute. The relationship of parent and child could be like that, where pain and anxiety are skilfully modified by an attentive physician and devoted nursing.

Isolation may be at its worst in the case of *neurological disease, degenerating slowly* over years with little or no verbal communication between parent and child and with all the added problems of feeding, fits and incontinence. Easson (1981) speaks also of the *Lazarus syndrome*: the resurrection phenomenon of a child whose death, for example, in prolonged coma, seems certain. The family prepares for the death, grieves, distances itself, reinvests emotionally, moves to future plans and then the child amazingly recovers. He may find that the family has left him emotionally and they, it is said, may find difficulty in reintegrating him as a family member.

In some cases (for example, *SIDS, accidents and overwhelming infections*) the task may fall on the accident and emergency department staff, and provision should certainly be made there for secluded grief and support, communication with relatives and humane transport. The hospital staff must not believe that they have discharged their full duties until they have the grief-stricken parents safely home and the home services have moved in.

In all these matters the single parent is likely to carry the greater burden. Not only does the possibly personal sadness behind his or her single state continue, but a new relationship may now be jeopardised, discussion may be impossible, employment may be sacrificed and a sense of personal guilt may become an obsession. What can scarcely be borne mutually by partners may break a single parent and it is often worst where the adult is least able. If there is a separated partner, he or she may share an even greater sense of guilt.

The Reactions of Others

Watson (1981) reports from the SIDS study that more than half the families mentioned behavioural problems with their other children after the death. They included insomnia, sleep-walking, nightmares, bed-wetting, regression in toilet training, impaired security, refusal to leave parents and fear of falling asleep. Those who had seen the baby being removed by ambulance were most upset. Immigrant families reported fewer disturbances, but whether this was due to language difficulty, reticence of a more fatalistic view of life was unclear.

In the slower deaths described by Easson (1981) schoolteachers noticed that other children in the family became listless and irritable. Although the other children experience the pain of impending separation from a brother or sister, the sad change caused to family circumstances may make them feel angry with the dying sib. This mourning anger may also be directed against each other. Where the child is dying because of an accident, the siblings may feel that they failed as protectors and all may remember with deep regret past quarrels or injustices for which they now feel responsible. Their thoughts may also turn anxiously to their own vulnerability. Why should the thing that killed their brother or sister not now turn upon them? They are unlikely to understand the process, but in genetic diseases such as Duchenne-type muscular dystrophy the inference is plain since their symptoms are shared.

Neighbours and friends may worry about the possible infectivity or alternative transmissibility of the fatal illness and the risks to their own children. They may also experience the natural reluctance to have theirs submitted to the emotional trauma of observing the dying process, even if their children do not recognise it until their friend has died. Teachers, too, may have similar anxieties about children in their care, should they know that a child in remission is returning to school. They may worry about what that child may do physically and academically, what he may eat and what is forbidden. Sometimes they may be assailed by guilt, where they have been hard on a child whose early symptoms they interpreted as idleness or naughtiness. They may be helped by a sort of medical 'absolution' — 'you could not be expected to know . . . your attitude did not contribute to the illness . . . even now that he is back, school rules must still apply'. Protection of the thrombocytopenic child from trauma, however, is essential.

Specific Management

Management is described in two sections. The first (specific) deals with particular situations and the second (general) with matters which are common to all; the latter is subdivided into longer-term management and to the final period when death appears to be imminent.

Newborn Babies

A natural conflict of view exists as to whether a mother should see her stillborn baby whom she and her husband have 'known' and loved throughout pregnancy. Its disappearance, even if malformed, may leave behind a feeling of disbelief and the comment 'it was abnormal, dear' may generate an exaggerated concept of the horror. Severe maceration is probably a good reason for disposal without the parents seeing the child, but thought should be given (and the parents consulted) before deciding that they should not see a 'fresh' stillborn baby, even if malformation exists. The baby's more frightening abnormalities may be covered.

The certifying of a gross malformation as 'stillborn' rather than neonatal death, even if a breath was taken or a heart-beat heard, has sometimes been intended as a kindness. It may, however, deprive the parents of important financial entitlement, since the Death Grant is never awarded to parents of a stillborn baby, but only to those whose baby has taken at least one breath or shown other evidence of life.

The baby struggling for life in a maternity hospital may still have his mother there. She should have free access to him and should, when it is unlikely to make any difference to the outcome, be allowed to touch him. Where the baby has been transferred to an intensive medical or surgical neonatal care unit elsewhere, the mother should be transferred as soon as possible, unless she clearly objects. Paediatric units should and normally do make every effort within the limits of sometimes archaic buildings to accommodate mothers and to provide not only 24-hour per day access to the baby, but a great deal of warm support and understanding. Explanation of and reassurance about the baby 'not suffering pain' among a mass of technological equipment is desirable too. The mother's chair should be comfortable, since she has not long been delivered, and she should be able to see as much of her baby as is visible in the incubator without having to stand to do so. A well-padded stool of adjustable height with a back and a foot rest is desirable. She may be given a theatre frock, partly for hygiene and partly to minimise discomfort in a very warm environment. Hopefully there should be a withdrawal room or two, where parents may rest and have tea or coffee. The comfort of non-smokers should be remembered, since hospital rooms of this kind can be made insufferable by anxious smokers.

During this period of waiting, the family doctor and his team and the community service (district midwife and health visitor) should be kept informed and they must be told immediately if the baby dies. Arrangements can then be made for appropriate support at home and for subsequent discussions with the parents. The importance of skilled autopsy by a paediatric pathologist is stressed, since it may reveal matters of great genetic or other management importance relevant to future pregnancies.

In traditionally Christian countries there is a wide demand for infants to be baptised before death and the belief may extend even to its application to the dead: for example, of the stillborn. Not all professionals, including clergymen, accept that such a need exists, but it is commonly of the very greatest importance to parents who make no other profession of religious belief or practice. Their need should be met immediately in such emergencies; it is not a time at which to discuss the finer points of theology.

The management of severe neonatal malformation received world-wide publicity in 1981 during and after the criminal prosecution of a paediatrician. His clearance by the court does not remove the problem from each doctor who faces it in future. The critical decision about terminating life has been advanced in Britain in recent years to the first part of pregnancy. A foetus with meningocele, adrenogenital syndrome, trisomy-21 or male sex with a haemophilic or muscle-dystrophic brother may be legally discarded up to 28 weeks of gestation, but not of course later without the risk of a murder charge against the doctor concerned. That is certainly so by the time the foetus reaches the so-called age of viability. Such a situation understandably provokes heated ethical debate, since the decision seems to relate more obviously to size than to sanctity. The majority view, however, is likely to remain in favour of present policy. Faced with a very abnormal baby of 28 weeks' gestation, the physician is not permitted to end its life and would operate hopelessly against the whole code of accepted professional practices were he to increase its suffering. I would include in that a policy of not feeding the baby or of permitting its dehydration. On the other hand, the physician's duty is to relieve suffering and should he fail to do so, then he is negligent. I favour the prescription of analgesia and sedation in the dose which is just adequate to provide real relief and not just a measure of amelioration. The recent controversy, however, makes desirable a well-documented consultative medical decision by at least two colleagues. The decision not to strive officiously to keep a baby alive is simpler. Faced with an infant which can only die soon, after greater suffering, the physician should be free *not* to intervene, answering parental questions carefully and leaving the way open for a second or third opinion and the possible intervention of a colleague who supports it.

There is at present a real danger of developing metaphoric tunnel vision in neonatal, as in other, medicine. Important as each new life is, the truth also is that no single patient should so absorb staff, equipment and time that the majority of special care babies are deprived and may suffer a greater morbidity and even mortality as a result.

Malformations and Inborn Metabolic Errors

The treatment of malformations and inborn errors is beyond the scope of this chapter, and the general management of weakness, boredom, discomfort and anxiety is described later. Whether the child dies early, as perhaps in proprionic acidaemia, or later, as in the lysosomal disorders, parents should know the genetic implications as soon as the diagnosis is made. There is nothing worse than the very early conception of another affected child in ignorance of the risk. The physician is most likely to find authoritative advice from a medical genetic clinic, but illustrated books of malformations and syndromes (for example, Smith, 1976) and paediatric texts about inborn errors should be in every hospital library. The mode of inheritance, where known, is described. If it is relevant, then the parents should be counselled and the greatest care must be taken to ensure that the meaning of, for example, a one-in-four risk is understood. Should they wish advice and help with family planning, these should be provided immediately. If pre-natal diagnosis is possible in future pregnancies, their views about it and about selective discard should be recorded. Pre-natal diagnosis by amniocentesis without the possibility of parental consent to abortion is pointless and cannot be justified simply to satisfy academic curiosity.

The mother's maternity record may be marked accordingly, but populations are very mobile and it is also useful to give the mother a note of the diagnosis, emphasising that she should keep it carefully and give it immediately to the doctor who deals with any subsequent pregnancy.

Accidents

Everyone knows how to prevent accidents and although not everyone is able to do so, the death of a child by scalding or fire, by poisoning, by falling from a height, by drowning in a canal or by a vehicle generates in most parents, guardians, baby-sitters or even older siblings the most terrible sense of guilt. 'If only I had . . .' Too often, of course, it is true and they must learn to live with it; the pain will dull with time. It may help, however, with the more sensitive (who are often those who have least with which to reproach themselves) to meet later with the physician. who can help create a sense of perspective. 'Children of even the best parents are at continuous risk . . . children are so quick at that age . . . before anyone can stop them . . . most of them escape of course . . . it usually takes some other factor . . . call it bad luck if you like . . . or the will of God . . . mothers and their families are often most vulnerable just before the monthly period . . . that's scarcely your fault.' Sensitively and quietly guided, parents can begin to find a sense of peace. Above all, they must be told not to place the blame on the shoulders of an older child who was 'left in charge'. I knew two teenage sisters who had a car crash. The one who was driving survived. She was reminded frequently by her mother, in company and out of it, that her beautiful sister would be alive had she, the survivor, not lost control of the vehicle. That is monstrous.

Malignancies

Malignancies introduce a new factor into this section, because remissions may be so successful that the child and the family must now live with health, knowing that death may be over the horizon. Indeed it shows its face from time to time, as the increasing confidence of prolonged remission is destroyed by relapse, only to be re-established for an unknown period and for an unknown number of times by further therapeutic attacks. The undoubted merits of an oncology clinic or at least of an oncology team (a highly desirable development) brings with it the sadness of a concentration of children who become aware of final casualties in their ranks. Faith, hope and love, however, create

tremendous fortitude and many of these children suffer much operative pain and medical side-effect because they are not dying that day,
although it may happen tomorrow or next week or next year. Any
physician who has been through the personal experience knows that
hope is difficult to kill. Even the traditionalist may in his desperation
turn to alternative medicine or to spiritual healing. The patient's
physician need not encourage false hope, but he will be a bad and sometimes sorry one if he tries to destroy it.

Even though treatment of solid tumours and of acute lymphoblastic
leukaemia are now much better than they were, the time comes for
some when the caring team must ask if more treatment is desirable, to
what end and for what quality of life. Thirty years ago the side-effects
of chemotherapy (aminopterin) were so unacceptable and even the
short-term results so poor that some paediatricians advised parents
against it, but toxic effects are now less and the chances of long-term
survival so much better that it is more difficult to take a clear decision
against continuing the fight. Each case must be decided on its merits,
but there comes a time for some when mutilation, organ removal,
intellectual damage, paralysis, ineradicable infection and psycho-social
deterioration compel a decision that 'enough is enough'. It is admittedly a subjective decision and physicians should consult together
before deciding against treatment and in favour of increasing analgesia
and sedation. They know that the submission of a child to more pain
and more distress in the course of therapeutic research study at a time
when the fight has been lost is a less moral decision than the prescription of relief. The parents cannot be asked to take this decision, but an
older child may volunteer the wish for peaceful death and that judgement should not be ignored. In her terminal illness from malignancy my
own wife opted to die with dignity without loss of hair or limb or
beauty. 'Do not make me suffer what you would not let the dog suffer'
is a powerful plea.

Slow Respiratory Deaths

In practice such deaths in north-west Europe and America result now
from cystic fibrosis, although there are exceptions (for example,
bronchopulmonary dysplasia and rare bronchiectasis). They occur more
now in older children, adolescents and young adults than in the past
when cystic fibrosis death was common in infants and toddlers. There is
naturally hope among patients and their relatives that new developments will some day clear the lungs of infection and restore an acceptable quality of life so that there is a natural desire to cling to life

rather than to surrender to death. Increasing weakness, exhausting cough and breathlessness even at rest can still create prolonged distress over many weeks before death brings final relief. These patients are naturally aware of what is happening. Many may have read about it for years or even helped raise funds for research. Some may have resigned themselves to death, but silently harbour an increasing fear of the manner of their going. Extrapolating from adult experience, I think it possible that a little information to adolescents about nature's kindness in providing progressive unawareness (carbon dioxide narcosis) may help. The relief of anxiety and the provision of sleep by medication are desirable and suppression of the cough and respiratory centres is not an acceptable contra-indication if survival is limited to days or weeks.

Duchenne-type muscular dystrophy shares these comments, since such patients also know much about their disease and its prognosis, may have seen a sibling die, suffer weak respiration, cough and infection and they are alert until near the end. Management of the closing stage should be, as for cystic fibrosis, generous. Everyone wants that including by that time the patient himself.

Renal Failure

Renal failure in children shares with malignancy an uncertain prognosis and a therapeutic programme (peritoneal or renal dialysis) which has difficulties and dangers ranging from interrupted schooling to hospitalisation, infection and death. It too, however, carries the greater possibility of future health and happiness if transplant becomes available, is successful and leads to newer and better developments in care. Other problems soluble only by successful transplant (for example, marrow) cause the same weakness made bearable by the hope that a tissue 'fit' for transplant will emerge. The length to which the patient and family will go and the suffering of the patient again decide the moment at which the long struggle should be replaced by kindly release.

The Dying Parent

The dying parent is naturally described in other sections of this book dealing with the primary illness. He or she faces not only the crisis of personal death, but also the problem of the family's future. This is unbearable if one of the children is handicapped or seriously ill with a bad prognosis. Provision for them helps relieve the patient's final anxiety.

General Management

Breaking the News

Bad news should be broken gently, in an appropriate place and at a suitable time. It should be based on the most accurate diagnosis that can be achieved and should not deny the possibility of recovery. The range of diagnosis offered at times by panels dealing with the pathology of childhood tumours and the rare spontaneous disappearance of malignancy encourage caution. Precise prognosis in days or weeks to death in children is very unwise.

Remission Possible, Death not Imminent

Comfort. The least that the dying child deserves in the acute relapse or not immediately fatal phase of his illness is comfort, for example, a bed to himself if he wants it or a parent to sleep with him if he needs that security, nice pyjamas or nightdress, a good mattress, clean bed clothes, good skin care and a fleece on which to lie if bones are prominent and bed sores possible. He should have fresh air in the room and a deodorant or perfume if the illness is associated with a bad smell. He should also have the means of achieving or of at least maintaining the position which he desires, for example, to read, write, see television or watch the family.

Some Self-pride. Loss of hair, bruising, pallor, mutilation, smell — all of these destroy confidence and a normal interest in self-appearance and they may isolate the patient further, first from his friends, then from his relatives, his family and eventually himself so that he looks at the mirror with increasing disgust. Always, but especially where remission is possible, morale and company should be maintained using, for example, a wig (if desired), cosmetics, clothes and deodorants. The caring team should be imaginative in creating the best environment in which the patient looks most normal.

Nutrition. Long spells in hospital or even at home, cut off from fresh air and exercise and stimulation, impair appetite. The art of old-fashioned 'invalid cooking' has been lost in institutional kitchens and even diet kitchens too often lack the imagination of a good mother in a good home. It is not in fact just a matter of an attractive and balanced diet on a tray, but the love that comes with it, the mother's or the nurse's company during the meal, her encouraging voice and the light in her eyes. The child with a fatal illness and one in temporary relapse needs small meals of what he fancies, nicely served, out of bed if possible and with a good bedside table if that is impossible.

Inactivity, toxic drugs, fever and a small appetite can cause constipation, which is distressing because it pains. The fibre content of the food should be maintained, but the child is unlikely to have a taste for bran products. Fresh fruits and salads should be encouraged. A mouth made sore by drugs or invading monilia can 'sting', however, if fruit or fruit juice is taken. Milk, yoghurt or synthetic food supplements are better, although too much milk may constipate. Proprietary viscous gels such as 'Isogel' or 'Fybogel' will prevent constipation and can be given in small amounts three or four times daily, sprinkled on a bland fizzy drink (even on soda water), stirred with a little sugar and taken before it froths over or gels. Vitamin syrups in an appropriate dose are wise and so may be such supplements as iron if intake is poor or blood loss is increased.

Communication. Communication with a child, with anyone, is not confined to speech. A parent sitting silently with a child, reading a magazine or sharing a television programme, communicates security and sympathy. That is why children should be in paediatric units with 24-hour visiting and facilities for a parent to sleep beside the child in hospital, if at all possible. That is also why a few fortunate hospitals have adolescent units or at least enough single or double rooms to accommodate those who are no longer children but who in these frightening circumstances are not yet adult. Where a parent's company is not practicable (for example, a single parent with inescapable domestic commitments), the child should certainly have the use of a telephone in order to talk to his family at home.

The best arrangement is, of course, to keep such children at home, to provide the treatment team's skills there by home visits and to so organise transport and hospital day treatment facilities that chemotherapy, irradiation and transfusion can be arranged without admission. In this way the unnatural conditions of hospital are minimised at a time when life itself is threatened.

Both in hospital and at home, continued contact with friends is also desirable and their parents may need reassurance that the patient's condition is non-communicable: so many children perished in the past because they were not excluded from continued close social relationship with a tuberculous family.

Diversion. There are many hours when immediate social contact is not possible (friends at school; parents are busy). A little radio, a cassette player and television are great distractions and the privileged enjoy electronic games, although they are better played in company. Crayons and paints and plasticine help pass the time and small children get great comfort from a favourite cuddly toy or from a properly looked-after pet. Book and toy libraries and occupational therapists who come to the home can help the young ones, and home teachers from the Department of Special Educational Services can help occupy the minds of older patients. The play leaders of children's hospitals make a wonderful difference to long-stay patients and their skills may be extended to the home through home-care personnel.

Although television brings the real and fantasy world into the home, little outings boost morale. The family should be advised as to what is wise and unwise. If they have no car, some local groups (the local church) or a neighbour may help: but seat belts must be worn if thrombocytopenia persists.

Behaviour. The emotional reaction of children has been described already. Their irritability, their 'ingratitude', their downright aggression must be interpreted in the context of the illness and of the handling of it. The need to maintain family rules and discipline is stressed. Misbehaviour should be treated sympathetically, but it cannot be condoned. Morale is likely to be best sustained when the familiar things remain, and that includes what is regarded as desirable, acceptable or unacceptable. Simple disciplinary reaction should not be avoided.

School. School attendance is wise where it is possible because it provides a familiar environment and friends and it occupies the mind. Intermittent absence is essential for clinic visits or intercurrent infections. If there are restrictions (for example, on football, physical education, swimming or corporal punishment, should that still survive), then these should be documented and made known to teaching staff and the school doctor. Catering staff too may need information, if diet is important.

Because children with malignancies are commonly given immunosuppressive drugs and because such simple infections as chicken-pox may prove fatal under these conditions, the schoolteachers and doctor should be very much on the alert for an outbreak at the school, should an immuno-suppressed child be attending at the time. A period of isolation at home is probably wise and this may have to extend to siblings, unless it is possible for the patient or the siblings to spend time with relatives.

Some children will go to school hairless and unconcerned after chemotherapy. Others will scarcely leave their house because they fear mockery. For them, two good-quality wigs should be prescribed so that one can be cleaned while the other is worn. Other children at the school should be warned in advance and their co-operation sought, since a school bully can make attendance impossible for the patient. I have known cases where the Director of Education has changed the child's school so that the patient may attend with those who have no idea that a wig is worn.

Eventually, or intermittently in the case of recurring remission, school attendance becomes too difficult, even if transport is provided. Special schooling, with its new and handicapped population, is best avoided and a home teacher should be sought. This may be enough to enable a child to keep up with the peer group and to re-enter his usual class if remission is established. Finally, of course, he may be too ill and too sedated to co-operate.

Home Care. The infrequency of death nowadays, especially in children who are unaware of the prognosis, deprives general practice teams and health visitors of this sad experience. As with some of the complex disorders of childhood (for example, diabetes, cystic fibrosis, phenylketonuria), there is great advantage in having a hospital outreach by a team of maximum experience: not to 'takeover', but to participate and to guide. Home Care sisters such as are based on the out-patient service of the Royal Hospital for Sick Children in Edinburgh have the advantage of close contact with the hospital service and bring to the community all the information and equipment needed. It is also an invaluable support to parents bereaved by an unexplained cot death at that time, in subsequent pregnancies and during the first year of a new baby's life.

Worthwhile Remission Excluded: Death Imminent

Now is death merciful. He calls me hence
Gently with friendly soothing of my fears
Of ugly age and feeble impotence
And cruel disintegration of slow years.

Am I going to die? At this stage of the illness prevarication is pointless and the truth is much better tolerated than a sham cheerfulness and shallow promise. The answer should be gentle and empathetic.

The time given is well spent.

How shall I die? The fear of death and the distress at parting are commonly less than the fear of pain, of choking or asphyxia. An honest and reassuring answer about the sort of sleepy twilight of carbon dioxide narcosis and skilfully given medicines do much to remove the terror of the unknown.

Where shall I die? The best place of course is at home among the family and among familiar things. The parents must be carefully consulted and may wish to prepare the other children in the family for this event before the patient is discharged from hospital. Some families find it quite impossible to plan for a child's death at home, and all will certainly need support from the local practice team and from the hospital Home Care Team, should such exist.

Raimbault's (1981) moving account of the 13-year-old boy whose mother was agitated by the late arrival of an ambulance to take him home quotes him as saying: 'I'll hang on till it arrives . . . I'll die at home.' This desire for 'togetherness' at the end may be intense, and the simple account by Cotton, Cotton and Goodall (1981), 'A brother dies at home', shows how preferable it may be where local circumstances permit.

If death is to take place in hospital, then the ritual of intermittently moving the bed and screens nearer to the exit should be avoided. Many of the nineteenth-century hospitals in Britain were not built to deal with rare cases of death today. Some effort should be made, however, to provide or improvise a room capable of accommodating child and parent and of permitting other visitors. Such arrangements may have been made in any case for the treatment of immuno-suppressed children with a view to reducing the risk of infection and so there need be little change between the admissions for treatment and the final admission for terminal care. Failure to provide such facilities constitutes a further argument in favour of discharge to a skilled caring service at home.

When shall I die? It is usually impossible to predict the time of death, even to the parents, since it is so easy to be wrong and it initiates a macabre countdown which has no point. It is usually enough to reply 'not yet awhile . . . certainly not today', since the dying child may find one more day quite reassuring. On such a day-to-day basis the patient may be lulled slowly into unawareness.

What happens after I die? The child's spiritual belief until early adolescence is likely to be that of the parents and if this includes a faith in happy immortality and family reunion, then the caring team must respect it and encourage the involvement of the family's clergyman and/or the hospital chaplain. This is true for all world religions. If, on the other hand, the parents have no belief and are entirely opposed to any attempt at religious education, then that view must also be respected, although motivated staff will have every chance to show the love of a living faith. There are, however, many families who have no strong feelings one way or the other and at this time they want simple advice as to what they may believe about a continued spiritual life. The hospital chaplain has a major part to play and if the child is discharged home, he should place the family in contact with the clergyman of their community and remain in contact.

Medication. Apart from the complex chemotherapy given to children with leukaemia and solid tumours, terminally-ill children should be assured of sleep, using whatever hynoptic is found to suit best and in a dose which achieves this end. Anxiety may be relieved with chlorpromazine and analgesia, with increasingly effective compounds ranging from dihydrocodeine tartrate to diamorphine used in low doses frequently. Antidepressants are given if there are true indications of depression and I suspect that too often they are given too late to have any effect. Since they are comparatively safe compounds to use and since they are non-addictive (in the case of remission), I believe their earlier use in terminal illness is fully justified.

Even when death is certainly close, it is appropriate to maintain hydration and to treat monilial infection of the mouth, which can cause great misery in the last few days of life. Otherwise it is not a kindness to treat a terminal pneumonia, only to have the patient live for another week or two.

Accommodation. As already stated, hospitals should do all in their power to provide a room for a dying child and an attending parent. At home there should be a facility for crisis relief — allowing the parents some time to sleep — achieved by supplying community nursing staff and social workers. The latter are also the most appropriate source of information about such things as financial entitlements, for example attendance allowance and death grants.

Follow-up

Contact should always be maintained with the family after the child's death so that feelings of guilt, of anger and of doubt can be discussed and rediscussed until a measure of restabilisation and adjustment has been reached.

Note:

1. A wide range of printed information for parents and professionals on unexpected infant deaths is available from the Foundation for the Study of Infant Death (Cot Death Research), 5th Floor, 4 Grosvenor Place, London SW1X 7HD.

References

Cotton, M., Cotton, G. and Goodall, J. (1981) 'A brother dies at home', *Maternal and Child Health*, Barker Publications, Richmond, Surrey

Easson, W.M. (1981) *The Dying Child*, 2nd edn, C.C. Thomas, Springfield, Ill.

Kubler-Ross, E. (1970) *On Death and Dying*, Tavistock Publications, London

Limerick, Lady S. (1981) 'The role of the Foundation for the Study of Infant Deaths', *Medicine, Science and Law*, 21, 112–16

Raimbault, G. (1981) 'Children talk about death', *Acta Paediatrica Scandinavia*, 70, 179–82

Smith, D.W. (1976) *Recognisable Patterns of Human Malformation*, 2nd edn, W.B. Saunders, Philadelphia, London, Toronto

Symposium on Cot Death (1980) *Medicine, Science and Law*, 21, 76–122

Watson, E. (1978) 'The inner North London study of Sudden Infant Death and its relevance for the community services', *Medicine, Science and Law*, 18, 271–3

Watson, E. (1981) 'An epidemiological and sociological study of unexpected death in infancy in nine areas of Southern England: III Bereavement', *Medicine, Science and Law*, 21, 99–104

Watson, E., Gardner, A. and Carpenter, R.G. (1981) 'An epidemiological and sociological study of unexpected deaths in infancy in nine areas of Southern England: II Symptoms and patterns of care'

Yudkin, S. (1967) 'Children and death', *Lancet* (special article 7 January), 37–41

Recommended Further Reading

Alexander, I.E. and Alderstein, A.M. (1965) 'Affective responses to the concept of death in a population of children and early adolescents' in R. Fulton (ed.), *Death and Identity*, John Wiley, New York

Anthony, S. (1940) *The Child's Discovery of Death*, Harcourt, Brace, New York

Bartholomew, S.E.M. and Bain, A.D. (1982) *Proceedings of International Research Conference on Sudden Infant Death Syndrome*, Baltimore, USA (June)

British Paediatric Association and British Association of Paediatric Surgeons (1980) *Report of the Working Party on Paediatric Oncology Services and on Training in Paediatric Oncology*

Evans, A.E. (1968) 'If a child must die', *New England Journal of Medicine*, 278, 138–42

Farrow, G. (1982) 'The soothing touch', *World Medicine* (7 August)

Gartley, W. and Bernasconi, M. (1967) 'The concept of death in children', *Journal of Genetic Psychology*, 110, 71–85

Green, M. and Solnit, A.J. (1959) 'Psychological consideration in the management of deaths on paediatric hospital services. Part 1, The doctor and the child's family', *Paediatrics*, 24, 106–12

Green, M. and Solnit, A.J. (1959) 'Psychological consideration in the management of deaths on paediatric hospital services. Part 2, The child's reaction (vica) fear of dying', in *Modern Perspectives in Child Development*, International Universities Press, New York, 217–28

Knudson, A.G. and Nalterson, J.M. (1960) 'Observations concerning fear of death in fatally ill children and their mothers', *Psychosomatic Medicine*, 22, 456–65

Knudson, A.G. and Nalterson, J.M. (1960) 'Practice of paediatrics – participation of parents in the hospital care of fatally ill children', *Paediatrics*, 26, 482–90

Richmond, J.B. and Waisman, H.A. (1955) 'Psychological aspects of management in children with malignant diseases', *American Journal of Diseases in Children*, 89, 42–7

Silverman, W. (1982) 'Hospital setting for humane neonatal deaths', *Paediatrics*, 69, 239–40

Stewart-Brown, S. (1982) 'Personal view', *British Medical Journal*, 284, 1628

11 PSYCHOLOGICAL ASPECTS OF THE TREATMENT OF CHRONIC PAIN

Michael Bond

> It is not possible to treat pain in isolation for we have to consider the whole person.
>
> Cicily Saunders, 1963

The management of chronic pain is an important part of the palliation and care of patients with both benign and malignant diseases, and it may surprise the reader to learn that it also forms an important part of the care of individuals with certain chronic disorders of personality and emotion, who suffer no less than those with proven physical illnesses. Therefore, it is clear that those caring for individuals with chronic painful illness should have, as Cicily Saunders pointed out twenty years ago, a broad-based understanding of the nature of pain and the means of controlling or relieving it; including those of the pyschological or social nature. Pain is not a disease in its own right, although it was thought to be so as recently as the eighteenth century (Lobb, 1739); it is one symptom experienced by suffering persons who may have several other hurts or discomforts, anxieties about being ill, and worries concerning the personal and family consequences of that illness. Therefore, it is obvious that some of the psychological and social complexities of illness must be considered, when analysing and treating pain problems. These issues and means for attempting their solution form the basis of this chapter.

Attitudes Towards Pain and Suffering

Most of us feel that the ability to endure pain and suffering with little or no complaint is an admirable trait and, accordingly, stoicism in the face of pain and suffering is almost always rewarded with admiration, sympathy and direct material support in the form of pain-relieving medicines. However, those thought to complain excessively are discouraged from doing so, often they are regarded as weak, especially if the sufferer happens to be a man, and disapproval tends to be shown

242

verbally or practically by the withholding of analgesic drugs or the administration of placebo substances. These attitudes are widely held in our society and deeply rooted in our religious and philosophical heritage (Bond, 1980). It is in our interest to examine the historical origins of these attitudes and their consequence as a basis for 'resetting' our own feelings about those in pain if necessary.

The high value we place on the endurance of pain and suffering appears to have originated in the beliefs of the school of the mystic Greek philosopher, Pythagoras, who lived in the sixth century BC. The same attitude also existed in the ancient Hebrew civilisation. The Pythagoreans praised moral purity and, in particular, regarded the bearing of pain as one of the most important and effective means of developing self-discipline and self-control. At a much later date, the Christian Church of the Middle Ages in Europe, which had absorbed much of the teaching of Greek philosophers at an earlier date, viewed pain as evidence of sin, punishment for spiritual misdemeanours and a beneficial form of preparation for salvation after death. Presumably, therefore, there was considerable tolerance of pain and suffering of all kinds at a time when treatment was often lacking or ineffective.

Although the attitude that pain should be bravely borne persists today amongst many of the population, it appears to be weakening in the face of several forces which tend to undermine this belief. There seems to be an increasing number of patients who feel that they should not have to be in pain and who express considerable dissatisfaction at times with medical care which does not bring complete relief. This may be due in part to evidence from papers, magazines, radio and television that scientific medicine has made enormous progress this century, bringing with it the belief that control of pain should be possible. It may be related to lessening demands within certain sectors of society for personal self-control in speech and behaviour, and of the almost ceaseless exposure to the pain and suffering of others at a distance brought to us by means of the media. Perhaps most important of all, it may be the result of the demystification of Christianity and the removal of a reason for suffering, thereby making chronic pain seem useless, pointless and unacceptable.

The Nature of Pain and Development of Associated Behaviour

Pain is a subjective experience which arises as the result of an interaction between biological, psychological and environmental factors

Figure 11.1: The elements of pain experience and behaviours

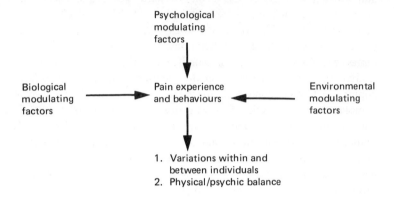

(Figure 11.1). Therefore, there are several ways in which pain problems may be analysed and treated; these are outlined in Table 11.1 from which it can be seen also that treatment may be provided in accordance with different approaches to pain and, of course, more than one approach and one treatment may be used for any given patient.

Table 11.1: Approaches to the investigation and management of chronic painful illnesses

Biological paradigm	Management techniques
Anatomy	Local analgesia
Physiology	Nerve blocks
Neurochemistry	Surgery
Pharmacology	Transcutaneous neural stimulation
	Acupuncture
	Analgesics and other drugs for pain
Psychological paradigm	
Personality	Psychotherapy
Mood	Behaviour therapy
Behaviour	Group psychotherapy
Interpersonal relations	Biofeedback
	Hypnotherapy
	Psychotropic drugs
Sociocultural paradigm	
Religio-philosophical concepts	Spiritual counselling

With very few exceptions, man is born with the capacity to react to noxious stimuli, and the behaviour associated with the experiences they produce, apart from the rapid reflex withdrawal of an injured part to an external stimulus, is learned and developed, especially during childhood and adolescence (Craig, 1980). Others, in particular parents and close relatives, mould attitudes and behaviour by acting as models when in pain themselves, by the directions they give and the reactions they show towards the child in pain. Pain due to any physical injury or disease experienced in childhood and personal methods of coping with it are carried forward into adult life in a modified form. In addition to coping with pain due to physical causes, the child also learns that complaints of pain may be used in one of several ways. For example, complaints of abdominal pain may serve to avoid unpleasant events — school tests or visits to the dentist. Children also learn that pain may be used to punish others. Boys learn that they must be brave in the face of pain and girls do so too, although they appreciate that less pressure to show fortitude is placed upon them. The use of complaints of pain to express distress is learned at an early age and the practice is common in adult life. This is only accepted to a limited extent by society and persistent use of the technique is regarded as abnormal. Therefore, patients who are deemed to complain unnecessarily are said to show 'abnormal sickness behaviour' and often pose difficulties for doctors faced with the problem of making diagnosis and prescribing treatment (Pilowsky, 1978).

One important therapeutic issue that arises from the comments made about cultural attitudes to pain concerns the attitudes of those who care for the person in pain, because they come from the same sources and are frequently reflected in the way in which they approach the pain sufferer. Therefore, the carer must be aware of his or her own attitudes and consider whether or not they are likely to bias treatment in a way that increases, or at best does not diminish, suffering. Despite the advances made in caring for the chronically ill, cultural attitudes already described exist and sometimes more negative effects may be compounded by ignorance of the psychological factors which influence pain and behaviour — a subject which is dealt with in the next section.

Coping with Chronic Pain

The Influence of Personality

Personality is that combination of mental traits which gives us our psychic individuality, and several personality characteristics are known to influence pain and associated behaviour (Bond, 1979). In addition, chronic pain produces changes in personality leading to exaggeration of some aspects and alteration in the balance of others. Also, basic personality characteristics are related to the ways in which individuals cope with distress, including chronic pain. As implied earlier, certain coping strategies are learned and developed in childhood, whereas others develop later, even in adult life.

The inborn traits of introversion and extroversion influence both pain intensity and complaint behaviour (Bond and Pearson, 1969). Put simply, those who are primarily introverted experience more pain than those who are extroverts, but complain less about their suffering. Therefore, complaint behaviour amongst patients is influenced to a considerable extent by this trait and reports of pain tend to be high amongst extroverts. These fundamental differences in the freedom with which patients complain about their feelings and suffering may well play a part in the noticeable difference in the way people respond to the administration of standard doses of analgesic drugs. For example, for a given body-weight dose an extroverted patient is more likely to complain of residual pain than an introverted person, and it may be felt that either the analgesic has been less effective for the extrovert or that he or she is complaining excessively, having been given what is regarded as adequate treatment (Bond, Glynn and Thomas, 1976).

It is known that a predisposition to emotional breakdown under stress is closely correlated with the ease with which individuals develop anxiety, and that levels of pain experienced in any given condition are related to levels of anxiety. Therefore, those who are most prone to develop anxiety are liable to do so more readily when they become ill and, if in pain, to experience greater levels of pain. Furthermore, in its turn the very presence of pain increases anxiety and it is easy to see how high levels of pain and anxiety may result and be accentuated by inadequate treatment. The latter may be the result of the use of inappropriate analgesics, doses that are insufficient to control pain and incorrect timing. Thus it is much better to anticipate increasing pain than to permit it to rise to high levels. Therefore, a regime tailored to patients' needs is the most effective method of combatting pain by pharmacological means. At the same time, other potential causes of anxiety, in other words the threats and dangers related to the illness and its treatment, or to social problems arising from it, must be dealt with in order to obtain complete treatment for pain. Failure to treat pain adequately is often related in the patient's mind solely to inadequate medication, and at times drugs will be asked for when they are not needed and be 'hoarded' for some future occasion. Amongst those with chronic illness, feelings of depression are quite common for several reasons. First, chronic illness leads to various losses; second, control of pain may be inadequate; and the appearance of new symptoms is a third and potent cause. The feeling that doctors and nurses have lost control over the disease or have lost interest in the patient adds considerably to anxiety and depression. Thus a patient's perception of staff attitudes to pain control, whether correct or not in terms of what the staff are really doing, is very important as a means of increasing or decreasing anxiety. At a practical level, adequate active reassurance that control is being sought and that interest levels are high are essential ingredients of treatment.

Those who are over-concerned with their health and bodily function, whether this is reflected in frequent visits to their family doctor with a series of trivial complaints, frequent self-administration of proprietary medicines or excessive concern about diet, weight and physical fitness, are regarded as showing evidence of a hypochondriacal nature. Kenyon (1976) proposed that, 'hypochondriacal traits, symptoms, ideas and fears should carry with them the implication that there is morbid preoccupation with mental or physical function or the state of health'. This trait is common and those who have it tend to be more anxious and introspective. In more general terms, increased concern about symptoms, especially pain, is a feature of illness of all kinds and it is particularly prominent amongst those who are hypochondriacal. For example, studies of women with cancer pain revealed increased levels of hypochondriasis when compared with a healthy population, but the levels did not reach those of individuals attending a psychiatric clinic (Bond, 1971). Another interesting aspect of this study was that further analysis of the elements of hypochondriasis as proposed by Pilowsky (1967) revealed that patients without pain exhibited a strong denial of serious physical illness, although they did accept the presence of somatic symptoms. Thus one of the commonest human responses to stress of a potentially life-threatening nature, namely denial, emerges as part of an attitude to illness which has associations with a preoccupation with the function of the body. The point being made is that intense focusing of interest upon symptoms thrusts their meaning and significance into the background and this point is taken up again later.

To conclude this section on the relation between personality and pain experience, consideration is given to the role of hysterical qualities in the personality. Individuals with hysterical personality traits, most commonly women, are immature, dramatic, extroverted and shallow in their affections. They seek excitement and attention, dress for effect and seem to enjoy emotional clashes with others who tend to retire hurt, angry or baffled. Symptoms of illness tend to be exaggerated by these characteristics and the main problems for the clinician are, first, placing the symptoms in their true perspective against the background of clinical signs detected, and second, dealing with the hysteric's intense desire for immediate relief and low capacity to cope with stress. Alternative consultations, medicines and treatments may be demanded and the doctor may feel propelled towards unnecessary investigations which will only result in more confusion and tension for the sufferer. A firm detached clinical approach is needed at such times!

Changes in Mood in Patients with Chronic Pain

The previous section dealt with ways in which pre-morbid personality factors influence pain levels and associated behaviour. Many of the changes described are most likely to be seen amongst those with relatively short histories and less serious conditions, whereas in contrast prolonged painful illness and the significance of that illness to the patient have a powerful influence upon the feelings and behaviour tending to some extent to overshadow pre-morbid personality factors. Moreover, chronic illnesses, especially those which end in death, are marked by groups of symptoms which change with time. Some of them, for example, vomiting, diarrhoea and breathlessness, are extremely distressing and occur at the same time as pain. Therefore, chronic illness, especially cancer, produces a state of mind marked by uncertainty and dread of the future. The sufferer is apprehensive about the eventual and often known outcome, commonly fearing increasing pain, perhaps mutilation by the disease or its treatment, and possibly death. There is evidence suggesting that pain heightens emotional responses to chronic illness, which include increased vegetative signs (impaired appetite, levels of activity and energy), mental changes including irritability, anger, hostility, anxiety, depression, withdrawal of interest, altered relationships with others and increased somatic preoccupation. Apart from fears about the actual suffering and its meaning, patients' moods are altered by the feelings of loss of vitality, usefulness, relationships, work and pleasure. The intensity of his or her feelings intensifies rapidly if the patient senses that the doctor has reached the limit of his power and when fresh symptoms occur. In fact, helplessness in the face of advancing disease and hopelessness induced by failure to halt its progress form a fertile ground for the development of depression and may hasten death. The difficulties in determining whether a patient is depressed in terms a psychiatrist would use, or in misery, are greatest in chronic-pain patients with many symptoms other than pain that are taken as evidence of the biological features of depression in psychiatric patients. Plumb and Holland (1977) examined this problem in cancer patients and found that they were not more depressed than their relatives and significantly less depressed than physically healthy patients admitted to hospital following a suicidal attempt. In fact, most cancer patients and their relatives were not depressed. Others have produced results indicating that radiotherapy produces depressive feelings, but not clinical depression. Hinton (1963) found that slightly less than half of a group of dying cancer patients were mildly to severely depressed and Hackett and Weissman (1969) and Craig and Abloff (1974) produced similar figures for terminally ill cancer patients. Plumb and Holland note that patients who were under 34 years of age reported more non-somatic complaints than older patients. They also observed that in adolescents loss of personal attractiveness, being different from peers, worries about career, spouse and family are more marked. Finally, none of the surveys reported showed any increase in the incidence of depression in relation to the nearness of death. It was concluded that a negative change in self-image in a cancer patient is the most urgent indication for a psychiatric consultation.

In the later stages of terminal illness many patients are aware of the approach of death, although few may mention this directly. At this time preoccupation with physical symptoms, especially pain, may become an unconscious means of dealing with the fear of dying or become a means of communicating increasing emotional distress about dying. There is also an interesting change in some patients' attitudes to pain at this time. Whereas at an early stage pain had been regarded as an integral part of the illness, the patients' comments show that it seems to have become an alien entity, as unwelcome though often commanding total attention, as invasive, malign, almost tangible and coming from without the self. It seems to overwhelm other psychic functions and this may be part of the process of dealing with an unavoidable experience which is physically and emotionally destructive. Having become a major preoccupation, paradoxically, the daily battle with pain may become essential for the preservation of life! This comment is based on the occasional observation that at times of sudden total relief of severe chronic pain in patients with advanced cancer, for example, by cordotomy, there is a period of complete calm that lasts only a few days and ends in death. Whatever its base, whether biological or psychological, the well-intentioned reason for removing the struggle for life appears to bring it to an abrupt but comfortable end.

Mental Defence Mechanisms

Methods of coping with pain are expressed in mental and behavioural terms. As stated at the beginning of this chapter, in an evaluation of suffering, pain cannot be considered in isolation from other physical aspects of the illness and the influence of external factors, including interpersonal relations and environmental conditions. Earlier comments indicate that the presence of chronic pain tends to enhance emotional responses to illness and, if severe, it tends to add significantly to physical incapacity.

At the mental level, responses to pain appear to relate chiefly to the underlying threats posed by the illness in terms of the losses it might cause — including, ultimately, the sufferer's death and disintegration of the self. Acute and chronic severe illnesses that are life-threatening evoke a series of reactions known as mental defence mechanisms. A mental defence mechanism is a specific intrapsychic process which operates unconsciously, relieving the patient from emotional conflict and thereby preventing overwhelming anxiety. The mechanism most often cited in the literature is *denial*. In the case of denial, an external reality or realities — for example, the threat of mutilation, prolonged suffering or death, any of which is likely to be consciously intolerable to the sufferer — do not emerge into consciousness. Denial is often marked in individuals who suffer acute illnesses; for example, the sufferer of an acute myocardial infarction may, if chest pain is mild or moderate, ignore it or regard it as being due to some form of gastric upset, in which case he or she may take antacids. However, the fact that there is an underlying concern about the possibility of a more serious cause for the pain is reflected in the patient's behaviour. For example, in the case of a man, he may carry out a number of 'press-ups' or run upstairs, just to prove to himself that the pain is not really serious. Denial operating in this form cannot be regarded as entirely protective, although its intention is to allay unconscious anxieties and fears. By contrast, in chronic life-threatening disorders the features of denial serve as a positive and protective reaction which waxes and wanes with variations in the disease process.

Other mental mechanisms which reduce anxiety are also a feature of both acute and chronic disorders and include *repression* — a process which leads to the banishment of unacceptable ideas from consciousness and which leads to the failure of information about the life-threatening nature of illness to merge into consciousness. This should be contrasted with *suppression* — a consciously determined process of avoiding consideration of the implications of the symptoms experienced. In this regard, concentration upon pain and the means of obtaining relief from it may be regarded as a positive feature, not due solely to its commanding nature, because focusing of interest and thought in this way directs the mind from more unpleasant and threatening issues, contemplation of which may do more harm than good.

The chief purpose of the mechanisms described so far is protection from stress and anxiety aroused by suffering and pain. However, this does not mean that patients in pain are not anxious; in fact their anxieties are considerable, but they are often focused upon symptoms and treatment, rather than the ultimate meaning of their condition. The disabling effects of painful chronic disorders lead to withdrawal from many activities of daily life. The extent to which this happens depends not only upon the degree of physical debility and disability, but also upon the individual's tendency to assume a more dependent role, in other words, his or her tendency to *regress*. Regression, another mental defence mechanism, is a process of retreat into a more childlike and dependent form of thinking and behaviour with the expectation that others will care and take over various responsibilities from the sufferer. The extent to which it happens varies and seems to be most marked in those with an immature pre-morbid personality. They develop considerable anxiety and are unwilling to take responsibility or make decisions. They seek attention and often make heavy demands upon medical services, involving doctors in frequent home visits and at the same time bombarding them with requests for powerful analgesics. If in hospital, the patient may rapidly become unwilling to leave its secure and supportive environment. These features are illustrated by the following case history.

Mrs A. A young married woman with several children, Mrs A. had a chronically painful and progressive but benign disease affecting her lumbar spine and sacrum. She had had many orthopaedic and neurosurgical investigations and several admissions to hospital. Her disorder was not amenable to surgical treatment and her pain was controlled adequately by regular use of analgesics of moderate potency (dihydrocodeine and Distalgesic). Unfortunately, a close member of her family developed breast cancer which progressed rapidly, placing Mrs A. in a position in which she was under considerable pressure to deal with her relative's domestic problems and basic physical needs. At this point, Mrs A. began to complain of considerable increase in her own pain. She called her family doctor frequently, often in the night, begging him to prescribe more powerful analgesic drugs, and her husband was obliged to take over almost all the household duties. His reaction was to drink heavily, and both withdrew from their few social contacts outside the home. Further neurosurgical investigations were performed which showed no evidence of progression of the disease process. Eventually psychiatric help was sought and admission to a psychiatric ward in a general hospital was arranged. Investigations revealed that Mrs A. was an immature anxious woman who had been moderately dependent upon various members of her family for several years, though for the most part equilibrium had been established. It had been noted previously that at times of stress Mrs A. became anxious, complained of more pain and needed more domestic help. A management programme was devised consisting of organised practical help for the sick relative, because it was unrealistic to expect Mrs A. to take on the amount of physical work needed or the emotional demands of the individual concerned. Psychiatric help was offered in the form of regular out-patient appointments for both Mr and Mrs A., the objective being to deal with practical difficulties and emotional problems that might arise at home. Finally, it was decided to keep the period of hospital admission as short as possible. Within twenty-four hours of admission, Mrs A.'s pain had decreased considerably and far less analgesic was required for pain control. She became cheerful and the relief of her husband's tension was also obvious. Longer-term plans for management were partially successful and during periods of greatly increased stress Mrs A. began to demand analgesics from her general practitioner as before, but these situations were dealt with fairly easily by additional appointments with the psychiatrist and further hospital admission was avoided.

This patient's case history demonstrates other aspects of an individual's failure to cope with stress and pain. For example, although never mentioned, Mrs A. was very angry with her family doctor because he was reluctant, or an occasions refused, to visit her home on the grounds that he could not offer her further help — a comment which aroused Mrs A.'s anger and, at the same time, made her feel very isolated and anxious about having to bear very severe pain. In other words, her behaviour led to a breakdown in the doctor/patient relationship, a matter only resolved by her admission to hospital. Thus, whatever adjustments Mrs A. achieved mentally, in her domestic and social life, collapsed when she was under severe stress and, in particular, her ability to bear pain was almost abolished.

The need for resourcefulness, planning ability and, above all, emotional stability in close family members is clearly necessary if a pain sufferer is showing signs of failure to cope with pain, other physical symptoms or adverse problems in life. Obviously Mr A. did not possess these qualities sufficiently to cope with the dual pressures of serious illness in two members of his family. His failure and consequent heavy drinking is a well-established response to stress.

It is clear that coping with chronic pain results in mood changes and, although often not as obvious as anxiety, depression, irritability and anger are important feelings which may differ from others by being expressed in terms of the failures of medical or nursing staff to provide relief or cure. In other words, patients' angry feelings about their own failures, frailties or frustrations are *displaced* to others – an example of yet another defence mechanism. The sensitive carer may feel very hurt by such accusations or implied feelings; therefore we should understand their origin and avoid any tendency to alienate the patient. Clearly, it is important to discuss a patient's angry feelings and hostility in an attempt to discharge this emotion and then to provide practical help.

Behavioural Reactions

Behaviours associated with different personality traits, behaviour changes accompanying alterations of mood and those developing as a result of the operation of certain mental defences have been outlined. Other behavioural changes occur specifically in relation to pain and two are of particular importance: namely, the development of behaviour directed towards obtaining ever-increasing amounts of analgesic medicines; and the development of behaviour which indicates that the sufferer has moved towards increasing his or her 'gains' from being in pain and, in particular, to increased dependency. The second of these developments is a particular problem in the management of chronic pain arising from benign lesions and both have implications for long-term management.

The development of habituation of addiction to drugs, in particular to narcotic analgesics, is a constant source of anxiety for many nurses and quite a number of doctors. In some cases this may lead to the with-holding of medicines of appropriate strength, to the administration of inadequate doses, or to early termination of treatment. The work of the hospice movement and, in particular, the studies of those at St Christopher's Hospice in London, led by Dame Cicily Saunders, and the Oxford group at Sir Michael Sobell House, led by Dr Robert Twy-cross, have advanced the techniques for handling problems associated with the control of pain in terminal illness to a very great extent and their accounts of the patient's last days and hours are a testimony to this. However, matters are less satisfactorily handled in other areas where caring for the chronically ill in pain takes place. The following case history illustrates this point.

Mrs B.   A 45-year-old married woman with breast cancer, Mrs B. had secondary deposits in her thoracic spine. She was admitted to a general surgical ward and it was noted that her emotional distress was extreme and that her complaints of pain were loud and frequent. The staff were at first sympathetic, but soon became angry with the woman because of her complaint behaviour. In a short time they resorted to the use of morphine and then to heroin, as a result of which the patient developed symptoms of addiction. Her demands for increasingly frequent injections were rebuffed and she would beg for treatment.

This very distressing problem must be an extreme example of failure to cope with an emotionally distressed person who, in this case, died without resolution of her emotional or pain problems. It illustrates a total lack of ability on the part of the nurses and doctors concerned to engage the patient in a therapeutic relationship and is somewhat unusual because of the way they appeared to prescribe powerful narcotic analgesics without regard for the consequences. It is almost certain that the incessant nature of the patient's complaints reflected her feelings of extreme anxiety about the outcome of her illness, a sense of isolation from those who might provide her with help and her anger with them for not providing the comfort she needed.

Initial success in treating the emotional and physical problems presented by patients with chronic pain may well lead to dependency and this is illustrated in the following case.

Mr C. A 60-year-old married man with advanced chronic chest and heart disease that might cause his death at any moment had, in addition, long-standing pain in his back, related to ageing processes in the lumbar spine. He was cared for at home by his wife and by his family doctor who visited regularly, but not frequently. Visits to a cardiologist were made at six-month intervals. The family doctor began to receive an increasing number of calls, including night calls, from the patient's wife who asked 'for something strong' for her husband's back pain. Palfium was prescribed and later taken by the patient in ever-increasing amounts until his family doctor felt that he had become addicted. The advice of the cardiologist was sought and the patient was referred to a psychiatrist at a pain clinic for assessment. As a result, he was admitted to a psychiatric ward for drug withdrawal and discussion of the problems posed for both him and his wife by his illness and, in particular, his pain. Withdrawal of the medication was achieved with remarkable ease, and both the patient and his wife expressed great relief at having been given an opportunity to discuss the significance of the patient's other physical problems and the fact that his life was drawing to a close. It was revealed that the calls to the doctor occurred at times when the patient or his wife began to feel considerable anxiety about the progression of symptoms of breathlessness and chest pain, and they were aimed chiefly at gaining reassurance from him that the disease was under control even though their requests for help came through the demands for analgesics. It is clear that the family doctor did not recognise the signals, or act upon them if he did, and the reduction in tension brought about by the development of a channel for discussion was the way in which a reduction in medication was achieved. The patient improved mentally and physically. However, it was noticed that his dependency moved from drugs to the ward staff and, as the time drew near for his discharge, his anxieties about leaving hospital increased very considerably and had to be dealt with by means of a series of discussions before he was able to return home. The main issue concerned the question of the availability of continuing care and the channel of communication through which anxieties might be dealt. The matter was discussed with the family doctor who took up the challenge and the patient's further care was successfully managed by him and the cardiologist.

This case illustrates how increasing anxiety about illness may be manifest in increased requests for treatment of pain and how, given an understanding and supportive environment, a fearful and anxious patient rapidly develops dependency. Mr C. was clearly very loath to leave the security of the hospital ward, a feeling that was increased by his experiences prior to admission.

Role of Psychotropic Drugs

Psychotropic drugs are used in the management of pain in three ways.

First, neuroleptic drugs (for example, chlorpromazine) are commonly used to supplement other medicines in the treatment of severe pain caused by physical diseases, especially cancer and certain chronic neuralgias. Next, anxiolytics are of value, especially in the short term, in the control of anxiety and tension associated with physical illness or disease. Finally, antidepressants are used to treat mental disorders in which pain is a major symptom, but this use of psychotropic drugs will not be considered further.

The Anxiolytics

The benzodiazepine group is the most common member of this family of drugs used for control of anxiety caused by pain, or anxiety reactions giving rise to pain (Herrington, 1982). They do not have a direct analgesic effect, and in higher doses cause mental slowness, drowsiness and induce sleep. It is clear that they reduce anxiety by inhibiting the diffusely projecting reticular system. In addition, some compounds act more peripherally, for example, diazepam relaxes striated muscle, and in any painful disorder in which local inflammation gives rise to muscle spasm, the drug both calms and reduces pain locally. All members of the group tend to produce habituation with both psychological and physical withdrawal symptoms developing under appropriate circumstances. Sudden withdrawal from patients who have been on high doses for some weeks may precipitate epileptic seizures, as the following case history demonstrates.

> *Mrs D.*   A 40-year-old woman, Mrs D. suffered from multiple sclerosis which was slowly progressive and which gave rise to severe pain in both legs. By nature she was an anxious woman with hysterical features in her personality, and her home life was gradually disintegrating as a result of the friction between herself and her husband. The family doctor prescribed analgesics and diazepam to control pain and the patient's emotional distress. Unfortunately she took far more tablets than he prescribed and became habituated. During a domestic crisis she was admitted to hospital, where nothing was known of her drug habituation initially. Diazepam was not prescribed and the patient developed status epilepticus within the next 24 hours. Fortunately the attack was brought under control and the woman survived the ordeal. Thus care must be taken when prescribing benzodiazepines.

Differences between these drugs are due largely to their variations in metabolism. A number of drugs have long half-lives because they are metabolised slowly via several intermediaries (for example, diazepam, chlordiazepoxide and medazepam) and have prolonged effects. Others are rapidly excreted by the kidney, have briefer half-lives and shorter effects (for example, oxazepam, lorazepam and temazepam). Flurazepam and nitrazepam have long-lasting effects and their plasma levels rise slowly; in the case of diazepam, it may take several weeks to reach a plateau level. Their differences in metabolism dictate the use of these drugs. Long-acting compounds like diazepam are of value where anxiety is severe, and chronic and shorter-acting drugs are useful in control of acute anxiety and panic attacks. Drugs used as hypnotics should act rapidly to induce sleep and be metabolised quickly to avoid hangover effects, and for this purpose lorazepam, temazepam and triazolam are indicated.

The propanediols are also anxiolytic and meprobamate, which is both a minor tranquilliser and a muscle relaxant, is a member of this group which is used occasionally. However, it belongs to a generation of compounds that produce marked drowsiness and is dangerous if taken in an overdose. It is also liable to cause habituation, with epilepsy on sudden withdrawal after massive doses.

The Antidepressants

Tricyclic antidepressants in their tertiary form (for example, imipramine and amitryptiline) have both antidepressant and analgesic properties. The former take up to two weeks to become effective and the latter become obvious within a day or so. As mentioned previously, many chronic painful illnesses produce misery, but the development of deep depression is far less common, especially in cancer patients (Plumb and Holland, 1977). True depression is typified by feelings of a very depressed mood, a sense of guilt, loss of self-worth and perhaps suicidal thoughts, although these are relatively uncommon. The feelings are unrelieved by changes in physical symptoms or changes in the environment designed to improve the patient's comfort or peace of mind. As mentioned previously, the evaluation of psychiatric patient is difficult because several of them (for example, weight loss, poor appetite and disturbed sleep) are commonly found in progressive and debilitating diseases. Therefore, the decision to use antidepressants should be made on the basis of the patient's mental state. As depression of mood is also associated with increased feelings of pain, satisfactory treatment of a depressed chronically ill patient should improve both his or her mental state and reduce the intensity of pain. The antidepressant selected should be used in the full doses, but unfortunately the tricyclic group have unpleasant side-effects related to their many anticholinergic properties and also they are cardiotoxic. Therefore it may be better to select a member of the newer tetracyclic group, for example, mianserin, which has relatively few side-effects and can be given once daily and at bedtime. It is not known whether this group of antidepressants has analgesic properties.

The Neuroleptics

This group of drugs is used chiefly in the treatment of major psychoses. The phenothiazines, which are related to the tricyclic antidepressants, have primary analgesic effects and potentiate the analgesic effects of opiates. This group of drugs is often used in physical medicine as a supplement to narcotic analgesics in the treatment of chronic pain. Chlorpromazine is favoured by many and should be given in doses of 25 mg in association with the selected narcotic. Two other members of the group, pericyazine and perphenazine, may be used in the same way. Fluphenazine, a fluorinated piperazine derivative of the phenothiazines, has been shown to reduce pain significantly in some patients with chronic pain due to diabetic neuropathy. Chlorprothixene, a thioxanthine analogue of chlorpromazine, gives relief from another, post-herpetic neuralgia, if given in high doses for only five days. Herpes Zoster occurs quite often amongst patients with cancer who have received radiotherapy, and this drug might be considered in the palliation of this aspect of the disease and its treatment. However, caution is needed because it produces drowsiness, tiredness and perhaps faintness or vertigo. In other words, the drug is only useful as a last resort in patients with intolerable levels of pain.

Use of Psychological Methods in Palliation of Chronic Pain

Fear, concern and a firm belief that, given appropriate physical methods are used, pain should be relieved lie at the heart of the feelings and thoughts of those who suffer chronic pain. Patients look to doctors, whom they see as parental or authority figures, for relief of symptoms in a way that may well place the doctor beyond his or her ability to produce the desired result; in other words, the doctor is invested with omnipotence by his patient. Those who are physically ill need to feel that doctors take their illness seriously, they expect action of some sort from him and, should interest fail or relief not materialise, angry feelings may be aroused. However, such feelings are seldom openly expressed, as patients tend to fear rejection and abandonment to their fate by the doctor.

Recognition of the fact that important emotional elements are present does not mean that a doctor can or will attempt to deal with them using psychological methods. All too often further investigation and drug treatments, that is, medical activity, take the place of an attempt to deal with emotions until eventually, unable to solve the patient's problem, the doctor passes him or her on to another colleague, and so a chain of referrals is established. This is, in part, related to medical training and attitudes, but it is only fair to point out that many clinics for sufferers of chronic pain are not organised in a way that permits doctors to attend to psychological problems, thus reducing the possibility of meeting emotional needs. Fortunately, dealing with emotions requires skills that are not solely in the possession of doctors. Others take up responsibility, often as part of a team which includes a doctor; the other members of the team may be nurses, psychologists, social workers and ministers of religion. The team approach to the management of chronic pain is established in certain areas of medicine. For example, the care of the terminally ill, and the development of psycho-social resources is taking place, albeit rather slowly, in pain clinics.

Psychotherapy

Psychotherapy, a means of helping patients overcome emotional distress by the establishment of a therapeutic relationship through the means of discussion, is a form of treatment used amongst those with painful physical illnesses. When using psychotherapy, it is essential to ensure that the physical needs of the sick person are met as fully as possible. This is what patients expect and deserve. Psychotherapeutic techniques must be used in parallel with physical treatments; in their simplest form they are practised consciously or unconsciously by many who carefully and sympathetically explain the facts of the disease and meet whatever needs the patients have to know about its investigation, treatment and prognosis. Considerable reassurance in these areas is needed, because of the many fears and fantasies patients have about their bodies, about illness and about medical care.

A more sophisticated approach is needed when dealing with the emotions, anxiety and depression, fear, frustration and anger, that may arise despite, or even as a result of, fairly simple discussions about illness. Ideally, these matters should be dealt with by a person who has training and experience in psychotherapy with the physically ill.

The aim of the therapist is to develop a relationship between him/herself and the patient by means of a series of discussions that can be used as a therapeutic tool. Brief psychotherapy involving 12 to 25 sessions of 45 minutes each is used widely in the world of psychiatry, but with the ill and seriously debilitated the duration of sessions and their number may have to be reduced. Therapy proceeds through several stages (Pilowsky and Bassett, 1982).

Assessment. In the first stage the therapist focuses upon the patient's pain and other physical symptoms, showing empathy and a strong positive regard for them. Although we tend to think that all complaints of pain are really physical matters, especially in those who have a definite organic illness, complaints may act as a means of expressing wider feelings of suffering, beginning with difficulties about bearing pain and extending into worries about matters beyond the self. If, as is also the case, the patient cannot express his or her feelings in words initially and uses somatic language for this purpose, acknowledgement of the fact usually leads on to discussion of emotional and interpersonal issues without difficulty. The fact that the therapist shows interest and concern about physical suffering is important, as patients often interpret discussions of emotional issues as an indication that their pain is being regarded as imaginary, or that they are losing their reason, or that there is no hope for them. For these reasons, anger is encountered at times and the therapist must be prepared to deal with it in order to move on to the next stage.

Intervention. Approaching emotional issues carefully, and having pointed out the psychotherapist's part of the team's approach to the illness, the therapist should explain that his role is to help the patient with emotional problems produced by being ill and in pain. The therapist must make it clear that there are limitations to what can be achieved, thereby removing the patient's fantasies or fears that his or her mind will be taken over and that the therapist has ultimate power to heal. So far, the approach has been to gain the patient's confidence; having been successful and identified the main area of emotional and interpersonal difficulty as seen by him or her, the therapist begins the main task of this phase – the exploration of problems. Interestingly, once this stage has been reached, patients often talk less and less about physical problems and pain, especially when the illness is chronic and not marked by suddern alterations in symptoms, and where pain intensity is related to emotional problems, as in the case of Mr C. referred to earlier.

Supportive therapy is probably the most common form of psychotherapy used amongst those who are seriously physically ill and in pain, and also those who have chronic benign disorders and do not possess a sufficient level of insight into their own inner life needed for more extended therapy. Having identified the patient's problems and means of coping with them, the therapist seeks to strengthen strategies which are positive and constructive, for example, use of methods for gaining distraction from pain and techniques for socialising. The therapist is very active, makes suggestions that will lead to emotional and social improvements, and encourages the patient to take up and try out the methods suggested. At this point, it may be an advantage to add a related psycho-physiological treatment – for example, relaxation – which increases the benefits of psychotherapy by giving the patient feelings of increased self-control over the body's functions. Improving self-control and ego strength are key matters in this form of therapy. The following example illustrates a number of the points made.

Mr E. A 40-year-old unemployed man, Mr E. suffered from chronic back pain and sciatica. He had had intermittent episodes of back pain only over a period of ten years and then suffered a severe attack of pain with sciatica. This was relieved by a period of bed rest at home, but was followed two years later by a further attack, which did not respond to treatment. He was admitted to hospital, where management included traction, followed by physiotherapy designed to improve the strength of his back muscles. However, the pain was not relieved appreciably, but the patient was sent home and further care was left in the hands of his family doctor who, after a brief period, stopped visiting the patient and gave every sign of having lost interest in him.

Mr E. was constantly in pain, he gave up all interest in his family, he gave up leaving the house and he moved into one room downstairs where, at night, he would sleep on the floor. He felt that his family showed decreasing interest in his plight and eventually became quite depressed. Eventually, twelve months after his last visit, the family doctor was called again as Mr E. would not eat, was depressed and talked of suicide. He was admitted to a psychiatric unit. Examination revealed that he felt abandoned by doctors at the hospital to which he had been admitted previously, by the general practitioner and by his family. He had become increasingly angry and resentful at first, but gradually his anger changed to feelings of depression and a belief that he faced a life of pain and isolation.

The therapist examined Mr E. and arranged for a series of physical investigations, after which he explained the results to him. Much to his surprise, Mr E. discovered that his physical deficits were relatively minor and that he was able to walk without crutches or even a stick with the therapist's encouragement. Physical treatment was continued by physiotherapists, whilst the psychotherapist discussed with the patient his feelings of anger concerning doctors and his family. At a later point the discussions, which included his wife on several occasions, became more constructive and involved a development of ways of repairing family relations and examining future prospects for work and leisure. After six sessions Mr E. had become cheerful, enjoyed his visits to physiotherapy and walked well, though with a limp. He was discharged home, following discussions with his general practitioner about the nature of the problems uncovered. At his first visit to the out-patient clinic a month later, Mr E. described his family relations as being transformed and proudly announced that he had been able to travel to hospital unaccompanied on a bus and without any form of mechanical support.

Completion. It is important to let the patient know in advance that therapy will be limited in time, but the therapist should not destroy his or her expectation of positive results − a key ingredient in therapy. Depending upon the therapist is the main potential difficulty, especially when neglect by other doctors has been a major problem in the past. Anxieties lessen if management brings significant relief from symptoms and emotional problems, making completion a relatively simple matter. Some therapists follow their patients for a further limited period, seeing them at intervals of three or four weeks, whereas others explain that it is necessary to hand over care to the team in charge of physical problems, having first discussed aspects of the patient's emotions with team members. Arrangements for this stage of treatment are so dependent upon the nature of the patient's problems and local resources and attitudes to care, that no hard and fast rules are possible.

Other Psychological Treatments

Apart from individual psychotherapy, the techniques available for the management of pain problems include group therapy, behaviour therapy, biofeedback and hypnosis. The first three are used almost exclusively amongst patients with chronic pain, especially those who have pain that has a trivial physical cause or those who have pain for which no physical explanation can be given; in other words, amongst those for whom being in pain has become a way of life. Group and behaviour therapies share similar objectives, namely, the correction of faulty behaviour (for example, the need for attention, rest or medication) by providing a combination of insight into the use of pain (group therapy), and a means of learning more appropriate forms of behaviour that lead to better relations with others, some capacity for work and for leisure (behaviour therapy). Biofeedback is essentially a technique used to obtain muscle relaxation amongst those in whom tension-induced pains (for example, muscle headaches) are a major problem. Hypnosis is of greatest value in the management of acute pain and has a definite place in the reduction or abolition of pain in childbirth, dentistry and other forms of minor surgery.

Of the four therapies, group therapy is the only one used to any extent amongst sufferers from chronic pain due to physical disease. For example, it is employed by those who care for haemophilic patients and sufferers of chronic arthritis conditions, especially rheumatoid arthritis. The main aims of therapy are to provide information about the disease process and its treatment and outcome, to deal with attitudes to suffering, and to provide some sense of mastery over the condition (Baptiste and Herman, 1982). The inclusion of individuals who have improved as a result of group participation in the past increases optimism, and a clear definition of group goals – for example, control of medication – together with realistically laying out the probable outcome of the disease, all enhance the chances of success. The realisation by the patients that they are not alone and that their problems can be seen in others, or by others, gives support and a sense that control of pain and emotion may be obtained. Self-defeating attitudes and negative self-regard may be dispelled, and irrational fears and beliefs removed by discussion and learning. Groups tend to become less dependent on the therapist with the passage of time and begin to exert their own authority. Usually they run for eight or nine weeks with meetings once a week, and on conclusion members often retain contact, which helps to reinforce the gains made during group therapy.

To conclude, the psychological aspects of chronic pain are many and varied. Attitudes, personality, mood state and behaviour all contribute to the clinical picture. Palliation is the theme of this book and it is clear that this objective can never be obtained amongst those who suffer chronic pain, unless there is knowledge of psychological processes involved and a willingness to apply psychological methods of management in appropriate circumstances.

References

Baptiste, S. and Herman, E. (1982) 'Group psychotherapy. A specific model', in R. Roy and E. Tunks (eds), *Chronic Pain, Psychosocial Factors in Rehabilitation*, Williams and Wilkins, Baltimore and London, pp. 166–79

Bond, M.R. (1971) 'The relation of pain to the Eysenck Personality Inventory, Cornell Medical Index and Whiteley Index of Hypochondriasis', *British Journal of Psychiatry*, 119, 671–8

Bond, M.R. (1979) *Pain, its Nature, Analysis and Treatment*, Churchill Livingstone, Edinburgh, London and New York

Bond, M.R. (1980) 'The suffering of severe intractable pain', in H.W. Kosterlitz and L.Y. Terenius (eds), *Pain and Society*, Dahlem Konferenzen, Verlag Chemie, Weinheim, pp. 53–62

Bond, M.R. and Pearson, I.B. (1969) 'Psychological aspects of pain in women with advanced carcinoma of the cervix', *Journal of Psychosomatic Research*, 13, 13–19

Bond, M.R., Glynn, J.P. and Thomas, D.G. (1976) 'The relation between pain and personality in patients receiving pentazocine (Fortral) after surgery', *Journal of Psychosomatic Research*, 30, 369–81

Craig, K.D. (1980) 'Ontogenic and cultural influences on the expressions of pain in man', in H.W. Kosterlitz and L.Y. Terenius (eds), *Pain and Society,* Dahlem Konferenzen, Verlag Chemie, Weinheim, pp. 37–52

Craig, T.J. and Abloff, M.D. (1974) 'Psychiatric symptomatology amongst hospitalised cancer patients', *American Journal of Psychiatry*, 131, 1323

Hackett, T.P. and Weissman, A.D. (1969) 'Denial as a factor in patients with heart disease and cancer', *Annals of the New York Academy of Sciences*, 164, 802

Herrington, R.N. (1982) *Anxiety and Depression*, Update Postgraduate Centre series, 2nd edn, Update Publications, London

Hinton, J.M. (1963) 'The physical and mental distress of the dying', *Quarterly Journal of Medicine*, 32, 1–21

Kenyon, F.E. (1976) 'Hypochondriacal states', *British Journal of Psychiatry*, 129, 55–60

Lobb, T. (1739) *A Practical Treatise of Painful Distempers*, James Buckland, London

Pilowsky, I. (1967) 'Dimensions of hypochondriasis', *British Journal of Psychiatry*, 113, 89–93

Pilowsky, I. (1978) 'A general classification of abnormal illness behaviours', *British Journal of Medical Psychology*, 51, 131–7

Pilowsky, I. and Bassett, D. (1982) 'Individual dynamic psychotherapy for chronic pain', in R. Roy and E. Tunks (eds), *Chronic Pain, Psychosocial Factors in Rehabilitation*, Williams and Wilkins, Baltimore and London, pp. 107–26

Plumb, M.M. and Holland, J. (1977) 'Comparative studies of psychological function in patients with advanced cancer: I. Self-reported depressive symptoms', *Psychosomatic Medicine*, 39, 264–76

12 THE PHYSICAL CONTROL OF PAIN

Derek Doyle

The psychological aspects of the treatment of chronic pain have been dealt with in Chapter 11, in which Michael Bond has eloquently stressed that one cannot even attempt to control chronic pain without due attention to the patient's personality, psychological coping mechanisms, attitude both to pain and suffering, and his total psycho-socio-spiritual needs. As will be demonstrated shortly, there are many possible reasons for failure to alleviate the pain of the dying patient, but in many such patients one of the principal reasons will often be the unscientific reliance on the purely physical methods to be outlined in this chapter. It cannot be stated too strongly that a purely 'pharmacological' approach, no matter how skilled, is bound to fail in many patients. Readers, both medical and nursing, are urged to study Chapter 11 before attempting to assimilate what follows. Although their pioneer physicians never intended it to be so, it is a fact that hospices have demonstrated such skill in using their pharmacological analgesic agents that some colleagues have chosen to believe that their success can be copied merely by emulating this pharmacological prowess to the exclusion of the profound and often highly complex psychological and spiritual needs of these patients. Such needs may be difficult to describe and even more difficult to meet, but are daily recognised in all good terminal care units. Put in simple language, *we are all challenged not only to alleviate the pain of cancer, but also the 'pain of dying'*.

The Problem of Chronic Pain

Most experienced doctors would agree that acute pain is easier to control than chronic and that, complex and challenging as it often is, cancer is often easier to control than chronic non-malignant pain. They would probably agree that in their training, particularly as undergraduates, most of their learning was with patients suffering from acute pains of trauma, infarction, infection and colic. Many doctors and nurses complete their training believing that chronic pain is merely a more protracted form of acute pain, with similar presentation and management, based on the same underlying neurophysiology. Nothing could be farther from the truth, and herein probably lies one of the reasons for our poor record of pain control and the widely-held belief of many patients that dying, particularly from cancer, must inevitably be characterised by agonising pain.

Acute pain, by definition, attacks suddenly and is short-lived, but often intense. So dramatically does it temporarily change the patient's life that he describes it vividly, willingly and often very accurately. One is left in no doubt that he has pain and by his eagerness to describe it he elicits immediate professional interest and care. It follows that in acute conditions, for doctors and nurses, 'no pain reported' means 'no pain present'.

Chronic pain has no clear beginning and no life-span. It is rarely described in any detail and even when the patient can be encouraged to talk about it, he usually does so without the use of his hands, devoid of graphic description, often appearing either depressed or apathetic. He seems to sense that it will not command much professional interest or activity and, in consequence, it is mentioned less and less the longer he suffers it. This is a puzzling picture to many professionals who are more comfortable dealing with acute pain syndromes and too often they infer that 'no pain reported' means 'no pain present'. In *chronic pain*, 'no pain reported' means only 'no pain reported'!

A commonly-met clinical example may illustrate this. In one bed in a general hospital can be a patient with renal colic. His description is so accurate and helpful and his suffering so obvious that every attendant feels for him and loses no time in relieving his pain whenever it strikes. In the bed bedside him is a patient with multiple bone metastases from carcinoma. He lies still, quiet and uncomplaining, a trifle 'uncomfortable' on being moved, but obviously 'depressed' because he takes no interest in his paper or radio, has poor appetite and sleeps badly. It is only after he has completed his palliative radiotherapy, had any nerve blocks necessary and become established on his regime of prostaglandin inhibitors and opiates (possibly as high as morphine 60-90 mg every 4 hours) that he is seen to be a different man – outgoing, interested, stimulating to be with, eating and sleeping well. Yet that man, in the present author's experience, may well have been said by doctors and nurses to have no pain, because 'he never told us he had any'. It is a useful rule in palliative care to *assume* that a patient has pain until proved otherwise. Not only may the presentation of pain be different, but it has to be remembered that the nerve fibres most responsible for the conduction of the 'nagging, aching' pain in cancer are the unmyelinated C fibres, which are susceptible to neurolytic blockade, rather than the fast-conducting A fibres with thick myelin coats.

Even the pharmacology appears to be different. One gains a strong clinical impression that some of the analgesics employed in acute pain have a shorter duration of action in chronic pain. For example, oral pethidine may be effective for 3–5 hours in acute conditions, but only 2–3 hours in chronic ones. Dextromoramide is said to work for 4–5 hours in post-operative patients, but is rarely effective for longer than 2 hours when taken orally for chronic pain syndromes. Pentazocine is a useful drug in acute medicine, but virtually useless in the chronic pain of malignant disease.

Finally, the principles of treatment of the two types of pain are vastly different. Because acute pain has a limited time-span, analgesics may safely be given on a p.r.n. (as required) basis. In chronic pain, which because of the underlying pathology may continue indefinitely, analgesics must be given regularly to prevent the *breakthrough of pain*, but the dose may often be smaller than in acute pain. With very rare exceptions, there is no place for p.r.n. prescribing in chronic pain; it is failure to appreciate this that can condemn the patient to a pattern of hours free of all pain, followed by intense pain before another dose is given. Twycross has coined the truism that in cancer pain 'p.r.n.' stands for 'pain relieved never'. Our aim in all such patients should be to achieve total relief of pain (by *all* means at our disposal) so speedily that we eradicate the memory of pain. Only then can the dose be reduced in some patients (though rarely discontinued) and attention be directed to his many other distresses which, by then, he is willing and eager to share with us.

Principles of Pain Control

Define the Site and Cause of each *Pain*

The eight principal pains are as follows.

Bone Pain. This often has two components. There is the persistent ache diffused widely and vaguely over the affected areas, unrelated to position or activity, and the intermittent piercing pain fairly clearly localised to a small area, often demonstrated with the patient's finger-tip, and (depending on the bone involved) related to position, weight-bearing and activity.

Visceral Pain. This is usually of a constant nature, demonstrated with the flat of the patient's hand over the offending organ, whether liver, kidney, bladder or even lung. Here it is worth remembering that even bronchogenic carcinomas are often said to be painful by patients, that liver pain is first experienced in the right lower ribs in the back before the hypochrondrium until hepatomegaly is marked, and oesophageal pain first presents under the left scapula tip before the anterior retrosternal area.

Headache. If due to a space-occupying lesion such as a primary or secondary tumour, the headache is characterised by early morning pain and is usually described by the patient gripping one side of the head with his whole hand, but then localised to one region with the tips of his fingers. Only occasionally does it persist all day or recur in the evening, or is it associated with vomiting and photophobia.

Colic. Colic may be described as it would be in acute pain (as with biliary or renal calculi), but often the patient does not double up with it, because the whole abdomen is also involved with tumour and such sudden flexing exacerbates that pain too. One has to rely on the history of intermittent, short-lived episodes of pain, accompanied by nausea and a sense of faintness or collapse.

Nerve Entrapment. As from vertebral collapse, scar tissue, tumour infiltration and post-operative or post-radiation fibrosis, nerve entrapment calls for special attention, because it is very painful, readily helped by nerve blocks and easily diagnosed. It is clearly localised to a few dermatomes which can be mapped out on the patient's body as he traces the radiation or area involved with his own fingers. Few examinations can be so satisfying for the doctor as when he uses his felt-tip pen to map the affected area and compares it with his dermatome chart to find that it involves, for example, D9-12 or L3-5 or S5.

Joint Pain. This differs in no way from that of any of the arthritides.

Muscular Pain. As at any other time in life muscle pain is felt in/over the affected muscle group and worse when these muscles are in use.

Skin Pain. Hyperaesthesia is the characteristic generalised supersensitivity reported by some patients with oat-cell bronchogenic carcinoma, Hodgkin's disease and melanomatosis. Nurses become aware that a firm grip on the patient is less upsetting than a gentle touch; that even the lightest bedclothes are too heavy and that even drying the patient with a soft towel is distressing.

Define the Emotional, Social, Spiritual Factors

See Chapter 11.

Define the Grade of each Pain

To many doctors this is a routine in acute pain yet not in chronic, where, in fact, such recording and reporting is more important, if management is to be effective and scientific. Pain may be graded as follows:

Grade 1:   Pain relieved by *occasional* low-strength analgesics.
Grade 2:   Pain relieved by *regular* low-strength analgesics.
Grade 3:   Pain relieved by *regular* medium-strength analgesics.
Grade 4:   Pain relieved by *regular* strong analgesics.
Grade 5:   Pain not relieved by regular strong analgesics.

It will be found that 65–70 per cent of cancer patients have some pain, but only in 13–15 per cent will it be grade 4 or 5, and only in about 10 per cent will specialist assistance be required for its management.

Prescribe an Analgesic Regime for each Type of Pain

This should be done, even if this means several drugs, nerve blockade, radiotherapy and chemotherapy to achieve success.

Review the Regime Regularly and Frequently

This review should be done according to the type of pain, stage of the disease, drugs employed and the individual needs of the patient. For some reason many doctors are disciplined in their care of patients with acute conditions, but ill-disciplined and unscientific in their care of the dying. They would never dream of keeping a patient on an antibiotic which was proving ineffective, yet not think of changing an analgesic failing to control chronic pain. Their knowledge of pharmacology should dictate that someone started on methadone will need to be reassessed after 36–48 hours, if not before, because of its long half-life and cumulative effect, whereas another put on to a morphine mixture will require *daily* assessment and review until the required dose is achieved.

Aim to Keep the Patient Alert, Dignified and as Independent as Possible

Fortunately doctors and nurses are increasingly recognising that few terminally ill patients either want or need to be heavily sedated and that skilled analgesia does not necessitate sedation.

Analgesia Checklist

A recommended checklist is given in Table 12.1. Daunting as it may appear, it is easily run through for each patient. The different groups of drugs and procedures are now considered in detail.

Table 12.1: Analgesic checklist

1. Drugs	Analgesics
	Antibiotics
	Anxiolytics
	Antidepressants
	Antimitotics (chemotherapy)
2. Radiotherapy	
3. Neurosurgery	Cordotomy
	Rhizotomy
	Myelotomy
	Electrode implants
4. Chemical neurolysis (nerve blocks)	
5. Transcutaneous nerve stimulation (TCNS)	
6. Barbotage	
7. Acupuncture	
8. Hypnotherapy	

Analgesics

These may conveniently be considered in three groups:

1. low-strength analgesics (including prostaglandin inhibitors);
2. medium-strength analgesics;
3. strong analgesics.

Low-Strength Analgesics (see Table 12.2)

This group includes: aspirin; paracetamol; codeine; dextropropoxyphene; phenylbutazone; oxyphenbutazone; mefenamic acid; indomethacin; benorylate; salsalate; diflunisal; fenoprofen; flurbiprofen; buprofen; sulindac; piroxicam.

Table 12.2: Low-strength analgesics

Names	Presentation	Dose range	Caution
Aspirin	Tablet, soluble 300 mg Tablet, enteric-coated, 300 mg, 600 mg Suppository 300 mg, 600 mg	300–1200 mg, 4 hourly	(1) GIT irritation (2) Enhances oral anticoagulants
Aspirin with codeine	Tablet, soluble, aspirin 300 mg with codeine phosphate 8 mg	1–2 tablets, 4 hourly	(1) Aspirin hazards (2) Codeine is constipating
Paracetamol	Tablet 500 mg Tablet, soluble, 500 mg	2 tablets, 4 hourly	(1) Hepatotoxic (2) Potentiates metoclopramide
Paracetamol with codeine	Tablet, soluble paracetamol 500 mg with codeine phosphate 8 mg	2 tablets, 4 hourly	(1) As for paracetamol (2) Codeine is constipating
Paracetamol with dextropropoxyphene	Tablet, and soluble tablet paracetamol 325 mg with dextropropoxyphene 32.5 mg	1–2 tablets, 4 hourly	(1) Sedation, dizziness, nausea, constipation (2) May enhance effects of alcohol
Dextropropoxyphene	Tablet, 65 mg and 150 mg	1 tablet, 6 hourly	(1) Constipation, sedation (2) Toxic psychosis and convulsions (3) Respiratory depression

Aspirin, in its many presentations, remains a most valuable drug in palliative care and its usefulness is restricted only by its tendency to gastrointestinal side-effects and the number of tablets needing to be taken. It is peripherally acting and probably cannot be bettered for headache and the hyperaesthesia ('flu-like' aches and pains) so often suffered by cancer patients.

Paracetamol and codeine are both centrally acting, the former having hepatotoxic properties and the latter its tendency to constipation and mild sedation. The combination of paracetamol and dextropropoxyphene (paracetamol 325 mg dextropropoxyphene 32.5 mg) has no proven advantages over paracetamol alone, but will probably continue to enjoy popularity with patients and have to be prescribed for that reason.

The dangers of phenylbutazone and oxyphenbutazone outweigh any advantages in the management of chronic pain. Indomethacin remains popular, but is a potent cause of mental confusion in the elderly; mefenamic acid, though a valuable analgesic, has a decided tendency to produce both nausea and diarrhoea.

Prostaglandin Biosynthetase Inhibitors. It is now well recognised that the pain of malignant secondaries in bone is produced by prostaglandin E1 release (PGE) and suspected that the pain of primary bladder cancer may have the same basis. It is therefore the first line of drug treatment (that is, after palliative radiotherapy for bone secondaries) to prescribe as an inhibitor − in maximum dose, supplemented if need be with a more potent analgesic.

The principal PGE inhibitors are shown in Table 12.3 Apart from consideration of price, the main points to choose between them are the frequency of administration and avoidable adverse effects. It is the author's practice to prescribe diflunisal 500 mg b.d. when attempting to keep all drugs on a b.d. basis for simplicity and patient compliance, and flurbiprofen 100 mg 4 hourly in all other cases. The incidence of gastrointestinal bleeding has been almost negligible.

It should be noted here that corticosteroids prevent the release of prostaglandins by their stabilising effects on cell membranes, rather than inhibition of synthesis. They do *not* help bone pain, but are undoubtedly effective in relieving pain due to nerve compression.

Table 12.3: Prostaglandin inhibitors

Names	Presentation	Dose range	Caution	
Indomethacin	Capsule 25 mg. Sustained release capsule 75 mg	25 mg, 6 hourly 75 mg once, twice daily	(1)	Headache, dizziness
			(2)	GIT upset
	Capsule, 75 mg Syrup 25 mg/5 ml Suppository 100 mg	100 mg suppository, nightly	(3)	Mental confusion
			(4)	Blood dyscrasia
Diflunisal	Tablet 250 mg, 500 mg	500–750 mg, 12 hourly	(1)	May enhance oral anticoagulants
			(2)	Renal failure
Flurbiprofen	Tablets 50 mg, 100 mg	50–100 mg, 4 hourly	(1)	Occasional GIT upset
Naproxen	Tablets 250 mg, 500 mg Suspension 125 mg/5 ml Suppository 500 mg	375–750 mg, 12 hourly Suppository: 500 mg, nightly	(1)	GIT upset
			(2)	Asthma and hypersensitivity
Salsalate	Capsule 500 mg	500–1000 mg, 8 hourly	(1)	GIT upset
			(2)	Salicylism
Benorylate	Tablet 750 mg Sachet, 2 g Suspension 2 g/5 ml	1–1.5 g, every 6–8 hours	(1)	GIT upset (less than most others)

Medium-Strength Analgesics

The commonest drugs in this range are listed in Table 12.4.

Dipipanone. It will surprise some readers that dipipanone is listed here, rather than in the list of stronger analgesics, but experience confirms that it is valuable only for grade 3 pain and for the early days of grade 4 pain. Were it not formulated with the anti-emetic cyclizine in the UK and only in the strength of dipipanone 10 mg, it might have much more usefulness. The sedation produced by the cyclizine is unacceptable when higher doses are used and the tendency to hallucinations when taken with the benzodiazepines, particularly nitrazepam, unnecessary.

Pethidine. As already stated, pethidine has a very limited role in palliative care and then only for colic. When taken orally it works for 3 hours, and when injected only for 1½ hours.

Nefopam. This was seen as a promising new non-addicting addition to our armamentarium when it was first released, but it is found useful only for grade 3 pain. By injection, it takes effect in 30 minutes, lasts 4 hours and a dose of 20 mg has an equianalgesic effect to morphine 12 mg. Taken orally, a single 30 mg tablet equals 300 mg aspirin only, but has a faster onset of action. Although it may be a rare event, nefopam can cause convulsions and must be avoided in patients known to be epileptic or with cerebral metastases. Doses higher than six tablets (that is, 180 mg) per day are not advisable.

Buprenorphine. This has an agonist/antagonist action and, like nefopam, is non-addicting and not euphorogenic. Its useful role in acute pain is becoming established, particularly in colic, and it has the benefits of minimal lowering of blood pressure or depression of respiration. Its place in chronic pain is not clear and its usefulness in any one patient unpredictable. The fact that it can be given sublingually avoids 'first pass' metabolism in the liver and makes it attractive for patients keen to avoid injections or many pills. In the author's view, its drawbacks lie in its not being antagonised by naloxone and the impossibility of giving it concurrently with an agonist, or indeed of being able to transfer a patient easily from buprenorphine to a member of the morphine group. These latter facts must be borne in mind before a doctor even starts a patient on the recommended sublingual dose of 0.4 mg b.d.

Table 12.4: Medium-strength analgesics

Names	Presentation	Dose range	Caution	
Dipipanone	Tablet, 10 mg with cyclizine 30 mg	10–30 mg, 6 hourly	(1)	Sedation (less than morphine)
			(2)	Hallucinations
Pethidine	Tablet 50 mg, 100 mg	50–100 mg, every 3 hours	(1)	Respiratory depression
	Injection 50 mg, 100 mg	50–100 mg, every 2 hours	(2)	Nausea
Dihydrocodeine	Tablet 30 mg	30–60 mg, 4 hourly	(1)	Constipation
	Injection 50 mg/ml		(2)	Sedation
	Elixir 10 mg/5 ml		(3)	Depression
Nefopam	Tablet 30 mg	Tablet: 30–90 mg, 6 hourly	(1)	Epileptogenic
	Injection 20 mg/ml	Injection: 20 mg, 6 hourly	(2)	Nausea, nervousness
			(3)	Blurred vision, sweating
Buprenorphine	Sublingual tablet 0.2 mg	Tablet 0.4 mg, 8–12 hourly	(1)	Sedation, nausea
	Injection 0.3 mg	Injection 0.3–0.6 mg, 8–12 hourly	(2)	Respiratory depression
			(3)	Not reversed by naloxone

Strong Analgesics

These are listed in Table 12.5.

Methadone. This is a valuable drug if its long half-life, cumulative effect and tendency to respiratory depression are borne in mind. It is marginally less nauseating than morphine and has less effect on the intestinal nerve plexus, making it a more useful drug than morphine in patients prone to subacute obstruction. Its marked ability to depress respiration condemns it for bronchogenic carcinoma and bronchitic patients.

It should be noted that in the UK it is also formulated as a linctus for cough suppression, but its low content of methadone (2 mg/5 ml) rules out much analgesic usefulness.

Dextromoramide. This is, in the author's view, the only drug which can, and should, be prescribed on a p.r.n. basis in palliative care. In acute conditions, it is said to work for 4–5 hours, but in chronic pain with malignant disease it works for no longer than 2 hours. It is therefore out of the question to ask a patient to take 12 doses a day, as would be necessary for suppression of pain! With such a short effect it is difficult to give its morphine equivalent, but at its peak plasma level it is probably three times that of an equivalent dose of morphine, that is, 5 mg dextromoramide equals 15 mg morphine. It must be emphasised that that equivalent is only relevant for a matter of minutes.

Its benefits lie in its being absorbed sublingually as readily as when swallowed, its lack of sedation, its low tendency to nausea and vomiting, and its speed of onset (10–15 minutes).

Dextromoramide has two indications in palliative care. First, it can be used as a short-acting analgesic during a painful procedure such as wound dressing, bladder lavage, effusion or ascites paracentesis, or marrow biopsy. General practitioners would find it useful to prescribe 5–10 mg to be sucked whilst the community nursing sister is preparing her equipment for the procedure. Second, it can be used as a 'bridge' for any occasional breakthrough pain occurring in a patient on morphine/diamorphine mixture not long before the next dose is due. If this happens frequently, it is an indication to step up the morphine dose rather than increase the frequency. If it is an uncommon event, dextromoramide (5–20 mg) sublingually happily tides the patient over until the normal medication time.

Paravaretum. This is little used nowadays, but has its place as an easily

Table 12.5: Strong analgesics

Names	Presentation	Dose range	Caution
Morphine	Powder (for solution) Injection Suppository 10 mg, 15 mg, 20 mg, 30 mg, 60 mg	Orally: 5 mg upwards, 4 hourly Injection: 5 mg upwards, 3 hourly	(1) Respiratory depression (2) Constipation
Morphine (MST)	Tablet 10 mg, 30 mg, 60 mg, 100 mg	10 mg upwards, 8–12 hourly	(1) Commence 12 hourly and increase to 8 hourly (2) Morphine side-effects
Diamorphine	Powder (for solution) Injection	Orally: 2.5 mg upwards, 4 hourly Injection: 2.5 mg upwards, 3 hourly	(1) Respiratory depression (2) Constipation (3) See 'equivalents'
Methadone	Tablet 5 mg Injection 10 mg/ml	5–20 mg, 6–8 hourly	(1) Respiratory depression (2) Cumulative effect (3) Mildly constipating
Phenazocine	Tablet 5 mg Injection 5 mg	5–20 mg, 6 hourly (sublingual or injection)	(1) Sedation (less than morphine) (2) Respiratory depression (3) Nausea, vomiting (4) Occasional excitement and fear
Dextromoramide	Tablet 5 mg, 10 mg Injection 10 mg Suppository 10 mg	Tablet: 5–20 mg, 2 hourly Injection: intermittent use only	(1) Short duration of effect (2) Occasional nausea

swallowed tablet, as well as the injectable form, with exactly the same pros and cons as morphine. Paraveretum 10 mg equals 5 mg morphine orally.

Levorphanol. This is longer-acting than morphine, making it possible to take t.i.d. or b.d., and less sedative.

Phenazocine. Phenazocine works longer than morphine, can be taken sublingually, orally or by injection, and is much preferable for any condition likely to cause colic, because it has less tendency to increase biliary and intestinal pressure. It produces more respiratory depression than any of the other analgesics, with the exception of methadone, and in elderly patients may be unacceptably sedative. For some reason its conveniently small, scored tablet form deceives some doctors into thinking it is less powerful than is the case, and the author has seen many patients who required naloxone for resuscitation. Phenazocine 5 mg equals 20–25 mg morphine.

Morphine/Diamorphine (Heroin)

These two drugs are the yardstick againgst which all other strong analgesics are measured and look likely to remain so for some time. All efforts to find equally effective substitutes without their addiction potential or tendency to tolerance have failed.

The experimental evidence need not be discussed here, but it can be taken as conclusively proved that there is almost nothing to choose between the two, provided the analgesic equivalents (see Table 12.6) are respected. *Both* constipate, initially nauseate and sedate, are capable of depressing cough reflex and respiration, produce euphoria, increase colic, are addicting and produce tolerance so that, under certain circumstances, the dose required to produce a given effect has to be increased.

What is there then to choose between them? There is much anecdotal evidence to support the long-held belief that diamorphine induces more euphoria than morphine does, and even in hospices, experienced nurses will sometimes suggest that a patient be transferred from morphine to diamorphine for better contentment. The principal difference is a practical and important one. Diamorphine is highly soluble, much more than morphine salts, and can be dissolved in exceedingly small volumes of water (or chlorpromazine), enabling very small injections to be given. Remembering that when taken orally both drugs *must be 4 hourly*, but given *every 3 hours by injection*, the need for the smallest-volume injections is obvious.

Table 12.6: Diamorphine/morphine equivalents

Oral	Diamorphine 10 mg = Morphine 15 mg (i.e. conversion factor 1.5)
Injection	Diamorphine 5 mg = morphine 15 mg (i.e. conversion factor 3)

The third difference is that diamorphine in solution is chemically unstable and is gradually deacetylated to morphine. Thus, although no hard and fast guidelines can be given, diamorphine solution can be considered stable for only two weeks or less. That is to say, any solution left on the shelf for longer than that is not, in fact, diamorphine, but morphine whose analgesic dose is different from morphine. In hospitals where the staff pharmacist is constantly reviewing ward drug cabinets this poses no problems. In patients' homes and surgery DDA cupboards, it is highly relevant.

It is therefore the recommendation of the author that for injections only diamorphine be used in countries where this drug is permitted. On all other occasions, morphine should be used.

Morphine Formulations

Morphine Solution (Mixture). The sooner we stop using the name 'Brompton's Mixture/Cocktail' the better. There are at least fourteen forms of it, some containing alcohol, some chlorpromazine, some syrup, some cocaine, some chloroform water. The content of the narcotic and the other constituents vary and nothing but confusion can follow! The best formula, and the one now used almost universally in palliative care units is:

Morphine hydrochloride 2.5-100 mg (the exact dose being specified)
Chloroform water: to 10 ml
Dose: 10 ml every 4 hours, day and night

Before leaving the question of morphine solution, it is worth stressing some points where confusion has arisen in the past.

1. Cocaine must never be added. It is not analgesic, has an unacceptable stimulant effect (presumably why it used to be added) often to the point of insomnia and hallucinations, is almost always incompatible with benzodiazepines resulting in frightening nightmares, is expensive and sometimes is difficult to procure!

2. Morphine in solution is nauseating in less than 50 per cent of patients (sometimes in as few as 20 per cent) and even then only for the first 3 or 4 days. Any anti-emetic needed must not be added to the solution, but taken separately. The best is probably haloperidol 0.5 mg t.i.d. or q.i.d., with prochlorperazine 5 mg q.i.d. a close second. When added to the solution, as *used to be* the author's practice, there is the risk of sedation when the dose is increased to give more narcotic and the real hazard of extra-pyramidal side-effects.
3. Morphine solution need not be sedative, if the dose is carefully, skilfully titrated to the patient's need. This is indeed one of the major advantages of the solution over tablets.
4. If the taste of the chloroform water is unpleasant, it may be replaced with ordinary water provided the amount of morphine does not exceed 100 mg/10 ml and the preparation is used immediately. The function of the chloroform water is to prevent the growth of algae.
5. Almost any flavouring agent may be added according to taste, but experience suggests that most patients prefer to take it unflavoured and follow it with a tasty drink of their choice.
6. The question is often asked of palliative-care teams if it is safe to leave the measuring and administration of such a potent narcotic to untrained patients and relations at home. Indeed this 'danger' is often given as a reason for not prescribing it until the last week or so of life! Every palliative-care physician will confirm that it is handled with the greatest care and precision by such people. The author has frequently been amused by listening to a patient, until recently vehemently declaring how he wished he was dead or should be given euthanasia, stressing to his wife how careful she must be in measuring out his mixture because 'it's very strong stuff and the wrong dose could do me harm'!

The dose of morphine will be discussed later in this section.

Morphine Tablets. In only a few hospital pharmacies are diamorphine tablets specially made, and their use will not be discussed here for that reason.

MST Continus Tablets (10 mg, 30 mg, 60 mg, 100 mg). These proprietary preparations are available in the .UK and are formulated for slow sustained release over 12 hours, are probably less nauseating than the solution, and easily swallowed. They represent a major advance in the presentation of this vital narcotic for palliative care.

When prescribing them, it has to be borne in mind that the drug is released over 12 hours. What may appear to be a large dose has to be divided by three to compare it with the more familiar 4-hourly regime. Thus MST 1 (that is, 10 mg) b.d. represents less than 4 mg 4 hourly — an exceedingly small dose. Some doctors appear alarmed at having to order MST 6 (60 mg) b.d., but this is only 20 mg 4 hourly, a middle-of-the-range dose for patients with advanced cancer, and one that few doctors would hesitate to provide as the mixture.

The drawback is the difficulty in titrating the dose to a patient's need when several tablets of different strength might have to be taken each time to achieve it; for example, the equivalent of 15 mg 4 hourly is difficult to give by MST tablets b.d. Initial titration and stabilisation on morphine is probably best achieved with the solution and the patient then transferred to MST Continus tablets.

Their ready availability, however, is an encouragement to employ low-dose morphine at an earlier stage in palliation than is usually the case. For example, the patient currently taking dipipanone (Diconal) 10 mg q.i.d. and likely to need steadily increasing doses over succeeding weeks is an ideal candidate for MST Continus 1 (i.e. 10 mg) b.d. — the exact analgesic equivalent of his dipipanone — and actually taking fewer tablets with better analgesia and contentment. In fact many patients can be put on to MST some twelve to eighteen months before the end of life, when it is seen that slowly increasing pain will be a problem.

Alternative Routes of Administration

Too readily do doctors and nurses change from oral to injectable forms of narcotics, in fact often from medium-strength analgesics to injection diamorphine, in their search for alternative routes of administration without due consideration of the sublingual and rectal routes.

Sublingual Administration. The drugs which may be given sublingually are shown in Table 12.7. Provided there is sufficient saliva, or its production is stimulated with citrus fruit drops or extract, this route is effective even in patients too ill to swallow.

Rectal Administration. The drugs that may be given by suppository are shown in Table 12.8. The advantage of oxycodone over morphine suppository is its longer duration of effect. Family doctors, in particular,

Table 12.7: Strong analgesics effective by sublingual route

Names	Presentation	Dose range	Comments
Buprenorphine	Tablets 0.2 mg	0.2–0.4 mg, 8–12 hourly	(1) Sedation (2) Respiratory depression
Dextromoramide	Tablets 5 mg, 10 mg	5–20 mg, every 2 hours	
Phenazocine	Tablets 5 mg	5–20 mg, every 6–8 hours	(1) Sedation (2) Nausea and vomiting (3) Occasional excitement, hallucinations

Table 12.8: Strong analgesics in suppository form

Names	Presentation	Dose range	Comment
Morphine	10 mg, 15 mg, 20 mg, 30 mg, 60 mg suppositories	10 mg upwards, every 4 hours	(1) 10 mg and 20 mg are available only on special order
Oxycodone	30 mg slow-release suppositories	30–60 mg, 6–8 hourly	(1) Available only on special order from Boots in UK (2) Longer effect than morphine (3) 30 mg equals 20 mg morphine PR
Dextromoramide	10 mg suppositories	10–20 mg, every 2–3 hours	(1) Useful only for analgesia during painful procedures

will appreciate the usefulness of this route for their patients. For example, a patient might be given two suppositories each night, oxycodone 30 mg and chlorpromazine 100 mg, with a guaranteed effect for each of 8 hours, carrying him through the night pain free and rested, without any need for his wife to be disturbed.

Injections. Most of the major narcotic analgesics can be given by injection, but, except in the case of diamorphine, the volume is large and, particularly when chlorpromazine is also needed, there is likely to be a problem in finding sufficient sites in patients. Methadone and phenazocine tend to be painful injections.

It must also be remembered, as stated already, that morphine and diamorphine injections must be given *every 3 hours*, round the clock. There is some evidence that the *intermittent* use of such injections accelerates the development of tolerance to these two drugs more than their regular use orally.

In hospice practice, it is usually found that no more than 5 per cent of terminally ill patients require regular injections, and then only when all other routes have been tried. When regular injections become necessary, consideration should be given to the employment of a syringe driver (resembling a small heparin pump), which can be carried around in a shoulder holster by the ambulant patient. The same injection site may be used for one or two days without reinserting the butterfly needle.

Epidural Morphine. It is increasingly recognised that morphine (in a purified form, free of all pyrogens, etc.) can be administered epidurally via a cannula left in the epidural space.

The cannula is inserted via an epidural needle in the routine way and either brought out of the back at the site of entry or brought round to the front of the patient buried in the subcutaneous tissue. Its end is fitted with a bacterial filter which must be changed weekly, and is firmly affixed to the patient's skin with adhesive tape.

The solution of morphine 2-4 mg is injected — initially by a nurse with medical approval and prescription, and subsequently by the patient after due instruction — every 6 hours. It is found that rarely is more than 4 mg 6 hourly required, even for patients previously on oral doses as high as 240 mg every 4 hours.

Undoubtedly valuable as this is proving in many patients, it has been found that the epidural cannulae tend to become dislodged and have to be reinserted, sometimes every two or three weeks; that analgesia may be total, but the central tranquillising/euphoric effect is lacking and many patients require the introduction of an anxiolytic into their regime; and finally, that many cannulae block for no apparent cause.

Nevertheless different studies have demonstrated their usefulness in patients who have had them *in situ* for up to 250 days with good analgesia and few, if any, of the unfortunate side-effects of oral morphine, such as constipation. In the case of an overdose, nalaxone is used, as would be expected.

Analgesic Equivalents

The analgesic equivalents of the principal analgesics are shown in Figure 12.1.

Duration of Effect of Analgesics

This is shown in Tables 12.9 and 12.10. The importance of this information is obvious. If, as has already been stressed, each drug must be prescribed *to anticipate pain*, on a regular basis, it is essential to prescribe according to the duration of effect. Thus morphine orally would be taken 4 hourly; phenazocine 6 hourly; methadone 8 hourly

Table 12.9: Duration of effectiveness: oral analgesics

Dextromoramide	2 hours
Pethidine	3 hours
Morphine Diamorphine Papaveretum Dipipanone	4 hours
Phenazocine Nefopam Levorphanol	6 hours
Methadone	8 hours
Buprenorphine	8–12 hours
Morphine-sustained release (MST)	10–12 hours

Table 12.10: Duration of effectiveness: injected analgesics

Dextromoramide	1–1½ hours
Pethidine	2 hours
Morphine Diamorphine	3 hours
Phenazocine Nefopam	6 hours
Methadone	6–8 hours
Morphine-microcrystalline	10–12 hours

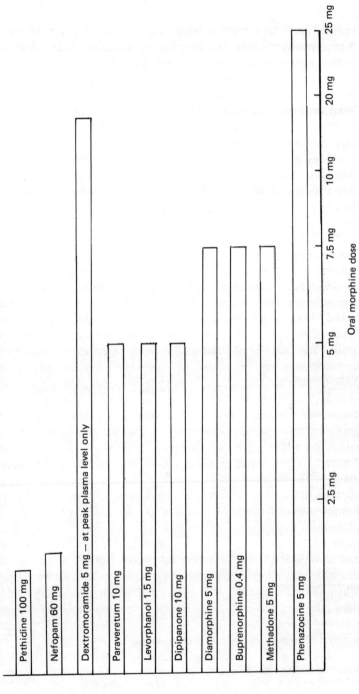

Figure 12.1: Approximate analgesic equivalents: oral route (with oral morphine as standard)

Pethidine 100 mg
Nefopam 60 mg
Dextromoramide 5 mg — at peak plasma level only
Paraveretum 10 mg
Levorphanol 1.5 mg
Dipipanone 10 mg
Diamorphine 5 mg
Buprenorphine 0.4 mg
Methadone 5 mg
Phenazocine 5 mg

Oral morphine dose

2.5 mg   5 mg   7.5 mg   10 mg   20 mg   25 mg

initially, but later 6 hourly; buprenorphine 12 hourly initially, though 8 hourly might later be required. Failure to follow this practice is one of the principal reasons for inadequate pain control.

What Drug and What Dose?

Having ascertained in the usual manner, by history-taking, examination and investigations, the probable sites and cause of *each* element in the pain, one chooses drugs appropriate for *each*, starting with the lowest dose of the low-strength analgesics, if possible. There is nothing to be ashamed of in employing aspirin, paracetamol or codeine in terminal care!

Thereafter, always using the grading of pain suggested, one transfers the patient to the next group of drugs until the maximum dose fails to control it, and finally one employs a member of the strong analgesics family. An example may illustrate this better. When the patient's pain is relieved with occasional aspirin, his pain is grade 1. When he requires 600–1200 mg 4 hourly and is pain free, it is grade 2; but when pain breaks through, this drug is no longer appropriate and his pain has progressed from grade 2 to grade 3. He may now need dipipanone 6 hourly or nefopam 6 hourly and, so long as he is pain free on that dose or a build-up to the maximum recommended, he is said to have grade 3 pain (that is 'pain controlled by regular medium-strength analgesics'). When, taking the maximum dose of these medium-strength analgesics, the pain recurs, he requires a change to a strong analgesic such as morphine (solution or MST), and the desired equivalent can be worked out from Figure 12.1. So long as he remains pain free, his pain can be graded as grade 4. The choice of drug for grade 4 pain will depend on his ability to take it, the need for 'middle-of-the-night' administration (as with morphine mixture), the availability of attendants to help him, his attitude to suppositories on a regular basis, and the physician's assessment of the speed of progress of the disease. When advancing slowly, and thus probably needing only occasional changes in dosage, such drugs as methadone or buprenorphine might be thought appropriate. When advancing rapidly, with a dosage alteration called for every few days, the best analgesic formula will almost certainly be morphine mixture, whose content can be changed unobtrusively every few days without changing the volume of each dose.

Morphine Dosage

The dose of morphine requires special attention. The rule is that the younger the patient the higher the dose, rather than a dose/body-weight formula. Only experience can equip the doctor here. For example, a young man in his twenties, no matter how emaciated, may eventually need 100–200 mg morphine every 4 hours for his pain from disseminated carcinoma. An obese old lady with equally widespread disease may be rendered pain free on as little as 2.5–5 mg every 4 hours.

There is no such thing as either a 'standard' dose or an 'average' dose. Certain guidelines, based on experience with several thousand patients, may help, however. Excluding the very young and the very old, about 80 per cent of patients will be rendered pain free on 20 mg morphine by mouth every 4 hours. Those with skeletal metastases, even when taking adjuvant prostaglandin inhibitors, require much higher doses. Thus a man with disseminated prostatic carcinoma often needs 60–90 mg 4 hourly.

The recommended increments are: 2.5 mg – 5 mg – 10 mg – 15 mg – 20 mg – 30 mg (at which point the addition of chlorpromazine as a narcotic-potentiator should be considered) – 45 mg – 60 mg – 90 mg – 120 mg – 180 mg – 240 mg – 360 mg. If pain control is not achieved by this time (and the use of such a dose is rarely required, even in specialist palliative-care practice), it is doubtful whether a higher dose will make much difference. Most likely, absorption is not taking place, potentiators need to be increased, and *much* more attention devoted to emotional, social and spiritual factors.

One of the secrets of effective analgesia in advanced disease is the skilled use of adjuvant therapy as follows.

Prostaglandin Synthetase Inhibitors. (see previous section, p. 272). These should be employed in maximum dose in all patients with bone metastases who are awaiting palliative radiotherapy or its benefit (remembering it usually takes 14–21 days to show any effect, but 7–10 days in myelomatosis), or when irradiation has failed to help.

Steroids. These are invaluable to reduce inflammatory reaction and, where there is nerve entrapment, their effect appears to be by lessening perineural oedema. The usual dose is EC prednisolone 15–30 mg/day in divided doses. Prednisolone is preferable to dexamethasone, unless the latter is being employed to reduce intracranial pressure (see Chapter 8).

Phenothiazines, Butyrophenones and Anti-depressants. 1. Haloperidol, chlorpromazine and methotrimeprazine have narcotic-sparing properties probably related to the dopamine-receptor blockade produced by them and the narcotics. Haloperidol is preferable, because it is less sedative than the other two and, contrary to the views of many doctors, patients in the advanced stages of disease rarely want or accept daytime sedation. The dose is haloperidol 0.5-1.0 mg t.i.d., chlorpromazine 25 mg t.i.d. up to 4 hourly, methotrimeprazine 12.5-25 mg t.i.d.

2. The tricyclics have a valuable place, but whether they act by raising the pain threshold, an intrinsic analgesic effect or by their action on serotonin is not clear. It certainly appears that this action is more than an antidepressant one, because they are useful in sub-psychiatric doses, for example, amitriptyline 50-75 mg at night.

3. A combination of amitriptyline and an anxiolytic such as per-phenazine has a distinct analgesic effect in its own right as well as aiding sleep and lifting mood. The best product is Triptafen-DA 2-3 at night.

Anxiolytics. Although in no way detracting from the principles laid down in Chapter 11 or suggesting that anxiolytics are a substitute for supportive psychotherapy and the fullest exploration and ventilation of a patient's fear, there nevertheless *is* a place for the use of anxiolytics. Occasionally one encounters a patient who, even to the most experienced and sympathetic attendant, does not appear to be in pain. He is now on a very adequate analgesic regime, sleeps well, eats better and moves more freely, but is obviously tense and apprehensive, frightened when nurses approach him and calls for a 'pain-killer' within a minute of a discomfort starting. The question is whether this is because of his memory of previous pain and the terror it produced in him, whether he will in fact benefit from even higher analgesic doses or more ventilation of his feelings, *or* should he be given a short course of an anxiolytic. Sometimes the latter is the line to adopt, so that as he relaxes he will regain confidence in himself and his attendants and better be able to gain from his pain-free state. The clinical judgement is a delicate one.

In such patients, one often finds a short-acting benzodiazepine such as lorazepam 0.5-1.0 mg t.i.d. better than chlorpromazine or even diazepam, whose metabolites linger in the body for so long. A drug to be avoided is meprobamate, because of its gastrointestinal effects and paradoxical excitement in some patients. The present author occasionally employs the β-blocker propanolol 40 mg t.i.d., when there are no dangers of cardiac decompensation or bronchospasm.

For emergency use, there is nothing better than IV lorazepam 1-2 mg or IV diazepam 5-10 mg, provided the physician is alert to respiratory depression.

Antibiotics. In Chapter 13, mention is made of the use of antibiotics in palliative medicine, particularly where inflammation is contributing directly to a painful lesion or otherwise increasing the patient's suffering because of a urinary tract infection, an upper respiratory tract infection, a secondary chest infection, etc.

Radiotherapy

For some reason many doctors and nurses continue to regard radiotherapy as a drastic measure, designed only to cure cancer, inevitably associated with malaise, nausea and vomiting, painful skin reactions and depression. How often the present author has been told by a general practitioner working far from a radiotherapy centre, 'Even if he was fit for the journey, my patient is far too ill for that sort of thing – what he needs is something for his pain!'

Palliative radiotherapy has much to offer, and failure to consider it for these patients borders on negligence. Many solitary secondary deposits will respond to it, either as single fractions or a very short course, and it is the *first line of treatment* for the pain of skeletal deposits and myeloma. It is worth considering for certain fungating tumours, always worth it for superior vena caval obstruction and spinal cord compression, and with modern regimes it is remarkably free of unpleasant side-effects after the first few days.

Chemotherapy

So rapid are the advances in medical oncology that no book such as this can be up to date. Not only does chemotherapy have a major place in the possible cure ('complete remission') of many of the rarer tumours, it is valuable in palliative medicine to effect tumour shrinkage, particularly in the pelvic organs, to reduce pleural effusion and ascites, to help superior vena caval obstruction and certain cerebral tumours. Unpleasant side-effects there certainly can be, but these are markedly fewer and less distressing than even a few years ago. (See Chapter 9.)

Surgery

Short-circuiting operations have a place in bowel cancer, where a defunctioning colostomy can make all the difference to the final year or two of life, and also in pancreatic tumours, where the relief of obstructive jaundice is so helpful. (See Chapter 9.)

Pathological fractures can be managed with permanent internal fixation, or occasional hip replacement in the case of necks of femur. Post-operatively, the patient may be given palliative radiotherapy with such good results that many patients resume active lives for months with multiple bone secondaries and unhealed fractures. The place of palliative neurosurgery lies in the following areas.

Laminectomy for Spinal Cord Compression

This is an emergency and must be carried out within 24 hours of its development. It is always worth seeking a neurosurgical opinion, but in many centres, because of the short prognosis, it will not be performed for bronchogenic carcinoma secondaries. After 24 hours the first line of treatment is radiotherapy after emergency IV methylprednisolone 250 mg or IV dexamethasone 8–16 mg.

Hypophysectomy

This is done either for hormone ablation for breast carcinoma or as an analgesic measure when, instead of an open operation, 1 ml absolute alcohol is injected into the pituitary gland via a special trocar and a cannula, introduced through the nose and sphenoid sinus into the pituitary fossa. Pain relief may occur almost at once or take up to 24 hours to develop. Some 50 per cent of patients will be rendered completely pain free and a further 30 per cent much improved. The technique is applicable for both hormone and non-hormone-dependent metastases.

This procedure has much to commend it, and requires a minimum of an overnight stay in hospital, although most neurosurgeons or ENT surgeons would ask for longer, both to prepare the nose beforehand adequately and to observe the patient afterwards for cranial-nerve lesions and the development of diabetes insipidus (10–15 per cent of patients). Hormone replacement with corticosteroids must be started at once, but thyroxine replacement may wait to see if the patient survives six months.

Cordotomy, Rhizotomy, Myelotomy

These highly specialised procedures are included here for the non-neurologist for consideration in any patient thought to have a 'long' prognosis of at least six months, where high doses of narcotics might cause more upset than the operation, period of recovery and any complications of the procedure.

Increasingly, cordotomy is now performed as a 'closed' percutaneous procedure. At the level of C1 and C2, a needle is introduced into the subarachnoid space under local anaesthesia and through it a fine wire is stereo-tactically placed in the antero-lateral column of the cord. As a current is passed through the wire, which is insulated except at its tip, the patient experiences a tingling sensation in the part of the body near his painful lesion; this can aid the surgeon for the very accurate localisation of the coagulating current until pain relief is total. An anterior 'open' approach can also be used and is more usual when a bilateral cordotomy is done. Post-cordotomy dysaesthesia (1 per cent of patients) occurs six months or more after the procedure and may be impossible to relieve.

Rhizotomy (section of the posterior nerve root as it enters the cord) is valuable for persistent pain in one or two dermatomes, rather than repeated chemical neurolytic injections, which become progressively more difficult to perform principally because of scar tissue.

Myelotomy requires deroofing of the cord and a vertical mid-line incision to cut the sensory tracts as they cross to the contra-lateral side to the spino-thalamic tracts.

Electrode Implant

Direct implantation of electrodes for dorsal-column stimulation may be done at laminectomy or percutaneously through epidural needles; cerebral stimulation is done under stereo-tactic control via burr holes.

Chemical Neurolysis (Nerve Blocks)

These relatively simple procedures are appropriate in at least 10 per cent of terminally ill patients with grade 4 or 5 pain. As with patients being offered drug regimes for analgesia, they are never a substitute for careful assessment of every factor in the patient's physical and emotional suffering, and for the most skilled support for him and his family. They are useful for patients in whom only the highest doses of narcotic would effect any relief, or when pain is so localised that, by its control, no drugs will subsequently be needed.

The solutions used are 5–7.5 per cent phenol in glycerine (the commonest), 2 per cent chlorocresol, and alcohol. The principal blocks used in palliative medicine are as follows.

Intercostal Blocks

Intercostal blocks are useful for rib secondaries and fractures, nerve entrapment, localised skin nodules and mesothelioma. The procedure takes minutes, can be performed even on patients in bed or in a ward treatment room, and may be expected to remain effective for 3–6 weeks. The danger is pneumothorax and the principal drawback is the scar tissue which makes for difficulty in subsequent injections in the same site.

Paravertebral Blocks

Useful for intrathoracic pain and certain bronchogenic carcinoma, this requires a specialist unit using X-ray or visual image-intensifier control.

Coeliac Plexus Block

This may achieve analgesia in up to 75 per cent of patients with pain from a posteriorly invading pancreatic carcinoma, but it is also useful for other upper abdominal lesions and the perineal pain from recurrence of rectal carcinoma, which is otherwise so difficult to control. Relief may be expected for up to six months.

The coeliac plexus block is done either via a posterior approach (under a visual image-intensifier) or transabdominally (under scan) with the patient lying on his back. Because of the likelihood of hypotension, the patient must remain under careful observation in hospital for 24–48 hours.

Pudendal Blocks

These are useful where pain is strictly localised to the perineum, and the use of the block will not further endanger bowel/bladder function. It is relatively simple to do and requires a similar technique for localising the nerve as in obstetric practice.

Sacral Blocks

Sacral blocks are useful for pain limited to one or two sacral dermatomes and performed by injecting through the sacral foramina. When they are done unilaterally and where no bladder dysfunction was previously present, the incidence of sphincter disturbance is only 5 per cent.

Brachial Plexus Blocks

This is a 'last-ditch' procedure, because of the mixed motor/sensory structure of the plexus with almost inevitable motor deficit after the block. It is therefore of use only in patients with intractable pain (grade 5), who have already almost no use in the arm, although it may be justified in someone with brachial neuralgia secondary to a Pancoast tumour or similar malignant infiltration into the plexus. Not only is there the real danger of motor loss, but there is also a high risk of puncturing the apex of the lung producing a pneumothorax.

Intrathecal and Epidural Blocks

These are now regularly done and can be expected to be effective for 8–10 weeks and 16–18 weeks respectively. They are indicated for any unilateral pain between the levels of D4 and L4 whatever the cause.

The principles involved are simple. The patient lies on the affected side if phenol in glycerine is used (being hyperbaric), or on the contralateral side if alcohol is used (hypobaric). The former is much the more common, because the addition of glycerine, in addition to increasing the density, delays the release of the neurolytic agent and permits a more leisurely and accurate positioning of the patient for the exact localisation of the injection. The needle is placed in the dermatome involved or the one above, and the solution injected either into the subarachnoid space (intrathecal) or into the epidural space where it bathes the sensory roots.

These procedures are almost painless and remarkably few patients decline to have them repeated. Initially, there may be a tingling sensation in the contra-lateral side, but this passes off within minutes. No more than 5 per cent of patients suffer 'light-headedness' and 5–10 per cent may report nausea. The patient is usually pain free within 4–8 hours and by that time ready to move around.

These neurolytic procedures are commended to readers as worthy of consideration for good palliative care. Patients considered suitable should be referred to pain-relief centres or hospices where specialist skills and facilities are available.

Transcutaneous Nerve Stimulators (TCNS)

One of the many by-products of Melzach's 'gate theory' was the recognition that additional sensory stimulation could block the transmission of noxious impulses to the higher centres. These devices, now readily and cheaply available, are the size of small pocket 'bleepers', equipped with two small electrodes, and under the control of the patient himself. The electrodes are placed over the offending painful area with electrode jelly and a low-frequency (20-100 Hz) pulse is applied. A tingling sensation is felt (in fact if it is not felt, benefit is unlikely to follow) and pain rapidly diminishes. The device can be used continuously or intermittently. In the UK these TCNS can be purchased by/for a patient and, provided a certificate is written by the physician, are VAT-exempt.

It is worth noting that TCNS are equally useful in many 'non-terminal' painful conditions such as post-herpetic neuralgia, fibrositis, lumbago, amputation neuroma, arthritis, neuralgia, etc.

Barbotage

Although Hitchcock first reported on this in 1967 and it is a useful technique, it is seldom used, possibly because of the difficulty in forecasting which patients may benefit. After the usual assessment and preparation of the patient, a lumbar puncture is carried out and 5-10 ml cerebro-spinal fluid (CSF) is slowly aspirated, then rapidly reinjected back into the subarachnoid space. A minute or two later the procedure is repeated; after about five barbotages, the patient is usually able to say if there has been any reduction in his pain. If so, and if the almost inevitable headache (for which he has been given an analgesic such as mefenamic acid in anticipation) is not too upsetting, a further five aspirations and reinjections are done. Thereafter he lies resting, as after any lumbar puncture. The analgesia is said to result from scattered demyelination. The technique is useful for thoracic and abdominal-wall pain and, it has been said, deep pelvic pain; it may remain effective for 8-12 weeks.

Acupuncture

Readers will know that acupuncture has been shown to release the body's own morphine-like substances, the peptide endorphins and encephalins whose action can be countered with naloxone. That acupuncture has a place in pre- and post-operative pain and many non-terminal conditions is now beyond dispute. Its place in the palliation of pain in far-advanced disease, in the present author's view, has still to be shown.

Hypnotherapy

Although hypnosis, like acupuncture, is clearly of value in many conditions, it has not been shown to be of value as an analgesic procedure for the severe pain of advanced cancer. It does, however, have undoubted value as a means of relaxing some patients, helping them to combat this pain or come to terms with it, in the management of fear and phobias, and for those with dependence on sedatives and tranquillisers. It is said to be easier to practise on the more intelligent, but must, at all times, be done only by those specially trained in it and possessing well-developed skills in personality and psychiatric assessment.

Recommended Further Reading

Bonica, J.J. and Albe-Fessard, D. (1976) *Advances in Pain Research and Therapy*, vol. 1, Raven Press, New York
Clarke, I.M.C. (1982) in E. Wilkes (ed.), *The Dying Patient*, MTP Press, Lancaster
Harcus, A.W., Smith, R.B. and Whittle, B.A. (1977) *Pain – New Perspectives in Measurement and Management*, Churchill Livingstone, Edinburgh
Lipton, S. (1979) *Relief of Pain in Clinical Practice*, Blackwell Scientific Publications, London
Lipton, S. (1979) *The Control of Chronic Pain*, Edward Arnold, London
Paul, R.P. (1979) *Chronic Pain Primer*, Year Book Medical Publications Inc., Chicago
Twycross, R.G. (1978) in C.M. Saunders (ed.), *The Management of Terminal Illness*, Edward Arnold, London
Twycross, R.G. and Ventafridda, V. (1980) *The Continuing Care of Terminal Cancer Patients*, Pergamon Press, Oxford

13 PALLIATIVE SYMPTOM CONTROL

Derek Doyle

Palliation is commonly defined as 'easing without curing'. Even in acute medical conditions we sometimes find ourselves unable to cure, but are aware that, given time and skilled therapy, the condition will right itself, become less of a hazard or less troublesome as it becomes chronic, and are still challenged to relieve distress when we cannot reverse a pathological process. One of the rewards of growing older in our profession is that of recognising that though remarkably few conditions are curable, many are self-limiting, and almost all are amenable to energetic palliation so that the patient may at least *feel* better. Nowhere is this better displayed than in general practice where, in spite of what the doctor may care to believe, most of his consultations are seen by the patients as oppertunities for relief and reassurance, and that only occasionally is there a discovery and cure of a life-threatening condition.

The challenge presented to every clinician, whether doctor or nurse, is to develop such a sensitivity to every patient's needs, whether spoken or unspoken, that he will devote his every energy to the easing of suffering. This chapter will suggest ways of achieving this in chronic conditions, particularly in their far-advanced stages.

General Principles

Quite apart from the underlying pathology, there are important differences between acute and chronic conditions. Failure to appreciate them can only lead to suboptimal awareness of a patient's needs and the consequent failure to relieve some of his distress. The patient's presentation of symptoms is different. In acute conditions he will usually recount every symptom, often in graphic detail, and with courteous encouragement can usually be relied upon to mention everything which seems significant to *him*, even though points of greater interest to the doctor, but omitted by the patient, may have to be drawn forth from him. This picture is so obvious that examples are hardly necessary.

The patient suffering a painful myocardial infarction will not fail to speak of the pain and describe its crushing nature, sense of foreboding and degree of dyspnoea, although he may not feel the necessity to describe the pain radiation. He will use his hands better to describe the sensation and terror it produced. The man with renal colic will, most certainly, grip his loin and point out the radiation of pain in his ureter, may mention haematuria and will probably demonstrate how he doubles up during each attack. Each symptom which concerns him will be mentioned in the implicit hope that the more he mentions, the better he describes, the easier will be the doctor's task of diagnosing, treating and hopefully curing. Most doctors gain their basic training and experience with such conditions and have learned that 'what matters to the patient will be described'.

Almost the opposite occurs in chronic conditions. The longer he endures the condition, the less will each distress be reported, the less graphic will be the description, the more he will suffer in relative silence. It is almost as though the patient recognises, sometimes better than his doctor, that repeated reporting either makes no difference to his condition or to the doctor's interest and enthusiasm, or to the eventual outcome. By the time the far-advanced or terminal phase is reached, 50 per cent of his distresses are not even mentioned; hence we would be wrong to refer to them as symptoms. Perhaps he feels they would be considered trivial or time-wasting. Perhaps he anticipates a label of hypochondriasis or exaggerating. Even when reported, they are usually not demonstrated or described in helpful detail. This in no way means that his distresses are to him unimportant or minor, imaginary or without fearful significance. The onus is upon the doctor to encourage the fullest ventilation of every single problem, followed by as careful a history-taking, examination and investigation as at any other time, and the giving of as much explanation of the significance of possible palliation as the patient is capable of understanding. Some examples here may be useful.

The patient with long-standing cancer pain will often sit or lie almost motionless, lose interest in his surroundings and attempts to mobilise him, sleep poorly, lose appetite, yet only mention pain when its presence is *specifically* questioned. Even then he may lie still and make no effort to localise it until every encouragement has been given to him. To the casual, insensitive observer, he is depressed and is regarded as having no pain, 'because if he had he would speak of it'! The patient with halitosis, no matter how aware he may be of his bad breath, rarely mentions it. Here, the questioning reveals that he thinks it comes from 'rotting flesh' inside (possibly a justified conclusion, if he has a fulminating bronchial or gastric tumour) or the odour is a reason for his wife and loved ones distancing themselves from him, when he needs their physical nearness more than ever before. To the doctor, excessive sweating may be seen as an inevitable concomitant of the patient's known cancer or Hodgkin's disease, and hardly worthy of mention for that reason. To the patient, it may signify 'consumption' (pulmonary tuberculosis), complicating the condition he already knows he has, an infectious disease which endangers his caring family. The significance of the symptom to the *patient* matters more than its significance to the *doctor* or *nurse*. Anorexia may be expected and understood by the doctor, quite a relief to the nauseated patient, but a cause of deep concern to relatives, whose final remaining act of love may be to prepare attractive meals in the forlorn hope of keeping him alive longer.

In far-advanced disease:

the patient's description of symptoms may be different;
the patient's perception of the significance of his distress may be different from his doctor's;
the patient's fears may have a different basis.

When the patient comes to appreciate as much as his professional attendants do that a cure is not realistic, then every energy should be devoted to the 'ease of suffering', that is 'palliation':

He fears the unknown more than the known.
He fears professional disinterest more than professional ineptitude.
He fears the process of dying more than the finality of death itself.
He fears isolation, whether physical or psychological.

Seldom, if ever, do such patients expect every distress to be removed or treated. They do ask that interest be shown in their distresses, that their significance be explained and the opportunity made available to them to speak of *everything* which, at any time, seems important to them.

Given a caring, loving, safe environment, the dying patient becomes ever more thoughtful towards his family and professional helpers, as he feels less need to be defensive and fight for his survival. As a result, his personality may seem to change. The selfish become thoughtful towards others, the abrasive become gracious, the restless become content, the demanding become generous. Consequently distresses caused by his suffering may take on a new meaning. They will now, more than ever before, affect relationships with others. If the faecal leak can be lessened, so will the embarrassment of his loved ones. Relief of his dyspnoea will not only reduce *his* fears, but also the all-too-evident fears of his family. Prescribing an appropriate hypnotic for him will enable his wife to get a much-needed restful sleep as well. Examples are legion. Only when the attending physicians and nurses recognise that, by this time, few patients are seeking a cure, but each is looking for compassionate recognition of their every suffering and putting as much enthusiasm and professional skill into achieving pallia-tion, will we be worthy of our reputation as 'caring' professionals.

This chapter is devoted to the commonest distresses encountered and the remedies that have proved useful when 'specific' therapy, as described in specialist chapters, is not possible or appropriate. *Obvious rules apply to palliation regimes.*

1. Each regime must be simple and readily understood by the patient and his attendants.
2. Each regime must be tailored to his rapidly and frequently chang-ing needs and ability to comply.
3. Each regime must be reviewed regularly and frequently.
4. Each regime must be explained to the patient and all his atten-dants as a simple honest explanation of the significance of each symptom or distress. This applies equally to the inter-professional communications between partners in general practice, doctors and nurses, doctors and paramedicals such as physiotherapists and occupational therapists, clergy and social workers. Nowhere is the need for team work more evident, more necessary and nowhere is the presence of a professional 'prima donna' more disruptive and divisive.

Anorexia

Common Causes

Oral Candidiasis. (This is present in 75 per cent of such patients, whether or not they are immune-suppressed or deficient.) In such patients the typical white plaque may not be found, but only a spongy, hyperaemic mucosa, particularly at the back of the palate where the upper denture plate presses firmly. Denture-wearers may have angular cheilosis and little other evidence of infection.

Chronic Constipation. Difficult as it is to explain why loading of the colon can produce anorexia, clinical experience confirms that its relief does aid return of appetite as well as patient comfort.

Uninteresting and Unimaginative Food. Sadly, we make too little use of the skills of dieticians and kitchen experts in our hospitals or have to accept the so-called administrative necessity of pre-served meal trays sent up from the kitchens, often with helpings so large that they discourage patients from eating undoubtedly good food. Colourless food, particularly the 'invalid' diets and liquidised meals, can be made attractive by the garnishing of parsley, mint, peppers or cherries. Bland flavours can be improved by the addition of a morsel of spice or herb or a dessert can be made tempting by a few drops of a fruit juice or liqueur.

The home cook can be advised to serve everything on a side plate to disguise the smallness of the helping, and special lipped plates can be used to lessen the embarrassment of chasing the last portions round a large dinner plate.

Meals Offered only at Traditional Times. The iller the patient the more he will usually enjoy his first meal of the day, often to the exclusion of all others. Attendants must be advised of this and helped not to feel a failure when the specially prepared mid-day or evening meal is rejected. In the same way, they must be told how food senses change dramatically, almost from day to day. The patient who has never liked ice-cream may now want it several times a day; another may ask for kippered herring late at night or prefer porridge for his supper. The old 'sweet tooth' may come to abhor all things sweet and crave for savouries and spices. Few will find it easy to adhere to traditional meal times, but enjoy mid-morning or mid-afternoon nibbles, often of the most unexpected foods.

Odours in the Environment. Sensitive nurses will make every effort to care for the anorexic patient away from others with foul-smelling wounds and colostomies, or endeavour to have the patient's own appliances changed long before his meal is brought to him. The smell of disinfectants may be homely to doctors and nurses, but a painful reminder to patients of their vomiting and wounds or dependence on these professional friends.

Nausea and Vomiting. Although self-evident, it is worth remembering that whereas vomiting is relatively easy to control, nausea — particularly in ovarian and gastric tumours — may remain the greatest challenge in palliative medicine.

Excessive Medication and/or Dry Mouth. In spite of a need to give drugs for several major problems, the physician must never forget that many cause anorexia, or sedation or a dry mouth. The obvious examples are analgesics, antidepressants and anxiolytics.

Depressive States.

Metabolic Causes. The principal causes are (a) hypercalcaemia (see the later section on p. 327), and (b) uraemia (see Chapter 5). The principle that no investigation should ever be carried out on a patient unless it might lead to an improvement or useful change in his care regime (or more accurate prognosis) is not a licence to omit the investigation of these two problems.

Post-radiation. The anorexia that follows palliative radiotherapy is self-limiting and no more need be done for it then preparatory explanation and reassurance that it will pass, given a few days.

Management

1. Try to remove or modify any of the offending causes already listed.
2. Offer all food either very hot or ice-cold. The nearer a patient is to death the colder he will prefer all food and drink, the more re-assurances will be required by relatives who fear that iced drinks will 'chill the stomach'. So common is this appreciation of cold drinks that it might almost be taken as a prognostic indicator of approaching death.
3. The only proven 'tonic' for impaired appetite is a steroid, either EC prednisolone 5 mg t.i.d. by mouth or injection methyl prednisolone 40 mg daily for one week. Dexamethasone already being employed for raised intracranial pressure will provide the same benefit.

Anxiety

Is it possible for anyone to go through a terminal illness without some signs of anxiety, if he has poorly controlled pain, recurrent vomiting, dyspnoea even at rest, bleeding, dysphagia or the look of fear or grief in the eyes of his loved ones or attendants? Even patients with 'normal' personalities and no history of anxiety neurosis would be anxious if:

(a) pain or any other distress is not taken seriously by professional attendants or given energetic treatment;

(b) the significance to the patient of each new distress is not explored and explained in simple, honest terms, remembering that the significance to him may be quite different from that to the professionals. Good terminal 'caring' requires that each attendant be on the alert for 'the final straw for the camel's back'. Palpitations may be thought of as cancer reaching the heart, sweating as a sign of tuberculosis, oedema as renal failure, poor visual focusing as incipient blindness, etc.

(c) different doctors and nurses give different and apparently conflicting explanations, prognosis and advice.

Management

1. No anxiolytic is as effective as time spent sharing a patient's problem and ensuring that he is as fully in the picture about his illness and its features as his intelligence, education and state of health will permit. This requires not so much quantity of time spent with a patient as quality of time. The dying are usually acutely aware of how little time is left to them and how busy are their professional attendants, and ask only that these attendants take them and their trouble seriously. A few minutes of serious, concentrated attention are more valuable to them than half an hour of light superficial conversation, when something is troubling them.

2. The best anxiolytics are those which relieve the distressing symptoms, whether appropriate analgesics for pain. steroids for anorexia, laxatives for constipation, or anti-emetics for vomiting.

3. When all else has been tried, only then should the true anxiolytics with the shortest half-lives be prescribed, preferably in the early morning and late at night when anxiety and pain are usually more evident and alarming.

4. When tablets cannot be swallowed, it is worth remembering that lorazepam can be taken sublingually or diazepam be given as suppositories (2 mg, 5 mg, 10 mg).

5. When pain is a feature of the condition, and of sufficient degree to merit consideration of an opiate, it should be borne in mind that morphine and diamorphine remain both the best analgesics, euphoriants *and* anxiolytics, particularly when combined with a steroid for its central effect.

6. It is sometimes forgotten that intramuscular benzodiazepines take longer to become effective than by oral or rectal administration.

Cough

Although, as might be expected, breathlessness and dyspnoea are often encountered in such patients, cough is remarkably uncommon. Even in palliative-care units treating hundreds of patients each year, months can elapse without seeing a patient distressed by cough.

Causes

Bronchial Obstruction from a tumour or mediastinal mass.

Secondary Bronchial Infection, pneumonia or infection in necrotic or atelectasis.

Paroxysmal Nocturnal Dyspnoea with characteristic dyspnoea and irritating cough, waking the patient.

Bronchial Irritation from inhaled irritants, particularly in a dry, centrally or gas-heated atmosphere.

Management

Patients with a productive cough are seldom as disturbed by it as those with a dry cough as in uninfected bronchial tumours, mediastinal obstruction and chronic bronchitis. The two will therefore be considered separately.

In Productive Cough.

1. The role of the physiotherapist in aiding expectoration and drainage is pre-eminent. Her undoubted skills will be used to most advantage if there is close co-operation with the physician, who can, by auscultation and X-rays, more accurately localise atelectasis, abscess or bronchial tumour. It is also the responsibility of the doctor to advise nurses about the optimum position for the patient in order to drain the affected areas.
2. Even in far-advanced disease, it is often worth having sputum cultured in case a specific antibiotic will clear secondary infection and facilitate a freer expectoration. Unscientific as it may appear when no pathogens have been found, the use of cotrimazole is often helpful.
3. Mucolytics such as bromhexine 8–16 mg t.i.d. may be useful, in spite of the paucity of scientific evidence to substantiate their use.
4. Expectorant cough mixtures are probably as effective as the syrup

base in which they are made and expensive proprietary ones offer no advantages over honey and warm water, glycerine or a hot 'toddy'. The doctor must be alert to relatives offering a sodium bicarbonate drink with its undoubted expectorant effect, but equally predictable electrolyte upset (see Chapter 6).

Dry Irritating Coughs.

1. Cough suppressants do work. Start with codeine or pholcodine linctus in warm water, progressing to methadone linctus and, finally, the ultimate drugs, morphine and diamorphine, in a syrup base, provided the lowest dose is used capable of alleviating cough without depression of respiration, and bearing in mind that each drug is capable of producing constipation to a greater or lesser extent. Experience convinces the author that in many patients with far-advanced disease, often characterised by other symptoms of pain, fear and dyspnoea, the skilled and judicious use of morphine has more to commend it than has usually been appreciated.
2. Humidification of the atmosphere frequently helps. It can be produced by commercial humidifers (expensive), steam kettles in the bedroom, steam inhalers, a Wright's vaporiser or, if oxygen is being employed, by humidification of the gas.
3. Steroids can reduce tumour and bronchial oedema and lessen bronchospasm. The most commonly used are EC prednisolone 5 mg t.i.d. or dexamethasone 0.5 mg t.i.d.
4. Bupivacaine aerosol used for 10 minutes every 4-6 hours promises to be one of the best remedies, but requires special equipment at present normally available only in hospital.

Nursing Measures

The need for close co-operation between doctors and nurses has been emphasised already. The former may too readily see cough as of minor importance only calling for a 'bottle', whereas it will fall to the nurse, whether a professional or a relative, to spend much of the day making the patient comfortable. The following guidelines also apply when the principal distress is dyspnoea.

1. Patients with *un*complicated bronchogenic carcinoma should be provided with two or three pillows and *not*, as in chronic obstructive airways disease, be propped bolt upright in bed. Both cough and dyspnoea in these cancer patients are reduced when nursed semi-prone or they are allowed to lounge in a comfortable chair.

2. Patients with pleural effusion, whether drained or not, should lie on the affected side in a semi-prone position. This underlines the need for any chest aspiration to be performed as painlessly as possible, if the chest wall is to be comfortable to lie on, and for the nurses to be fully informed about the side and size of any effusion.

Depression

Many terminally ill patients will be profoundly depressed, but will not be suffering from a 'depression state' requiring an antidepressant, the inappropriate use of which may lead to unnecessary sedation, worse constipation, uncomfortable dry mouth and halitosis and possibly urinary retention on top of all their other problems. Doctors and nurses, and indeed many clergymen, must train themselves to differentiate between 'depression' and 'misery'.

The principal features of a depressive state are no different in a terminal illness than at any other time in life; namely, early morning wakening; a disturbed sleep pattern; poor concentration and appetite; a sense of guilt and being a burden on others; and diurnal variation. In both young and old it may present as agitated anxiety. It is obvious that many of the features are also to be found in many other types of serious illness, making the diagnosis very difficult. Readers are here referred to Chapter 11 by Professor Michael Bond, where he so clearly describes the pattern of depression in patients with chronic pain and the change in clinical picture as their distresses are removed.

It is useful to regard the salient diagnostic features as (1) the changes in sleep pattern, and (2) impaired concentration and interest, and to look for them before embarking on a therapeutic trial of antidepressants. Even when features of anxiety are also present, it is preferable to use an antidepressant with anxiolytic properties, rather than a 'pure' anxiolytic. Although there is little to choose between the many tricyclic antidepressants, certain features are worthy of note.

Amitriptyline. Antidepressant/anxiolytic and mildly sedative when taken at night.

Imipramine. Antidepressant and mildly stimulant, therefore never taken after 4.00 p.m. Because it has been reported as epileptogenic, it is probably best avoided.

Protriptyline. Stimulant antidepressant with no anxiolytic properties.

Clomipramine. Antidepressant, useful when obsessional ruminative neurotic features are present.

Trimipramine. Antidepressant with sedative properties, useful in depressed, chronically insomnic, older patients.

Doxepin. Antidepressant with good anxiolytic properties.

The newer tetracyclic antidepressants (for example, mianserin) appear to have fewer side-effects and may produce a speedier effect, although this remains doubtful. Nevertheless, these features make them useful drugs for patients with enough to bear already. The dietary restrictions essential for the monoaminoxydase inhibitors (MAOIs) rule them out for most patients with advanced disease when there are better alternatives.

Clinicians will, quite rightly, continue to debate whether the many symptoms listed above should be regarded as inevitable features of terminal illness in many patients or evidence of depression necessitating antidepressants. In the author's opinion, it would certainly not be wrong to give a two to three-week trial of one of these drugs in adequate dosage. However, it cannot be stated strongly enough that the principal prescription must be sympathetic support for the patient, with an obvious willingness to encourage him to ventilate his every emotion and express his every fear, furnish him with full information, make every attempt to remove his pain and other distresses, and learn to sit with him when there is 'no more to be done'.

Dysphagia

The importance of this relatively uncommon symptom is obvious – it lies in the patient's fear that he will either choke or starve to death. That this rarely happens and peaceful death usually intervenes before such a horrifying event may be well known to doctors and nurses, but is seldom believed by the sufferer.

Causes

Pharyngeal Obstruction, from tumour, fibrosis, extrinsic pressure from neck glands, etc.

Oesophageal Obstruction, either intrinsic from carcinoma and oesophagitis or extrinsic from mediastinal masses.

Neuromuscular Failure as in motor neuron disease.

Plummer-Vincent Syndrome (Paterson Kelly syndrome in North America).

Management

1. The utmost energy must be spent on treating the primary cause, where possible.
2. A cilestin tube should be inserted in all but those already within days of death from a total obstruction of the oesophagus. Nurses, in particular, should be aware of the size of lumen, so as to advise on the bulk of food the patient may take, rather than enforcing a fluid or semi-fluid, liquidised diet. Before each meal he should drink soda water or tonic water, preferably with 1 teaspoon of honey in it, and repeat the procedure after each meal. It is often helpful to show a patient and his family a tube, so that they may be reassured about the type of food possible.
3. Dexamethasone 8–12 mg a day may be tried for mediastinal obstruction not amenable to palliative radiotherapy or chemotherapy, but the danger, if given for any length of time, of dexamethasone-induced myopathy must be borne in mind, particularly in the previously ambulant patient.
4. Adequate hydration, correct positioning after meals and advice to reduce air swallowing are the priorities for nursing attendants.

Dyspnoea

This symptom is present in all patients with chronic obstructive airways disease and is severe in 50 per cent of men with bronchogenic carcinomata and 25 per cent of women with this malignancy. There must be few more frightening symptoms. Not only are many of the normal activities of life curtailed, but the steady, inexorable difficulty in breathing convinces most patients that they will finally die of suffocation. It is therefore important for all attendants to know both how to palliate the distress and, by every means at their disposal, reassure the patient and family that when life comes to its end, it is usually peaceful and often during sleep. In fact no more than 1 per cent of patients suffer a frightening death associated with mental alertness, uncontrollable pulmonary oedema and panic-filled dyspnoea.

Whatever the underlying pathology, professional attendants must demonstrate the most sensitive interest in the patient's problem and his fears, which more often than not exacerbate his dyspnoea more than he probably realises, particularly in bronchial tumours. Specific management of respiratory failure is dealt with in Chapter 6, but the principal general causes of dyspnoea are summarised below.

Causes

Airways Obstruction. Caused by tumours of the nasopharynx, larynx, thyroid and enlarged cervical and mediastinal nodes. All may produce a degree of *stridor*. Obstruction by bronchitis, bronchial tumour and asthma will produce *wheeze*.

Loss of Lung Elasticity. Caused by lymphangitis carcinomatosis, emphysema, post-radiation fibrosis and interstitial fibrosis.

Loss of Lung Tissue. Caused by pleural effusion, tumour infiltration and secondary deposits or abscess.

Defect in Neuromuscular Control. As in motor neuron disease (MND) cerebral vascular accidents (CVA) and certain rare neuropathies.

Non-pulmonary Causes. Such as cardiac oedema, anaemia, mediastinal obstruction, elevation of the diaphragm by massive ascites or hepatomegaly, anxiety state or interruption of the phrenic nerve anywhere in its course.

Management

In spite of the multitude of possible causes and mechanisms capable of producing the dyspnoea, the principles of care can be stated simply.

1. Make very effort to reduce the cause and contributory factors by antibiotics where appropriate, tumour shrinkage by radio- or chemotherapy, reduction of oedema, expectoration of sputum, and judicious tapping of effusions and ascites.
2. Reduce bronchospasm and, to a lesser extent, bronchial tumour mass by *steroids*, for example, EC prednisolone 20–30 mg a day or dexamethasone 2 mg b.d.
3. Relieve bronchospasm with salbutamol orally or by inhalation.

4. *Morphine solution* 4-hourly day and night, in the lowest dose needed to relieve tachypnoea; remember that the dose is dictated by the age, rather than the size, of the adult patient. A young thin man will require a proportionately higher does than an elderly obese patient.
5. Many patients appreciate a simple fan on the bedside table, particularly if they can control it for themselves. Its benefit can only be psychological, but in the author's experience few measures have been found more helpful.
6. The question must inevitably arise whether oxygen should be employed. Its use in chronic bronchitis is fully dealt with in Chapter 6, but in most other patients, unless they specially request it because of faith they have gained from previous experience, its use is often more frightening than useful.
7. Alarming as dyspnoea can be, anxiolytics (even short-acting benzodiazepines) are seldom as helpful as skilfully used opiates.
8. Aminophylline suppositories, though principally of value for bronchitis and bronchospasm, do have a place for the dyspnoea of bronchogenic carcinoma.

Fungating Tumours and Odours

Can we begin to imagine what it must feel like for a patient to see part of his body 'rotting' and to have to live with the offensive smell from it, see the reaction of his visitors (including doctors and nurses) and know that it signifies lingering death? Denying the existence of a bad smell will never comfort a patient who is acutely aware of it.

Management

1. *Radiotherapy* should be *considered* for fungating tumours.
2. *Antibiotics* have a real place for reducing secondary infection and, in the case of abdominal sinuses and deep sloughing sores with overhanging edges, the insertion of a daily tablet/pessary of metronidazole may make all the difference to the smell.
3. Nurses will be aware that oxygen blown directly into a deep sore, even when no anaerobic organisms have been cultured, may speed its healing.
4. Plain yoghurt applied to a deep ulcer/fungating tumour may assist in de-sloughing and healing, and frequently reduces odour. It has to be reapplied daily.
5. The following preparations are said to help in de-sloughing, and price

seems to be the only thing to choose between them:

(a) chlorinated lime and boric acid solution;

(b) chlorinated soda solution;

(c) benzoic acid, malic acid, propylene glycol, salicylic acid solution or cream;

(d) Debrisan, mixed into a paste with glycerine or, alternatively, honey;

(e) streptokinase-streptodornase solution;

(f) Bismuthiodoform paste smeared on gauze before it is packed into the cavity or tumour.

Probably the most important thing about their use, apart from ensuring viability of surrounding tissues, is for *continuity* of a regime, rather than the indiscriminate changing from one to another according to which nursing sister is on duty.

6. The skin around fistulae may be protected with:

(a) barrier cream;

(b) carboxymethylcellulose gelatin paste;

(c) Complan applied locally when digestive enzymes are thought to be in the leakage;

(d) stomahesive;

(e) egg white applied once or twice daily.

7. The most effective deodorisers are charcoal pads applied on top of all the other packs and dressings on the tumour or wound. With these it is possible to remove all odour even for the patient himself.

The small aerosol air fresheners available commercially may be modestly effective, but their scented smell comes to be associated with painful memories for the relatives for years to come.

8. The smell from gynaecological tumours may be reduced with:

(a) pessaries hydrargaphen b.d.;

(b) pessaries povidone-iodine b.d.;

(c) bismuthiodoform paste, gently packed into the vaginal introitus.

Halitosis

This is rarely reported, but frequently suffered. It embarrasses the patient and his attendants, and may further isolate him from his loved ones.

Causes

Bad Oral Hygiene. Because of candidiasis, dental sepsis, dentures, loss of saliva, mouth bleeding.

Sinus and Naso-pharyngeal Infections.

Cess-pool Halitosis. Because of delayed gastric emptying or gastric carcinoma, particularly with linitis plastica.

Chronic Pulmonary Pathology. Particularly bronchiectasis, lung abscess and necrotic malignancy.

Management

1. Energetic attention to oral hygiene in all patients. This is an example of the attention to detail that is essential in good palliative care and something easily taught to attending relatives at home. Dentures must be removed and cleaned regularly, preferably in 0.2 per cent chlorhexidine or half-strength domestic bleach. When any infection has been cleared, the mouth may be kept fresh by sucking paper-thin slivers of iced pineapple in the buccal pouches (employing the proteolytic enzyme action of its ananase) or by 2-hourly swabbing with lemon and glycerine mouth swabs.
2. Gastric emptying may be accelerated with metoclopramide 10 mg t.i.d. or domperidone 10-20 mg t.i.d., the latter being preferable because of the absence of extra-pyramidal effects.
3. Peppermint or 'Amplex' sweets and lozenges occasionally help or, provided such an ill patient can take them, charcoal biscuits.

There is no cure for the highly offensive odour from some bronchial tumours, but occasionally antibiotics are helpful, even when sputum cultures fail to reveal a significant secondary infection.

Hiccups

The occasional short-lived attack does not need attention, but when it persists, sometimes for days or weeks, it disturbs sleep, rest and eating and can be very distressing or even alarming.

Causes

Irritation of the Phrenic Nerve by tumour involvement in the mediastinum.

Irritation of the Diaphragm by infection, tumour infiltration or after pleurodesis for recurrent pleural effusion.

Uraemia.

Dyspepsia, especially with hiatus hernia or reflux oesophagitis.

Elevation of the Diaphragm, especially with gross hepatomegaly from any cause.

Management

1. If it is indicated for other reasons, such as mediastinal obstruction, radiotherapy may occasionally relieve irritation of the phrenic nerve and reduce hiccups.
2. Interruption of the phrenic nerve may be achieved by:
   (a) surgical crushing in the neck under local anaesthetic;
   (b) 5 per cent phenol in glycerine infiltration around the nerve at the same site.
3. The following drugs are worthy of trial before a final decision is made to interrupt the nerve:
   (a) Haloperidol 0.5 mg q.i.d. orally or 1.5 mg intramuscularly to abort an attack.
   (b) Chlorpromazine 25 mg q.i.d. or a single injection to abort an attack.
   (c) Perphenazine 2-4 mg t.i.d.
   (d) Metoclopramide 10 mg q.i.d.
   (e) Hyosine hydrobromide 400 μg p.r.n. bearing in mind the distressing tachycardia which may follow.
4. Nurses will wish to help the patient rebreath his own CO_2 from a paper bag held over the face, but, in practice, this seldom helps unless the cause was simple flatulent dyspepsia.

Hyperhidrosis (Excessive Sweating)

This is another example of a symptom regarded as either inevitable or unimportant by professional attendants, but often deeply distressing and worrying to the patient, because he fears he has an infectious condition in addition to his main disease. For this reason alone, it is worth investigating it so as to reassure.

Causes

It should be noted that often no specific cause can be found to account for it.

Cachexia from rapidly progressive cancer of any type.

Bacteraemia or other serious infection (except in the *final* days of a terminal illness, it is usually worth while treating an intercurrent infection, if by so doing the patient's comfort is improved).

Hodgkin's Disease or Oat-cell Bronchogenic Carcinoma.

Anxiety State.

Management

1. Deal with cause, if possible.
2. Indomethacin 25 mg q.i.d. orally after meals or by suppository 100 mg b.d. The possibility of this drug producing mental confusion in such patients has always to be borne in mind.
3. Plasma exchange in Hodgkin's disease or the reticuloses.
4. Propranolol 40 mg t.i.d., if not contra-indicated because of bronchospasm or cardiac failure.
5. Any benzodiazepine with a short half-life.
6. Rarely is there an indication for surgical excision of the axillary sweat glands in such patients.

Most patients are more assisted by skilled nursing, frequent sponging and appropriate advice about clothing and bedding than by any medical measures.

Insomnia

Exactly why this is statistically more common in cancer patients than those with non-malignant terminal disease is not known. It is a cause of much distress to both patients and relatives, and can readily become a reason for hospital admission, if relatives become exhausted through their own loss of sleep. Although it is undoubtedly true that at many other times patients, particularly the psychoneurotic, too readily demand hypnotics, their skilled use in terminal care is justified if, by enabling them to sleep restfully, their pain threshold is raised, their anxiety tension is relieved and their attendants and, in particular, the relatives can care better.

Causes

The exact cause is seldom found, but is usually bound up with one or more of the following, each of which demands attention.

Poorly Relieved Physical Distress. This may not be reported as such by the patient, and is particularly the case with pain (see Chapter 11).

Anxiety. Sometimes this is so sub-clinical that it is not apparent during the day.

Depression. Disturbed sleep pattern, particularly in the elderly, may be the only feature for some time and failure to explore this and/or prescribe the therapeutic trial of an antidepressant is a common error.

Nocturnal Frequency. This may occur in either sex and (in the absence of benign prostatic hypertrophy) may respond to emepronium 200 mg on retiring.

Night Sweats. (See hyperhidrosis.)

Dependence on Barbiturates or Benzodiazepenes which, for some reason, have recently been discontinued.

Management

All that can be done is to give guidelines. Nothing, however, can be a substitute for companionship and a carefully created atmosphere of peace and safety.

1. If barbiturates have been regularly used until recently, they are best resumed, provided the patient is not now on anticoagulants or doxycycline.
2. When no cause can be found, it is wiser to *assume* that depression is responsible and to prescribe an antidepressant with sedative and anxiolytic properties such as amitriptyline, doxepin or trimipramine at bedtime.
3. The agitated patient will respond better to pericyazine 5-20 mg at night and to either chlorpromazine or a benzodiazepine.
4. The ruminative, obsessional patient may be tried on clomipramine 25-75 mg at night, the dose being increased gradually.

5. Long-acting benzodiazepines such as nitrazepam, chlordiazepoxide, diazepam, triazolam, flurazepam are to be avoided. Too frequently they leave the patient sedated next day, may actually induce fear in some patients, rather than being anxiolytic and any blurring of intellectual acuity may further distress these patients.
6. An alcoholic drink, particularly in the elderly and those not accustomed to much daytime alcohol, is often helpful. It would not be appropriate in a patient taking metronidazole, nor a tricyclic antidepressant.
7. The simple remedy of a low-wattage lamp, preferable a pink one, left burning in the room often helps to dispel some of the primitive fears of the dark.
8. Chlormethiazole is a justifiably popular and much-used hypnotic, but it cannot be prescribed with either a benzodiazepine or haloperidol, yet the latter are frequently necessary in terminal care. This underlines the need for the most careful review of the drugs being prescribed for such patients.

Finally, let it be remembered that, particularly in patients with cerebral neoplasms, there may be a reverse of sleep pattern with daytime sleep and night-time alertness. This must be left alone and every effort made to reassure the patient that his behaviour is not, as he may imagine, a manifestation of a neurotic or psychotic state.

Nausea and Vomiting

These two symptoms, singly or combined, are suffered by 25–40 per cent of the terminally ill. Although pain may be the most dreaded symptom, it is often much easier to control than nausea, the persistence of which, in spite of all anti-emetics now available, can be one of the most humbling yet challenging experiences when caring for the dying. Although nausea may not always be accompanied by vomiting, the two are best considered together.

Causes

Drug-Induced. Almost any drug can produce it, but the worst offenders are the analgesics, antimitotics, digoxin, oestrogen-like drugs and most syrup-based medicines. Contrary to widely-held beliefs, the opiates rarely continue to produce nausea after the first three or four days of their use. Doctors have as high a responsibility at this time as at any other to review regularly the drugs the patient is on, if by so doing they can reduce adverse effects, eliminating incompatability and effect economy.

Gastric Pathology. Although thinking here principally of carcinoma, it has constantly to be remembered that the dying may continue to suffer from their hiatus hernia, ulcer, etc. that they have had for so long.

Sub-acute Intestinal Obstruction.

Raised Intracranial Pressure.

Hypercalcaemia. (p. 327.)

Ovarian Carcinoma.

Uraemia.

Anxiety State.

Infection.

Idiopathic. There remains a small number of patients in whom, after as thorough and as exhausting investigations have been carried out as seem appropriate in those so ill, no cause can be found, but who may yet respond to dexamethasone 8-12 mg a day. Its mode of action is unknown in these cases.

Management

1. Remove or correct the cause (before prescribing an anti-emetic). Self-evident as this may sound, it is not often done because of the professional inertia and indiscipline sometimes displayed in terminal care. Infection can usually be treated with minimal upset and much benefit. Electrolyte imbalance or hypercalcaemia can be righted, bowels evacuated, diet manipulated, nauseating drugs be changed to lesser offenders, dexamethasone be prescribed for raised intracranial pressure, etc. What is required is the positive, energetic approach, which should be the hallmark of good palliative care.
2. Prescribe appropriate anti-emetics. This is easier said than done.

In theory, one ought to be able to choose one from the two groups — centrally acting and those acting upon the gastrointestinal tract — but in 15 per cent or so of cases two different drugs may have to be employed concurrently, and in 5 per cent of cases even three at once. For this reason it is worth reviewing the principal anti-emetics in current use.

Anti-emetics Acting on the Central Nervous System (centrally acting).
Prochlorperazine: Modest anti-emetic, some sedation and tranquillising
Chlorpromazine: Good anti-emetic, but some sedation and tranquillising
Promethazine: Modest anti-emetic, but marked sedation
Trifluoperazine: Modest anti-emetic, but marked sedation
Cyclizine: Good anti-emetic, minimal sedation, useful anti-vertigo
Dicyclamine: Modest anti-emetic
Perphenazine: Good anti-emetic, less sedating than chlorpromazine
Hyoscine hydrobromide: Modest anti-emetic, rapid development of tolerance, distressing palpitations
Haloperidol: Good anti-emetic, modest anxiolytic
Droperidol: Good anti-emetic, short acting, very sedative

Anti-emetics Acting on the Gastrointestinal Tract.
Metoclopramide: Good anti-emetic, no sedation
Domperidone: Good anti-emetic without extra-pyramidal effects
Cimetidine: Anti-emetic only in gastric hyperaemic conditions
Ranitidine: Same as cimetidine.

How does one select the right drug? Decide whether the patient would also benefit from an anxiolytic or mild sedation, what are the risks of producing extra-pyramidal effects (because almost all, including metoclopramide, are capable of producing them), whether vertigo is also a problem (in which case cyclizine or prochloperazine might help), whether the root cause of the vomiting would *appear* to be within the gastrointestinal tract itself (where metoclopramide, domperidone or cimetidine would be indicated). At the end of the day, the best advice is to know a few in each group and restrict prescribing to them, never hesitating to use two concurrently, but being ever alert to incompatibilities in the effects on the utilisation of other drugs.

For example, metoclopramide (to accelerate gastric emptying) would not be given with propantheline, emepronium or hyoscine. If given with analgesics, it would have to be remembered that movement through the upper gastrointestinal tract would be speeded up, and if given with aspirin or paracetamol, the latter would be potentiated. Neither should metoclopramide be given with haloperidol or any of the phenothiazines, because of the increased risk of extrapyramidal effects. Cimetidine would not be prescribed with diazepam, nor with propanolol, because of potentiation of the latter drug as a result of decreased hepatic metabolism.

3. *Anxiolytics.* When all else has failed, even without marked evidence of anxiety, it is often found to be worth while prescribing short-acting benzodiazepines (for example, lorazepam 1 mg t.i.d.), for a few days' trial.

4. Experienced doctors and nurses will not need to be reminded that patients suffering persistent nausea with occasional vomiting from abdominal carcinomatosis are usually symptom-free when lying flat in bed, but much worse when the abdominal contents drag on the mesentery as they stand up. Putting on abdominal binders or light-weight foundation garments have no benefit. Sadly, such patients may well have to spend their last weeks or months in bed most of the time.

Oedema of Limbs

Unilateral Upper Limb

Lymphoedema is best treated, not as is so often suggested by slinging the arm from a drip stand, which is usually too uncomfortable to bear, but by the use of a Flowtron (British) or Jobst (American) intermittent compression pump, starting with 20 minutes twice daily and increasing to four-hourly. In many parts of Britain, these may be borrowed for home-based patients from local physiotherapy departments, but there is much to be said for large group practices or health centres possessing their own, as they are useful both for cancer patients with lymphoedema and in the prevention of deep venous thrombosis (DVT) in bed-bound patients.

Bilateral Upper Limb

The clinical picture of a superior vena caval obstruction (SVC) with its venous distention, infra-orbital pouches of oedema and upper limb cyanosis must be learnt by all doctors and nurses caring for the dying.

The florid picture can hardly be missed, but those in attendance must be alert for its warning feature of visibly distended jugular vein when a patient stoops down to tie his shoelaces or pick up something from the floor. Its management with radiotherapy, chemotherapy and/or high-dose dexamethasone are dealt with elsewhere.

Unilateral Lower Limb

The three principal causes in terminal care are as follows.

1. *Venous and lymphatic obstruction*, because of tumour mass alongside the internal iliacs and in the inguinal glands. This is an indication for radiotherapy and chemotherapy.
2. *Deep venous thrombosis (DVT)* managed in the usual way, although it is seldom justified to use anticoagulants, unless there is estimated to be a relatively long prognosis and few secondary hazards of such drugs.
3. *Infection*, whether cellulitis, lymphangitis or deep tissue infection from nearby tumour, treated usually with appropriate antibiotics, bedrest, limb elevation and analgesics as required.

Bilateral Lower Limb

The three principal causes in terminal care are described below.

1. *Inferior vena caval (IVC)/pelvic obstruction*, often helped temporarily by radiotherapy, but less successfully so with dexamethasone (12 mg a day) than in SVC obstruction.
2. *Cardiac failure*, treated in the usual way. Although the diuretics of choice for efficiency and speed are the loop diuretics such as frusemide and bumetanide, the need to take potassium supplements with them means even more tablets for a patient suffering polypharmacy, and the first opportunity should be taken to change to an aldosterone antagonist with its potassium-sparing properties (for example, spironolactone or triamterene). The possibility of myalgia with bumetanide must be borne in mind when high doses are employed.
3. *Hypoproteinaemia*, either from dietary deficiency or loss of ascitic fluid. Whether such protein should be replaced in such desperately sick patients, if need be by IV infusion, is one of the difficult ethical problems frequently encountered in terminal care.

Pleural Effusion

Though not strictly a symptom, this complication of so many conditions can pose a problem to the clinician. It should be tapped only for the following reasons:

1. for diagnostic purposes;
2. if by so doing, it is expected to relieve incapacitating dyspnoea; that is to say, if it is considered the principal cause of the dyspnoea and not a coincidental clinical finding;
3. if any residual chest-wall discomfort after the procedure is not likely to make the nursing more difficult.

Obviously the clinical judgement is a fine one. If the patient has been told that he has 'fluid in his chest' and it has been tapped with some symptomatic improvement, the patient will inevitably expect the procedure to be repeated when dyspnoea returns, and will find it difficult or undesirable to appreciate that the effusion is only a part of a far more extensive disease process. The general practitioner must pause before sending such a patient back into hospital for tapping, and remember the effect of the journey, the anxiety for patients and family, the 'obligation' upon the junior doctor to tap, and the profound disappointment to the patient if the benefit he expected does not materialise.

It is worth remembering that, particularly with malignant disease, effusions tend to be loculated and the pleura so thickened that even the confirmation of effusion can be difficult and the procedure of tapping even more so. Junior doctors, in particular, need to be reminded that repeated aspiration of effusion, secondary to mesothelioma, leads to tumour seedlings in the needle track and chest-wall pain that usually requires nerve-block procedures to control it.

When the malignant effusion is likely to recur and the life expectancy of the patient will give him time to benefit from it, it is worth considering the instillation into the space of bleomycin, thiotepa, C-parvum, talc powder or tetracycline. With each, except tetracycline, there may be a brisk reaction with pyrexia and slight nausea, but the results frequently justify it (see Chapter 9). Finally, it has to be remembered that whereas in bronchial tumours an effusion heralds a short prognosis, in breast cancers the patient may still have eighteen months to two years of life.

Pruritus

Causes

Obstructive Jaundice.

Anxiety State.

Allergic Reaction, particularly to bed linen and soap powders used in laundering.

Melanomatosis. Here the condition is more one of hypersensitivity to light touch, even of bedclothes.

Management

1. In obstructive jaundice it is worth trying the following.
   (a) Haloperidol 0.5 mg t.i.d. or 2 mg at night. In theory, because of the long half-life, once daily administration should suffice, but it seldom does. Larger doses may prove hepatotoxic and certainly sedative.
   (b) EC prednisolone 30 mg daily in divided doses, reducing to 15 mg daily when relief is obtained.
   (c) Methylprednisolone 40–80 mg daily by injection for one week, and oral prednisolone or weekly 'depot' solution of methylprednisolone.
   (d) Cholestyramine 1 sachet b.d. if the patient can tolerate the taste, which may be improved by dissolving in tonic water.
   (e) Norethandrolone 10 mg t.i.d.
   (f) Methyltestosterone 25 mg sublingually b.d.
   (g) Cimetidine 200 mg t.i.d., 400 mg at night may be helpful in Hodgkin's disease.
   (h) Surgical management is described in Chapter 3.
2. General non-specific measures including the following.
   (a) Antihistamines such as chlorpheniramine 4 mg t.i.d., trimeprazine tartrate 10 mg t.i.d., but their sedative effects make these drugs unacceptable to many patients.
   (b) Sodium bicarbonate washes, as often as desired by the patient. These are made by dissolving 1 tablespoonful of powder in the smallest volume of water required to dissolve it and it is dabbed on with a piece of gauze. Few measures are more effective or more acceptable to the patient.
   (c) 1 per cent phenol calamine lotion as required.

(d) Crotamiton lotion or ointment as required. (Weak topical steroids such as hydrocortisone are seldom effective.)
(e) Cold fans playing on the exposed skin or eau-de-cologne sprays.
(f) In melanomatosis a β-blocker such as propranolol 40 mg t.i.d. occasionally helps.

Sore Mouth

Anything which makes eating, swallowing or speaking difficult is worth treating.

Causes

Oral Candidiasis. See also Anorexia.

Aphthous Ulcers. Much less common.

Vitamin Deficiency. Particularly of the B group.

Ill-fitting Dentures.

Chemotherapy. Where, in extreme cases, de-epithelialisation may occur.

Management

Candidiasis must be treated energetically or not at all. There is no point in asking a patient to take unpleasant-tasting medication without advising him on the supporting measures that are essential for eradication or control of the infection. Nothing is superior to Nystatin oral suspension 1 ml q.i.d., provided: (a) it is put in the mouth with dentures removed; (b) dentures are left out all night soaking in 0.2 per cent chlorhexidine or half-strength domestic bleach.

Superior Vena Caval Obstruction

This complication, neither a symptom nor common, merits mention because of the distress it produces and its dramatic response to therapy (see Chapter 9). Untreated it heralds death, within weeks usually, but, once treated, the patient may survive three months and have no further suffering from the obstruction. It occasionally presents as one of the genuine emergencies of palliative care, and its features should therefore be known to community nurses, who may be visiting the housebound patient more often than the doctor.

Management

1. Emergency radiotherapy.
2. Dexamethasone.
   Emergency: IM 8 mg t.i.d. for 2 days, and then orally in descending daily doses of 20 mg, 16 mg, 12 mg, etc.
   Maintenance: 8–12 mg daily in divided doses.

Urinary Symptoms

So interrelated are they that it is appropriate to consider here incontinence, retention, frequency, strangury and catheter problems. Urinary incontinence is found to be a problem in 20 per cent of the terminally ill with non-bladder cancer. Causes and management will be considered together.

Incontinence

Urinary Tract Infection (UTI). This is always worth treating if, by so doing, comfort and dignity can be restored. As in geriatric medicine, it is a common cause of confusional states in the terminally ill.

Structural Changes in the Bladder. For example, tumour, post-operative scarring for which even catheterisation may not be wholly successful.

Obstructive Retention or Neurogenic Bladder. This will also require catheterisation, though emergency neurosurgery or radiation may make this a temporary expedient for the latter.

Excessive Sedation. For example, hypnotics, tranquillisers, opiates. Being iatrogenic this is reversible, but when it is only a problem at night it may occasionally be helped by emepronium 200 mg on settling.

Urinary Retention

1. *Drug-induced*, particularly with anticholinergics, tricyclic antidepressants, opiates and sympathomimetics.
2. *Neurological causes* (as in incontinence).
3. *Faecal impaction* in the lower rectum.
4. *Pelvic masses* obstructing the bladder neck.

In all except (1), where it may be possible to withdraw the drug, and (3), where rectal evacuation is called for, the patient will require catheterisation.

Dysuria and Strangury

1. *UTI*, already referred to.
2. *Carcinoma of bladder or prostate*, particularly affecting the trigone.
3. *Calculi or retained blood clot.*
4. *Tumour infiltration* into the bladder from nearby organs (rectum, cervix, vagina).

In all except (1) catheterisation will usually be necessary to perform washouts and deal with the incontinence or partial retention often associated with it.

5. *Generalised bladder pain* (primary carcinoma bladder) is helped by maximum doses of a prostaglandin inhibitor with or without stronger analgesics such as opiates.
6. *Strangury* is occasionally helped by flavoxate 2 q.i.d., propantheline 15 mg q.i.d., emepronium 100-200 mg t.i.d., but failure is common and resort may have to be made to permanent silastic catheterisation and phenol blockade of the relevant nerves.

Urinary Catheterisation

So degrading and upsetting are dribbling incontinence or recurrent retention that, perhaps surprisingly, many terminally ill patients would prefer to have an indwelling catheter. Those who, with good reason, may resent it are patients who have been incapacitated following certain neurolytic or neurosurgical procedures for intractable pain.

Palliative-care physicians frequently encounter patients whose quality of life could have been markedly improved by catheterisation, but it had not been done, either through oversight, or more usually because it had been wrongly thought that the possible infection, haemorrhage, embarrassment or supervision problems outweighed any possible benefits. This is another example of the need for all who are caring for the dying to look most carefully and sympathetically at the whole picture of the patient's distress.

Guidelines for Catheter Care.

1. When it is anticipated that the catheter will be left in for a matter of days to a week, a soft rubber Foley catheter should be employed. When it is likely to be left in place for up to six months a silastic

catheter should be used.

2. Protect against introduced infection with cotrimazole 2 b.d. for the first two days, or ampicillin 1 mg stat., and thereafter maintain sterility with tablets hexaminehippurate 1 g b.d.

3. Do not inflate/deflate the bulb or reinsert different sizes of catheter to combat urine bypassing. Such manipulations do not help.

4. It is illogical to use expensive, dangerous or difficult-to-monitor antibiotics in an attempt to eradicate an organism in the bladder affected by a tumour or holding the catheter.

5. The simplest bladder washouts are the best in most cases:

    (a) chlorhexidine 1 in 5000 strength, daily for infection and weekly for maintenance;

    (b) saline for debris, deposits and clot-removal;

    (c) silver nitrate 1 in 10 000 for distressing bleeding from bladder tumour or mucosa;

    (d) Noxytiolin daily, only if all else fails, yet active antibacterial therapy is called for.

6. Deposits may be lessened or prevented by swallowing 1 g daily of effervescent ascorbic acid.

7. The pain (and fear) of catheterisation can be avoided by using an anaesthetic gel (lignocaine), rather than a simple lubricant, and the prior administration of lorazepam 2 mg sublingually or swallowed, or diazepam 5 mg suppository, if swallowing is impaired, or dextromoramide (Palfium) 5 mg sublingually, if severe pain is anticipated.

Weakness and Lethargy

Inevitable as both might appear to be for patients in the most advanced stage of fatal illness, they are worth reviewing. Occasionally one comes across a cause which is found after minimal non-invasive investigation and, corrected, makes all the difference to the quality of life remaining. It is therefore worth looking for the following.

Boredom

One of the many unsolved problems of terminal care is how to prevent boredom, sense of purposelessness, unproductive inactivity, the frustration of wasted time. Too readily do busy professional attendants, fulfilled in their roles, forget what it feels like to have to sit or lie all day, dependent on others, satiated with radio and television, often unable to concentrate for long and feeling of no real use in the world.

In caring for such people it is obligatory for doctors and nurses, at as early a stage as possible, to learn about the patient's interests and hobbies, to provide not only a range of reading material, radio, television (remote control, if possible) and cassettes, but simple work to do — work which is useful, helpful to others, creative and imaginative. Here one cannot too highly rate the importance of a skilled occupational therapist, particularly if she is oriented to craft work, and all the facilities of a day hospital/hospice. Anyone who thinks that occupational therapy means no more than tapestry and weaving is ill qualified to care for the dying.

Hypercalcaemia

This is found in 12-15 per cent of patients with advanced cancer, usually in the 2.6-3.2 mg per cent range and always worthy of attention. Management consists of:

1. maximum fluid intake, without which other measures may have little effect, along with a loop diuretic;
2. EC prednisolone 30-45 mg a day for dexamethasone 4-6 mg a day in divided doses until serum calcium is normal; or IM methyl prednisolone 80 mg a day;
3. mithromycin 1.5-2.0 mg slow IV injection or infusion;
4. effervescent sodium acid phosphate for maintenance, 1 tablet b.d. or t.i.d.;
5. calcitonin for short-term use or salcatonin for long-term therapy.

Hypokalaemia

This arises from the usual causes and is again worthy of correction.

Adrenal Failure

This occurs because of secondary deposits in the gland, failure to take replacement therapy or failure by the doctor to diagnose and treat the infection in a patient immune-deficient or suppressed. It is remarkably easy to be misled into thinking that the rapid decline of a patient is directly caused by the acceleration of his malignant disease when, in fact, it is adrenal failure secondary to septicaemia and good treatment restores the patient to a happy life, often for very many months.

Excessive Sedation or Analgesia

Depressive State

See section on pp. 306-7.

Miscellaneous

Many other topics could have been included in this chapter, but for limitations of space. Three final topics which merit brief mention are:

Constipation. This affects not less than 75 per cent of the terminally ill and is a cause not only of abdominal discomfort, nausea and lethargy, but also of considerable anxiety in many patients who feel that yet another basic bodily function is failing. Too readily it is overlooked by doctors or left to the nurses who are powerless to do much until a doctor has defined the cause, site and degree of faecal impaction and prescribed appropriately. An equally common fault is proclaiming that there is no impaction because no faecal mass was found on rectal examination forgetting that an empty but *ballooned* rectum signifies impaction *beyond* the examining finger.

Confusion. At some time or other this affects 30 per cent of terminally ill cancer patients and is, of course, a feature of encephalopathy, cerebral anoxia, bacteremia and septicaemia, of hypercalcaemia, of sodium imbalance and of dehydration, and of cerebral metastases. It is often recognised by the patient himself and the cause of untold distress to his relatives who may see it is the stigma of mental illness on top of all else he suffers.

Diarrhoea. Though close on 25 per cent of patients admitted to hospices are said to suffer from diarrhoea, only 5 per cent are found to have true diarrhoea, the balance having spurious diarrhoea or faecal leak from impaction. It is a good rule in palliative care that 'diarrhoea' should be regarded as spurious until proved otherwise and, on no account, should constipating agents be prescribed until the doctor has convinced himself from observation of the motions, examination of the abdomen and rectum that there is no constipation. What may also be described by the patient as diarrhoea is sometimes the mucous discharge from a rectal carcinoma.

Recommended Further Reading

Breckman, B. (1981) *Stoma Care*, Beaconsfield Publications. Beaconsfield, Glos.

Capra, L.G. (1972) *The Care of the Cancer Patient*, William Heinemann Medical Books, London

Chalmers, G.L. (1980) *Caring for the Elderly Sick*, Pitman Medical, Tunbridge Wells

Downie, P.A. (1978) *Cancer Rehabilitation*, Faber and Faber, London

Price, L.A., Hill, B.T. and Ghilchik, M.W. (1981) *Safer Cancer Chemotherapy*, Ballière Tindall, London

Saunders, C.M. (ed.) (1978) *The Management of Terminal Illness*, Edward Arnold, London

Saunders, C.M., Summers, D.H. and Teller, N. (1981) *Hospice: The Living Idea*, Edward Arnold, London

Stoll, B.A. (ed.) (1977) *Breast Cancer Management – Early and Late*, William Heinemann Medical Books, London

Tiffany, R. (ed.) (1978) *Oncology for Nurses and Health Care Professionals*, vols 1 and 2, George Allen and Unwin, Boston and Sydney

Twycross, R.G. and Ventafridda, V. (1980) *The Continuing Care of Terminal Cancer Patients*, Pergamon Press, Oxford

Wilkes, E. (ed.) (1982) *The Dying Patient*, MTP Press, Lancaster

14

NURSING: PRINCIPLES AND PRACTICE

Elizabeth A. Edwards, Jennifer M. Henderson and
Mary Parker

In order to obtain information for this chapter a number of patients
and relatives were interviewed by an experienced nursing sister. Ex-
tracts have been taken from some of the interviews, which provide an
opportunity to focus on the patient as a human being, to include him
in the dialogue concerning the plan for his care and to learn from him.
He is the teacher who can teach nurses and all who care for him about
the problems encountered in palliative care. In the authors' experience,
all patients and patients' relatives stress the need for compassion and
understanding from nurses. It is hoped that these interviews will encourage carers not to shy away from the 'hopelessly' sick, but to get
closer to them, to understand and to help them as their dependency
changes. Carers who do this emerge from each experience enriched.
Patients and relatives benefit as carers gain knowledge and confidence.
In this chapter the separate nursing, social and medical problems can
be drawn out, but these also interrelate and overlap, and therefore no
attempt has been made to separate them. Readers will be able to see
the care which is provided essentially by nurses. The nurse's role is in
observation, in initiating and co-ordinating care by others, in facilitating
communication between patients' families and carers, and in carrying
out the medical prescription. The importance of accurate observation
must be mentioned, as this provides feedback to doctors in order to
obtain the appropriate medical treatment, for example, continuation
or change in drug regime.

Interview 1

The first interview concerns Mrs I., a 67-year-old lady who became
paraplegic following a neoplastic invasion of her spine. The site of the
primary cancer was unknown. Until six months before the interview
Mrs I. had been a village postmistress, leading a full active life. The
following conversation took place four weeks after she had been
admitted to hospital.

Mrs I. Nurse, whatever is to become of me?

Interviewer (I) What do you think is wrong with you?

Mrs I. I was told I had arthritis but I don't believe it . . . You don't have radiotherapy for arthritis do you? I thought I was going to have an operation . . . but it's the other thing.

I What do you mean by 'the other thing'?

Mrs I. . . . the doctors are always saying to the other patients I have good news for you . . . but never to me.

I Have you ever asked the doctors to explain?

Mrs I. No, I always feel they are too brief, anyway I am afraid . . . I don't really know if I want to know the truth . . . half of me does, but then I don't think I could really cope.

I What does your husband say?

Mrs I. He tells me I must ask the doctors . . . Nobody is really talking to me at all.

It was obvious during the conversation that Mrs I.'s mind was in turmoil; she was distressed and tearful.

I How do you feel about being unable to walk?

Mrs I. Well, I am hoping it will improve, it should do, shouldn't it?

I Only time will tell, but even if it doesn't, you will be able to get around in a wheelchair won't you?

At this point the interview was interrupted by an occupational therapist, whom Mrs I. had not met before. She asked Mrs I. for details, as she said that aids would be required in Mrs I.'s home and she would need to measure the width of doors for Mrs I. to get around in a wheelchair. Mrs I. broke down and wept bitterly . . . she had not accepted the idea that she would not walk again and would be confined to a wheelchair.

A few days later:

I How are the plans coming on for you to go home?

Mrs I. Why couldn't it be a simple break? I cannot see any future at all . . . Just look at me . . . overweight, dependent . . . How can he possibly manage?

I Have you talked to your husband about it?

Mrs I. I dare not mention it . . . they are talking about sending me home for a weekend.

I Why are you afraid to talk to your husband?

Mrs I. I don't want to upset him . . . I know he won't be able to cope.

Comment

Many difficulties in communication emerge from this interview. The ward sister informed the interviewer that the husband had talked to the doctor and said he did not wish his wife to know her diagnosis. Despite this, it would seem that the doctors and nurses caring for Mrs I. had not planned Mrs I.'s treatment with her and her husband. If discussion had taken place with them, Mr and Mrs I. might have realised the facilities that could have been available to help with the activities of living such as washing herself, going to the toilet and how the use of a wheelchair would help. Mrs I. had not lost all hope and much more could have been made of this so that she would have been looking forward to the visit of the occupational therapist. A wheelchair would help her to regain some independence. The village community nurse might have been invited to visit Mrs I. in hospital, which would have helped Mrs I. to discuss how she and her husband would cope at home and what support they could expect from the health and social services. She need never have been told her diagnosis, but Mrs I. could have been occupied with plans for the immediate future. Her husband, who was tearful and upset when talking to the ward sister, might have been able to talk over his problems and work out the part he could play to help his wife.

Interview 2

The following discussion took place while Mr Mc. was in hospital, having been readmitted for control of severe pain. This a good example and shows how, through careful assessment, observation and treatment by doctors and nurses, plans were made which enabled Mr Mc. to have a much better quality of life for the last few weeks. He was discharged and looked after by his wife and the district nurse. He remained pain free, as careful assessment and readjustments were continued to his drug regime. He was able to enjoy life at home. His wife was pleased that she was able to cope and grateful for the support of the community staff, her minister, friends and neighbours.

Mr Mc. was a 52-year-old farm-worker who, like his father before him, had carcinoma of the bowel. Two years before this admission, he had had an abdominal perineal resection, he was able to work for some time, but unfortunately developed metastases.

I Where is your pain?

Mr Mc. Right across the base of my back and into my groin . . . It never goes away . . . it really wears you down.

I You also have a discharge from your back passage; does that cause you any additional discomfort?

Mr Mc. No, not really . . . it's just a nuisance.

I Are there any problems with your colostomy?

Mr Mc. No, I look after it myself.

I Good, I understand you also have a leaking sinus?

Mr Mc. That's right, the sinus drains into a bag . . . it smells a bit like a slurry tank . . .

I I'm sure we can give you something to take the smell away. How are you sleeping?

Mr Mc. Thank you, that would be an improvement . . . now, about this sleep, you can't sleep when you are in pain.

Mr Mc. was commenced on a morphine mixture and the dose adjusted until he was alert and pain free. The interview helps to illustrate the nature of chronic pain and the importance of careful assessment.

Mr Mc. It's good to be able to walk about again, and I do so much enjoy my daily bath . . . I wait until everybody else has had theirs, then soak and soak for about an hour.

I How are you sleeping now?

Mr Mc. Much improved . . . I just feel stiff in the morning . . . but it soon passes.

I Is the colostomy still working well?

Mr Mc. Yes, it's fine.

I That's good . . . the mixture can sometimes cause constipation. How is your appetite?

Mr Mc. Now that really is a problem . . . not very good I'm afraid. My mouth is very dry and sore . . . The food just goes into balls and sticks in my mouth . . . I chew and chew but it just won't go down.

On inspecting Mr Mc.'s mouth it was apparent that it was very dry and he had frank thrush. It was explained to him that it could be improved with medication and increased mouth care and that it was contributing to his eating problems.

At a further interview a few days later:

I How does your mouth feel now?

Mr Mc. Better, but I am still not eating . . . look at all the weight

I am losing.

I Have you talked to the dietician?

Mr Mc. Yes . . . but those puréed diets. Ugh!

I Did you have this problem at home?

Mr Mc. Not so bad . . . I could eat what I wanted and when . . . that was important . . . my wife's lentil soup!

I Why don't you ask her to bring some in until you go home again?

Comment

In summary, Mr Mc. was able to retain his self-respect and personal dignity, his pain was successfully treated, he had the companionship of his wife and family at home, and in this way his loneliness and isolation were reduced. He and his wife were able to talk about their problems, which helped both of them to face up to the physical separation of Mr Mc.'s subsequent death.

Mr Mc. was able to spend his remaining days at home, looked after by his wife and the district nurse. Continuing and careful assessment and adjustments to his drug regime enabled him to be free of pain. His quality of life was further improved by the treatment of the oral thrush infection and by the free choice of foods he was able to have at home, such as milk straight from the cow! This is a good example of how, with careful assessment and thought, a treatment regime was established for Mr Mc. A better quality of life was achieved for his last few weeks.

Interview 3

The interview that follows is with the eldest daughter in a family of three – two daughters and a son. The mother, Mrs E., had been living with her eldest daughter for 2½ years. She had gone to her daughter to convalesce following a right hemicolectomy for carcinoma of the caecum, but later suffered a cerebral vascular accident.

Families find palliative and terminal illness disruptive to their lives. Daughters frequently feel a sense of responsibility towards their parents and feel guilty if they seem to be unable to cope as well as they would wish. The interview is with Mrs E.'s daughter.

I When did you start looking after your mother? What were the problems at that time?

R Oh, it must have been 2½ years ago . . . before the operation, when she started having uncontrollable diarrhoea . . . that was the worst part.

I How did you cope?

R Well the house wasn't very suitable, you see my daughter had to share a room with my mother . . . if she was ill at night my little girl found it difficult to sleep and often had to spend the night in our bed. After the operation it was much improved, my mother was much better and we all had a good summer together.

I Were there any problems when she was discharged after her operation?

R Oh yes . . . lots, hospitals do seem to push patients on to their relatives far too soon . . . if only they had kept her in hospital a little longer . . . she was very incontinent when she first came home . . . we had redecorated the bedroom and had a new carpet laid . . . it was soon stained.

I Are you an only child?

R No, I have a sister and brother . . . actually I am a little bitter . . . they never helped, not even when she was well. They never took her for a holiday . . . it would have been nice for her, wouldn't it?

I Why do you think they didn't help? Did you ask them?

R I don't think they wanted the responsibility, but in fairness I suppose I didn't really ask them . . . I felt they should have offered.

I What was the reason for this admission to hospital?

R We were no longer able to cope, you see my mother had a stroke. For the last few weeks she was incontinent and unable to walk. We had to carry her up and down stairs, and on to the commode. I think she found it very humiliating, especially when my husband was helping.

I What other problems were there for you?

R It was difficult to cope with the washing and we didn't like to leave her so we worked alternate shifts so that she was never left on her own.

I This must have had a great effect on your lives.

R Yes, it was a tremendous strain on our marriage and I think it definitely had an adverse effect on the children.

I Would you be prepared to have your mother home again?

R Perhaps, but I would be afraid the situation would get out of control again . . . it was so difficult to get her back into hospital again.

I Did you have any outside help?

R No, just my husband.

I No district nurse or laundry service?

R I felt I could do as much as the nurses, after all I am an auxiliary nurse.

I How do you feel about your mother being in hospital?

R We did all we could . . . I don't feel guilty.

Comment

Mrs E. lived another 2½ months; she never went home again, despite frequent discussions about discharge with the relatives. It may be that Mrs E.'s daughter was difficult to help, but it does seem as if there should have been help and support provided by the community nurses when Mrs E. was discharged. This could easily have been initiated prior to Mrs E.'s discharge. Incontinence is an extremely difficult problem for any family to cope with, whether or not they have any nursing background. Perhaps the general practitioner could have provided support, by taking a firm line with the daughter and her husband when they were showing signs of stress. Had this been the case, Mrs E. may have been able to go home for a time before she died and the family would have suffered much less stress.

Interview 4

The next interview has been quoted in full because it provides so many insights, not least of which is the courageous way in which one couple coped. It describes their depth of caring and understanding of each other, and illustrates the high quality of life which can be enjoyed. The problem of continuity does not arise, as it is the spouse who is providing the nursing care until the last ten days of the illness.

Mr R. was in his early thirties and had been married for about two years. He and his wife had one baby and were looking forward to their future life together when the diagnosis which was to transform their lives was made . . . multiple sclerosis. Mrs R. had some wartime nursing experience and was able to care for her husband for all but the last ten days of his twenty years of illness.

I When were you told what was wrong with your husband?

Mrs R. Well, he had been having problems falling over and dropping things and had difficulty riding his bicycle . . . he had been investigated first in hospital. But it was on a subsequent admission, for repair of a hernia, when I was told. The doctor stopped me in the corridor and gave me the diagnosis.

I What was your reaction?

Mrs R. I was shaken, but I suppose it had been at the back of my mind. I dreaded telling my husband, and waited for an appropriate moment. I kept it as simple as possible and avoided using the term multiple sclerosis.

I Why did you do that?

Mrs R. I was afraid that he would look it up in a medical textbook and find out all the problems that may occur.

I How did you feel when your husband was discharged?

Mrs R. Pleased to have him home, but he was so much better I really couldn't believe the diagnosis . . . In fact I went to my doctor and asked him if it was true.

I How did you see the future?

Mrs R. I did not appreciate that we would have so many happy years together.

I How did your husband accept it?

Mrs R. Superficially he seemed to adjust quite quickly, at first he was uncertain and afraid, but very soon he began to overcome his disabilities, finding different ways to do things . . . he went through a period when he thought nobody could help, and the doctors had 'written him off', he appeared much quieter than usual, it probably lasted about a fortnight . . . but we were able to talk about it.

I Did you tell the family?

Mrs R. No, not straight away, I was afraid it was hereditary . . . I didn't want to worry them . . . of course, I eventually told them.

I Was your husband able to work?

Mrs R. Yes, he had a light job for about 18 months, but I realised I would eventually have to be the breadwinner and I returned to full-time work.

I What was the reaction to that?

Mrs R. I felt generally the family disapproved . . . but I don't regret it, I found it was a help to me and broadened my outlook. It also allowed us a few luxuries . . . a colour television.

I How did you cope with a sick husband, a child, full-time employment and a home to run?

Mrs R. I was very lucky we had support and help from the family and the community and of course my husband was able to help a little.

I Did your relationship change?

Mrs R. Yes, initially, I tried to protect him . . . a mother–child relationship but not quite, but soon I realised I was wrong, I was very dependent upon him as a person and relied on his companionship – he was still master of the house.

I Was there any change in your sexual activity?

Mrs R. At first it was intensified . . . it was a way of expressing our emotions in a physical way . . . but I was afraid I would lose him sooner, or rightly or wrongly I discouraged him . . . I perhaps regret it now. Of course later on it became more difficult . . .

I Did you ever discuss this problem with your doctor?

Mrs R. No, it was never that important and of course we were able to talk about it together . . . that helped.

I How mobile was your husband?

Mrs R. For most of the time he was able to get around the house and garden. His balance was poor and he tended to fall a lot and he was always dropping things. Of course for the last year he was confined to a wheelchair.

I Sometimes your husband must have been on his own when he fell?

Mrs R. There were always friends and neighbours who would rush to help him, but he preferred to wait until he could get himself up. The helpers were very understanding and just stayed and chatted with him.

I How did your husband adapt to being confined to a wheelchair?

Mrs R. Quite well, I was no longer able to cope without it . . . so it was a blessing. It gave him a mobility he didn't have before.

I How did you manage to get your husband up and down stairs?

Mrs R. It was very difficult . . . to come down I would sit on the stairs behind the chair and bump him down, I needed help to get him upstairs.

I Were you afraid?

Mrs R. Yes, I was very scared, it was also not good for him, it jolted him on each stair. Before we had the chair it was even worse . . . I used to help him and once or twice we both fell . . . he remained calm, but I became tense and afraid.

I Did you ever think of rearranging the house so that you didn't have to keep going up and down stairs?

Mrs R. The bathroom was upstairs so it was easier to use the bedroom as a lounge . . . we moved the television and his friends would visit him there. The lounge had two doors and it would have been difficult to protect him from draughts. It was also easier to see that he hadn't too many visitors at a time when he was upstairs!

I Did you ever think of moving to more suitable accommodation?

Mrs R. It was suggested once or twice and I was offered a single-storey house, but we both considered the help and friendship of the surrounding family and community were important.

I From time to time your husband had acute illnesses, how often did these occur?

Mrs R. Yes, that's right . . . often months went by, when he was ill it was usually chest infections which responded to antibiotics.

I How long was he ill for when these episodes occurred?

Mrs R. It could be just a few days or as long as 7-8 weeks in bed.

I How did you feel at these times?

Mrs R. I was very uptight and afraid he would not get better.

I Was it the same each time it occurred?

Mrs R. Exactly the same.

I Did you involve the family in your fears?

Mrs R. No, I had a lot of practical help, but never expressed how I was feeling.

I Did you ever say anything to your husband when he had recovered?

Mrs R. Not really, perhaps I would say, it's good to see you your old self again, but we never really talked about how I felt or about dying.

I Did you manage to keep your husband's skin intact?

Mrs R. He developed a small broken area once when we were on holiday . . . he sat on a plastic-covered seat for too long . . . I was very upset about it.

I Why were you upset? Was it because there was a pressure sore?

Mrs R. No, it was because he tried to hide it from me, he didn't want my holiday spoilt. It could have been prevented if I had known sooner that he was uncomfortable . . . However, we managed to heal it.

I Did he often try to hide things from you?

Mrs R. Sometimes perhaps . . . he didn't grumble very much.

I Were there any problems with incontinence?

Mrs R. We had a careful plan for his bowels, this was where my nursing experience was useful. We managed to control them . . . there was only ever one accident . . . My husband was extremely grateful for that. Towards the end when his mobility was poor he was sometimes incontinent of urine . . . it was more frequent towards the end.

I How did he adapt?

Mrs R. At the beginning it was very infrequent and he was able to use a urinal, eventually he became so floppy and was unable to manage. We tried some appliances but they were not always satisfactory, he could cope much better in bed than in a chair.

I What happened if you were working and he was incontinent?

Mrs R. Latterly he stayed in bed until I came home at lunchtime, and I was able to put an appliance on when I got him up.

I Was he ever wet when you came in?

Mrs R. Not really, sometimes his underpants were a little damp, but he was never soaking wet.

I How did he feel about being incontinent of urine?

Mrs R. We never really talked about the urinary incontinence, but I would think it came on so gradually that he adjusted to it.

I What happened if he was incontinent when he had visitors?

Mrs R. This was difficult for me . . . it was a problem trying to protect his dignity. Some were very understanding and would only stay a couple of hours, but others we had to ask to wait in the kitchen . . . he was very embarrassed at having to be assisted.

I How much was your daughter able to help?

Mrs R. She was of course grown up and living away from home by this time. She must have known her father was incontinent, but I tried to protect her Dad's dignity. I think perhaps the protection was for me. She would never have been involved . . . although she was capable of helping.

I How did you protect his dignity?

Mrs R. I never discussed with anyone his intimate problems . . . he was very much the most important person in the house.

I How long was he acutely ill in the last year?

Mrs R. It must have been over a period of months, he seemed to go from one chest infection to the next and having repeated antibiotics . . . each episode left him a little weaker. This continued until he had the worst one about 10 days before he died.

I Were you still working?

Mrs R. Yes, but the last week happened to be a week's holiday.

I Was it a very difficult decision for you to let him go into hospital?

Mrs R. Yes it was, because I knew in my heart that in his condition he could not go on indefinitely. He told me that this time he felt quite different from all the other attacks and he was going to die. He asked me if I loved him enough I would not try to prolong his life, he said he could not fight any more. This was where it was very difficult for me.

I Was this the first time you had talked in depth about dying?

Mrs R. Yes, in depth . . . we had spoken of it lightly but this was very different . . . we cuddled each other . . . and cried a great deal.

I What were you thinking?

Mrs R. I really didn't believe it was the terminal stage . . . but I understood when he said he couldn't fight any more.

I Did you feel you had let him down when he went into hospital?

Mrs R. No, because it was his decision . . . but afterwards I was sorry . . . he did it to make it easier for us . . . I wish I had realised that when he decided to go . . . maybe deep down I was hoping he was wrong and that the hospital could have done something.

I Did your relationship change when he went into hospital?

Mrs R. Yes, it was certainly different, our conversation became superficial . . . perhaps we had said it all before.

I Would you have liked to have been involved in his care when he was in hospital?

Mrs R. No, I don't think so, I was hoping he could come back home . . . stupidly . . . it was soon apparent he was far too ill.

I Did you find visiting tiring?

Mrs R. I was completely shattered . . . it was much harder than caring for him at home . . . you never knew what he would be like when you went back.

I How did you feel when it was all over?

Mrs R. I never realised how bad it would be. I knew I would miss him, but I'd never really adjusted to the idea.

I Do you think it was worse because you had done so much for him?

Mrs R. No, I think it was just the normal loss of a husband. Suddenly I hated having to register his death . . . under status I had to write 'widow' . . . he wasn't there any more . . .

I Did you find it difficult to make the other arrangements?

Mrs R. No, not so difficult . . . the undertaker was very helpful and could answer all my questions. The minister was also a great support. I had a great deal of comfort from the service and the letters I received.

I What was the hardest thing for you to adjust to?

Mrs R. It was not the caring for him . . . but the loss of his presence . . . his companionship I suppose.

I How did you fill your time?

Mrs R. I think I slowed down, helped lots of little organisations . . . even now I do not like being on my own very much, but it does get better . . . suddenly you find that you do not go into the house and think he's not there . . . it becomes just a house again.

Comment

This interview provides much insight into the day-to-day problems that surround any long-term chronic progressive illness which can only be dealt with palliatively. None of the carers in any team can ever have a complete picture of a patient and his family. Yet it is the aim of carers to enable patients to achieve as high a quality of life as possible within the limitations of their particular situation. It is hoped that readers will find inspiration from this interview.

Nursing Skills

These four interviews illustrate that the role of the nurse includes not only excellence in performing nursing tasks, techniques and procedures, but also a sensitivity to each patient's feelings and emotional needs. The tasks in nursing are for the most part simple and are not dealt with here, as they can be found in many textbooks on nursing. The care, often seen in terms of tasks, is extremely complex. Communication is the crux of effective care and communication consists of much more than the spoken word. Words are, of course, important. It is essential for nurses to be able to converse easily with patients and families, to ask the right questions and to hear and understand what is being said. But not all patients can speak, and many people find it difficult to articulate their problems. There is another aspect of communication which provides additional clues to another human being's feelings; this is termed non-verbal communication and relates to behaviour.

We become aware of non-verbal communication through facial expression, posture, body movements, tone of voice and appearance. Together with the spoken word, non-verbal communication can support, emphasise or contradict what is being said by one person to another. No two people live exactly the same lives or feel exactly the same, so it follows that no two people will react the same in palliative care, have the same fears or face death in the same way. We are all different, so there will be many different ways in which nurses obtain information from patients to help them to assess each patient's needs and plan their care with them.

Patients are alert to a nurse's attitude and nurses can bring much comfort to patients through their own non-verbal behaviour and responses. Sometimes patients will say: 'The nurse was so busy I did not wish to bother her.' This sort of remark indicates a lack of awareness on the nurse's part and that she is giving a patient the impression that she has not got time for him. The nurse may indeed be very busy, but this should only occasionally be communicated to a patient. It is important in establishing trust and confidence with patients that a nurse gives her full attention to each patient for whom she is caring. She may sit beside the patient, meet his eyes while chatting or listening to him. In this way, the patient will know that he is amongst friends, with all the comfort and security friendship brings, conscious always of the nurse's concern and understanding as she gently touches his arm or squeezes his hand. His relatives will be reassured and strengthened by her expressions of concern for him, and may well look to her for help in making the same overtures. A loved one can suddenly become estranged in frightening and unreal surroundings, and it will be a comfort to observe and learn from the nurse that expressions of love and concern are still possible and valuable. The patient, aware of the nurse's empathy with his nearest and dearest, will find solace in knowing that they too are being looked after.

The same empathy and understanding will be required when a patient is nursed at home. The security felt by patient and relatives at remaining in familiar surroundings can be replaced by fear and anxiety when the nurse is not there. Nowadays in most parts of the country the community nursing services are strengthened by evening and night nurses, who help to prepare the patient for sleep and can return during the night to give any necessary nursing care and drugs.

It is often necessary for hospital and community staff to share in the provision of care. Hospices have made excellent advances in developing this type of co-operation and in some areas specialist teams are available which may include MacMillan nurses. These teams can advise and support staff caring for terminally ill patients in both hospital and community. Marie Curie nurses are available to nurse patients with cancer and sometimes a night-sitter can support a patient and allow tired relatives to get a rest.

Co-ordination of Care

Good communication is essential, if the skills of all carers are to be complementary to each other and their activities satisfactorily co-ordinated. Although the patient will not need every professional all the time, there will be periods when many nurses will be involved in his care, as well as the general practitioner and his colleagues, hospital doctors, clergy, social workers, psychologists and others. There may also be students involved, and if co-ordination of care is effective, not only will patients and their families benefit, but all members of the team will find they are supporting each other.

The Needs of the Carers

In the past, nurses, and no doubt other professionals, were taught that they should not become emotionally involved; they should remain detached for their care to be effective. Yet each carer is human and has human reactions to the sufferings of a patient and his family. The ability to demonstrate the empathy which can effectively enhance professional skills can also drain the emotions of the carers, and they too are likely to need support at times. Much mutual support can be found when carers, through dialogue with each other, share each other's burdens. Students are particularly vulnerable and will be helped to cope if their supervisor discusses the various issues and problems which arise with them. Sometimes it is useful for someone who is not directly involved in the care of a patient to become involved in discussions with the carers or to listen to them.

We learn from many anecdotes told by patients and relatives how much comfort is derived from the presence of nurses and other carers, especially when a closeness has developed through expressions of consideration and concern. Emotion may be shown in times of particular joy or sadness, yet the balance between professional demeanour and personal involvement must be maintained, if carers are to fulfil their true functions. There is therefore much need for carers to be aware of this and to help each other.

All carers/nurses are human and there are times when a carer/nurse may find that she herself is unable to cope in a particular situation, as she may come to realise that some of her colleagues could be more helpful to a particular patient and family. Such situations only occur occasionally, but when they do there should be no sense of failure, instead recognition of the fact that someone else could do better in that particular situation.

Summary

This chapter clearly shows that nursing is carried out successfully by nurses who feel a personal responsibility for their actions and whose care for each patient is competent, understanding, compassionate and comforting.

Recommended Reading

Blondis, M.N. and Jackson, B.E. (1977) *Non-verbal Communication with Patients. Back to the Human Touch*, Wiley, New York
Doyle, D. (1979) *Terminal Care*, Churchill Livingstone, Edinburgh
Kubler-Ross, E. (1969) *On Death and Dying*, Tavistock Publications, London
Lamerton, R. (1973) *Care of the Dying*, Penguin Books, London
Saunders, C. (1960) *Care of the Dying*, Macmillan, London
Zorza, R. and V. (1980) *A Way to Die*, Trinity Press, London

15

NURSING CARE OF THE DYING CHILD

Marion Buchanan

A well-rounded life should have a beginning, a middle and an end, and this is just as true of a dying child's short life. There is a tendency for adults to feel that a child's life has only just begun, has everything in the future and no past. This is almost a denial of the child's very existence and causes distress, anger and bewilderment in the child. The age-range of children facing death is very varied, from very young to teenage and adolescent. The nurse has an important contribution to make to improve the quality of the quantity of life left. The needs of the different age-groups can make this very demanding for nurses, but there is a common core of nursing needs for most of these children, regardless of the diagnosis. There is much to be learned from the 'specialist nurses' who are hospital-based and provide home care for children with fatal and progressive diseases. Their experience has shown that with motivation, insight and nursing skills many of these children can be cared for at home with their family to the end. The following short case studies are included to help readers to appreciate the problems encountered by two children and their families and to illustrate the help which was provided.

Case Study 1

John – 14 years – Cystic Fibrosis

Initially, the only problems John had experienced with this disease were mild respiratory infections and 'smelly' stools. He was a keen footballer and played regularly with his brother Ian and friends, accepting the nuisance of Pancrex, twice daily physiotherapy, and clinic visits as part of his life.

In his thirteenth year the disease progressed and life changed for the family. John's chest infections became more frequent and less responsive to therapy and his activities became restricted. School and sport were fading into the background and even family outings by car were too tiring. The monthly visit to the cystic fibrosis clinic was traumatic and morale was low.

Over the years the home-care team and the social worker had formed

345

good relationships with John and his family, and now there was need for active support. The family wished to keep John at home and this was agreed. As stairs proved a problem for John, the downstairs living room was adapted with a bed, an old-fashioned armchair with wide arms and a bedside locker which contained a urinal and bedpan inside, and his portable television on top. The 'lobby press' had an opening window and the press was emptied to contain a commode and mechanical air freshener, both of which were greatly appreciated. John helped to choose a triangular pillow from a catalogue and sheepskins were obtained, money coming from funds available to the patients. Fluids were in bright containers and pop-star posters were in profusion. Mother encouraged his friends to visit and he entertained royally from his chair.

Over a period of many weeks, he weakened and spent a lot of time sleeping in his chair. His bouts of coughing frightened his brother Ian, but he still wanted to be near John. He came into hospital for re-assessment and had a course of intravenous antibiotics, which gave temporary improvement. Mother slept for nearly 24 hours. He went home with a Ventolin nebuliser. He was by now pale and emaciated, with a haunted expression, abdominal pain and nausea adding to his misery. He began to talk about his impending death and no attempt was made to deny this either by the family or the nursing team. He had things he needed to put 'in order'.

One week later, a readmission because of depression and breathlessness again allowed mother to sleep and revive. Ventolin was increased and he went home again. Now he always slept in his chair and mother moved in beside him. The nurses came several times a day to support the family, and three days later he died peacefully at 10.00 a.m. in his chair with his parents beside him. His brother Ian saw him soon after death and was distressed, but reassured to see John at peace.

Case Study 2

Donald – 8 years – Nephroblastoma

Donald changed in a few weeks from a happy, energetic little boy to a pale, sick miserable child. After diagnosis, he had immediate surgery and chemotherapy was started. The prognosis was poor, due to the spread of the cells, and the parents had been honestly told that life expectancy was not more than two or three months.

He went home and maintained his improvement, eating well and being active. Mother gave the impression of calm control and the parents tried hard not to spoil him, but nursing staff felt concerned about the mother. There were other younger children and a strong supportive extended family. Donald's hair came out and he was very philosophical about this and took a positive interest in the colour and style of his little woollie caps — 'to keep my nut warm'. Suddenly the pains started again and he was admitted to hospital with mother. He commenced 'Brompton's Cocktail' and obviously was not going to improve again.

Mother decided she wanted to have him at home, so a programme of care was planned by the home-care team. Relief of pain, nutrition, hygiene — especially mouth care and skin care — were planned, and mother was determined to cope. The home-care team visited very frequently, but Donald's condition deteriorated rapidly. He could not tolerate handling, and mouth care was not controlling the breakdown of his mucous membrane. Mother was distraught and totally exhausted, and the decision was taken by the nursing team to readmit Donald to hospital. Granny took the two other children and father and mother stayed with Donald until he died, unconscious, two days later.

This family had a strong religious faith and the parents were very hostile to the home-care nurses because they had 'taken Donald away' at the end. The nursing officer in charge of the team had been very involved with this case and she went to see the parents some time after Donald's death. The hostility had gone, but still they felt 'guilty' about having 'allowed' him to go back into hospital, when he should have died at home. This family will be followed up, as it is obviously helping them to talk it through.

Comment

These two case studies show the importance of assessing problems and making short-term plans to assist each child to live as normal a life as possible. These plans were evaluated frequently and adjustment made as each child's physical condition deteriorated. Relationships were established with the parents, families and school. The recognition of the mother's needs are clear in both case studies. Admission to hospital was as much to assist the mother as the child.

The staff evaluated each child's care some time afterwards. In John's case they felt satisfied and in Donald's case they examined whether more could have been done to allay the hostile and guilt feelings the parents experienced after their child's death.

Nursing Skills

In the ideal situation the hospital, family and community 'carers' would meet at an early stage in the progression of the illness. In paediatrics, it often does start from the moment of diagnosis and the links in the chain of care are formed. It may be a 'specialist nurse' or it may be a community nursing sister from a rural area who will be the main nursing link with child, family and hospital, depending on the locality or other circumstances.

Assessing the Home Situation

This has to be done realistically and there cannot be rigid guidelines. It can only be done by suggestion and invitation, and nurses are very sensitive to the dangers of appearing to be 'inspecting' the home, but most parents welcome this help and a relationship can be formed. The needs of the child at home can be discussed with mother — for example, stairs, lavatories, bathrooms. If the child is to be nursed downstairs and the lavatory is upstairs, practical advice can be given, as is illustrated in one case study. Experience has shown that most problems can be overcome with help and support. It is important to show the parents that although this is a 'small' patient, their child is not a 'small' problem to the nurse, but a real person to be cared for at home. The nurse can co-ordinate appointments to different hospital departments so that no unnecessary visits are made and this relieves so much strain.

Family Involvement

This is always relevant and can be very constructive and supportive, if there is understanding. Grandparents and siblings can suffer needlessly and be counter-productive if they are excluded from the care. The nurse can give valuable help to them in explanations, when parents are unable to communicate because of their own emotions and grief. There is a fine line between confidentiality and giving sufficient information to the extended family to avoid misunderstanding. The nurse may be the first 'carer' and may be the one to ensure that the family have access to all the help available to them. Other 'caring' professions may have to be alerted by the nurse.

Nursing Care

This may start early in a terminal illness, when the child is still able to attend school. Teachers may have anxieties and preconceived ideas about the child and his illness which can be allayed by an informal discussion. Older children with diseases which create anti-social problems — for example, offensive stools in cystic fibrosis, or unsightly problems such as baldness in leukaemia — can suffer a great deal from the unkindness of other children. With co-operation from the school, an informal chat from the nurse in one particular case transformed the scene to such an extent that the classmates came regularly to visit at home, when the patient could no longer attend school. The following examples may illustrate how attention to detail may make all the difference to a dying child's life and happiness.

1. Children who have to take regular medication find that tablets are less conspicuous in fancy tins, there is no need to take bottles.
2. Extra fluids which are essential to some children can be carried in light-weight bottles obtainable from camping shops.
3. Schools are often inadequate in small details, and mothers can be advised to keep the child well supplied with paper handkerchiefs and toilet paper in discreet containers.
4. Smells can be overcome. There are excellent pocket-sized aerosol sprays now available to dispel even the most offensive odours.
5. Hair loss is a tragedy for a child, especially the older ones, and much thought should be given to appropriate disguise. Wigs can be a source of ridicule for boys, but modern caps of all kinds can be worn unobtrusively. Girls can cope better with wigs, but sometimes little scarves are cooler and more appropriate.
6. Humidifiers may be necessary, especially in centrally-heated homes. Double-glazing creates problems for children with cystic fibrosis.
7. Ordinary activities and family outings should be encouraged, and play with friends is essential when the child is well. It is a natural reaction for the parents to wish to shield the child and in so doing isolate the child from his peers.
8. Thought has to be given to alternative interests and amusements for the children when they can no longer attend school or take part in games. Hospital play ladies have been a source of wonderful ideas for painting, typing, bed-bound table tennis, and the nurse will have to encourage and help the mother who has not been in the habit of playing with her child.
9. Clothing is important to children, and mothers should be encouraged to allow the child to dress in the current fashion — regardless of problems. It may look inappropriate to adults, but the child's self-image is vital and how he appears to his peer group. The 'pigeon chest' and painful thinness of a teenage girl is not noticed by her

peers when she has velvet knickerbockers and a frilly blouse for a disco. Only the adults are aware of any incongruity.

10. Nutrition is often a great anxiety for the mother, and parents sometimes feel that only 'proper' food will help the child recover. The nurse can reassure on this issue and fluids can be given in a great variety of ways. Most children do not care to have jugs of water near their beds, especially at home, and flavoured drinks in colourful containers can be regularly produced. Iced lollies are a great source of fluid, soothe sore mouths and maintain a semblance of normality. Small quantities of favourite foods can be given whenever a child wishes and special treats or forbidden foods occasionally.

Conclusion

The link between hospital and home is usually strong in paediatric terminal cases, and this includes many different carers. Recent experiences have shown the need for support for the carers themselves, in facing the stress and distress inherent in these situations. The sharing of problems as early as possible should be the goal for any 'team' approach, and it may be the community nurse or the specialist nurse who initiates this.

The concept of a nursing admission to relieve stress at home is illustrated in the second case study. Continuity of care and good communication can be achieved, especially through the logical approach of the nursing process. The assessing, planning, implementing and evaluating of each step, either in hospital or at home, ensures the best possible care for the child.

Nurses have had to learn to adapt their role to the needs of the families, and not all visits need to include clinical care. A cup of coffee and a chat is reassuring for both carers and parents. This is especially important in paediatrics, so that the child does not always associate the nurse with procedures and may see his parents being comforted and helped by her. Home-care nurses have observed that a friendly, informal visit by the hospital consultant means much to parents and child, and is recalled with gratitude long after the death of the child.

Much has already been written about children's reactions at this time, and the insight many of them have into their own affairs. They have thoughts about pain, and fear, and loneliness, and separation which they may wish to express. Every case is different and individual, and the nurse must be aware and receptive when the time comes.

16 NURSING MANAGEMENT

Jennifer M. Henderson

Patients suffering from progressive disease have much suffering to endure and have to cope with many distressing problems. The nurse's main aims are to alleviate the suffering and find solutions to the problems.

In this chapter, two experienced ward sisters attempt to determine what the most significant problems are likely to be, and suggest solutions which may help to alleviate them and bring comfort to the patient. None of the ideas or solutions is new; some are as old as Florence Nightingale. We hope to help nurses who may feel inadequate and unable to cope with what is, for them, a new and frightening experience, as much by suggesting the approach which might be taken to patients' problems as by offering solutions. We aim to help develop the nurse's awareness of the patient's needs and the ability to respond to these needs. In the case of the child, the nurse will find herself assisting the mother in the care of the child.

To this end, we have set out the various stages involved in this problem-solving approach in what we hope is a logical and jargon-free fashion. The problems are presented in aiphabetical order, for ease of reference, but each in its own right could be the most distressing problem for the patient. As for the solutions, they are essentially nursing solutions to nursing problems. We cannot stress strongly enough that the nursing approach to the control of symptoms should be seen as an integral part of treatment, not a second-best if time permits.

Although this chapter might rightly be regarded as primarily for nurses, it is our hope that it will help medical colleagues to understand better the discipline and skills of good nursing and so to contribute to the 'team caring and team sharing' so vital in good modern palliative care.

351

Anorexia

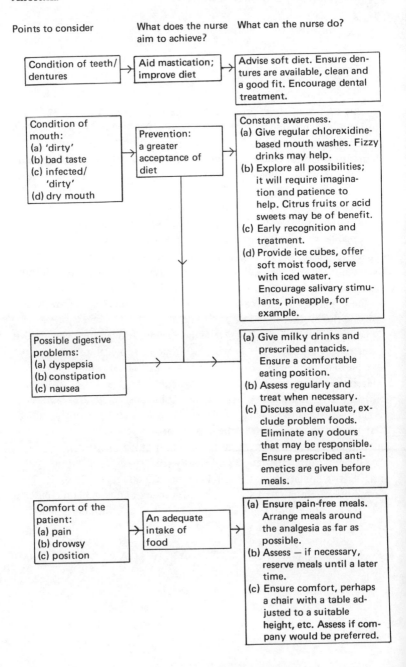

Points to consider	What does the nurse aim to achieve?	What can the nurse do?
Condition of teeth/dentures	Aid mastication; improve diet	Advise soft diet. Ensure dentures are available, clean and a good fit. Encourage dental treatment.
Condition of mouth: (a) 'dirty' (b) bad taste (c) infected/'dirty' (d) dry mouth	Prevention: a greater acceptance of diet	Constant awareness. (a) Give regular chlorexidine-based mouth washes. Fizzy drinks may help. (b) Explore all possibilities; it will require imagination and patience to help. Citrus fruits or acid sweets may be of benefit. (c) Early recognition and treatment. (d) Provide ice cubes, offer soft moist food, serve with iced water. Encourage salivary stimulants, pineapple, for example.
Possible digestive problems: (a) dyspepsia (b) constipation (c) nausea		(a) Give milky drinks and prescribed antacids. Ensure a comfortable eating position. (b) Assess regularly and treat when necessary. (c) Discuss and evaluate, exclude problem foods. Eliminate any odours that may be responsible. Ensure prescribed antiemetics are given before meals.
Comfort of the patient: (a) pain (b) drowsy (c) position	An adequate intake of food	(a) Ensure pain-free meals. Arrange meals around the analgesia as far as possible. (b) Assess — if necessary, reserve meals until a later time. (c) Ensure comfort, perhaps a chair with a table adjusted to a suitable height, etc. Assess if company would be preferred.

Anorexia *(contd)*

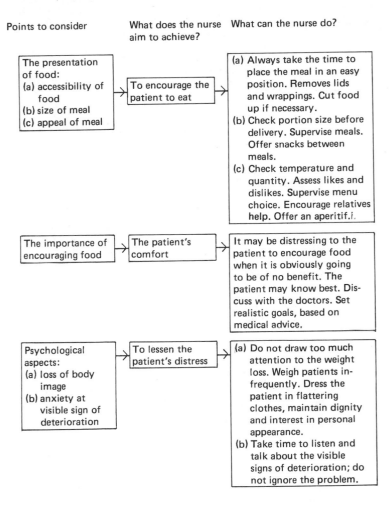

Points to consider   What does the nurse   What can the nurse do?
                       aim to achieve?

| The presentation of food: (a) accessibility of food (b) size of meal (c) appeal of meal | To encourage the patient to eat | (a) Always take the time to place the meal in an easy position. Removes lids and wrappings. Cut food up if necessary. (b) Check portion size before delivery. Supervise meals. Offer snacks between meals. (c) Check temperature and quantity. Assess likes and dislikes. Supervise menu choice. Encourage relatives help. Offer an aperitif.i. |

| The importance of encouraging food | The patient's comfort | It may be distressing to the patient to encourage food when it is obviously going to be of no benefit. The patient may know best. Discuss with the doctors. Set realistic goals, based on medical advice. |

| Psychological aspects: (a) loss of body image (b) anxiety at visible sign of deterioration | To lessen the patient's distress | (a) Do not draw too much attention to the weight loss. Weigh patients infrequently. Dress the patient in flattering clothes, maintain dignity and interest in personal appearance. (b) Take time to listen and talk about the visible signs of deterioration; do not ignore the problem. |

Confusion

Points to consider	What does the nurse aim to achieve?	What can the nurse do?
The cause: (a) acute brain syndrome (delirium)	To understand the reason for the confusion	Carefully observe and assess behaviour. Discuss with relatives, check notes. Observe for signs of agitation, fear, hallucination, rambling incoherence or attempts to escape. This will be the picture of delirium.
Needs of the patient	To maintain hygiene and bodily functions, reduce fear and prevent harm to the patient	Assess, implement and evaluate the basic needs of the patient. The patient's fear is probably greater than that of the nurse. Care for the patient in a quiet well-lit room, involve as few people as possible. Take time to orientate the patient. Adopt an imaginative approach. Cot sides are sometimes used, but it is unlikely that they help. The doctor may prescribe a tranquilliser.
The cause: (b) chronic brain syndrome (dementia)	To understand the reason for the confusion	Observe for signs of superficial labile and inappropriate behaviour. This will be the picture of dementia.
Needs of the patient	To maintain hygiene and bodily functions, reduce fear and to prevent harm to the patient	The care of the patient will be the same as for a patient with delirium. There is one exception: sedation will reduce the function of already-damaged brain cells.
The cause: (c) mechanical	A normal patient	Check for a full bladder or for pain. The patient will not be able to complain. Treat the cause appropriately.
Unrelated physical problems: (1) infection	To understand the cause of the confusion	Observe for a minimal rise in temperature in the elderly, as this may induce confusion. Inform the doctor.
(2) metabolic		The doctor will check electrolyte imbalance, for dehydration, etc., and will advise on the care to be implemented.

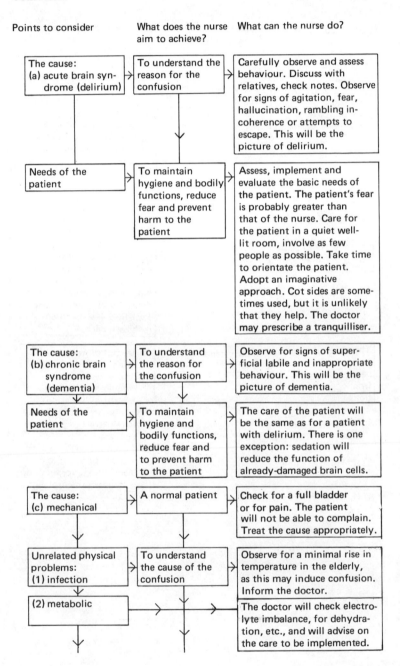

Confusion *(contd)*

Points to consider	What does the nurse aim to achieve?	What can the nurse do?

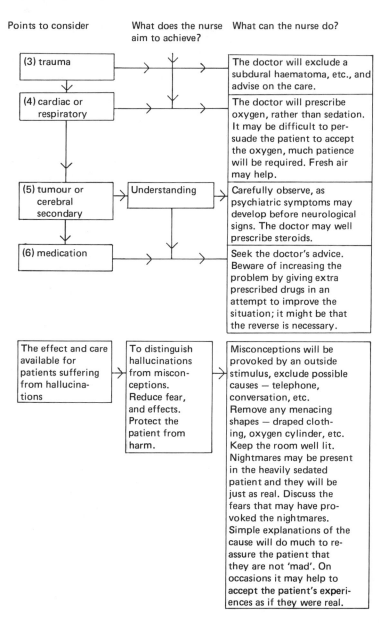

(3) trauma		The doctor will exclude a subdural haematoma, etc., and advise on the care.
(4) cardiac or respiratory		The doctor will prescribe oxygen, rather than sedation. It may be difficult to persuade the patient to accept the oxygen, much patience will be required. Fresh air may help.
(5) tumour or cerebral secondary	Understanding	Carefully observe, as psychiatric symptoms may develop before neurological signs. The doctor may well prescribe steroids.
(6) medication		Seek the doctor's advice. Beware of increasing the problem by giving extra prescribed drugs in an attempt to improve the situation; it might be that the reverse is necessary.
The effect and care available for patients suffering from hallucinations	To distinguish hallucinations from misconceptions. Reduce fear, and effects. Protect the patient from harm.	Misconceptions will be provoked by an outside stimulus, exclude possible causes — telephone, conversation, etc. Remove any menacing shapes — draped clothing, oxygen cylinder, etc. Keep the room well lit. Nightmares may be present in the heavily sedated patient and they will be just as real. Discuss the fears that may have provoked the nightmares. Simple explanations of the cause will do much to reassure the patient that they are not 'mad'. On occasions it may help to accept the patient's experiences as if they were real.

Confusion *(contd)*

Points to consider	What does the nurse aim to achieve?	What can the nurse do?
Care of the uncooperative patient	→ To gain the patient's co-operation	→ It may be necessary to repeat the instructions in simple terms many times. Individualised care will help, and much patience required. When coaxing a patient, beware of insulting them. If there is any suggestion of paranoia, do not disguise tablets, etc. If one person is trusted, use this to advantage. There is usually a way round the problem, rather than resorting to force, which should be avoided at all costs. One person, sitting rather than standing, should deal with the situation. Another member of staff can provide back up, if violence is feared. The key words are *time* and *patience*.

Constipation

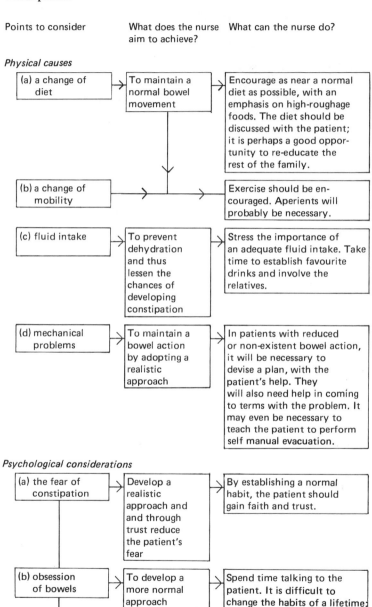

Points to consider	What does the nurse aim to achieve?	What can the nurse do?
Physical causes		
(a) a change of diet	To maintain a normal bowel movement	Encourage as near a normal diet as possible, with an emphasis on high-roughage foods. The diet should be discussed with the patient; it is perhaps a good opportunity to re-educate the rest of the family.
(b) a change of mobility		Exercise should be encouraged. Aperients will probably be necessary.
(c) fluid intake	To prevent dehydration and thus lessen the chances of developing constipation	Stress the importance of an adequate fluid intake. Take time to establish favourite drinks and involve the relatives.
(d) mechanical problems	To maintain a bowel action by adopting a realistic approach	In patients with reduced or non-existent bowel action, it will be necessary to devise a plan, with the patient's help. They will also need help in coming to terms with the problem. It may even be necessary to teach the patient to perform self manual evacuation.
Psychological considerations		
(a) the fear of constipation	Develop a realistic approach and and through trust reduce the patient's fear	By establishing a normal habit, the patient should gain faith and trust.
(b) obsession of bowels	To develop a more normal approach	Spend time talking to the patient. It is difficult to change the habits of a lifetime; try to find the origin of the obsession. It might then be possible to help the patient.

Constipation *(contd)*

Points to consider	What does the nurse aim to achieve?	What can the nurse do?
(c) unfavourable lavatory conditions	To provide a relaxed and comfortable environment	Tact and consideration are most important. If at all possible, avoid a commode at the bedside, be sensitive during visiting. Take time to provide privacy. Bedpans are uncomfortable and extremely difficult to balance on and should be avoided.

Diarrhoea

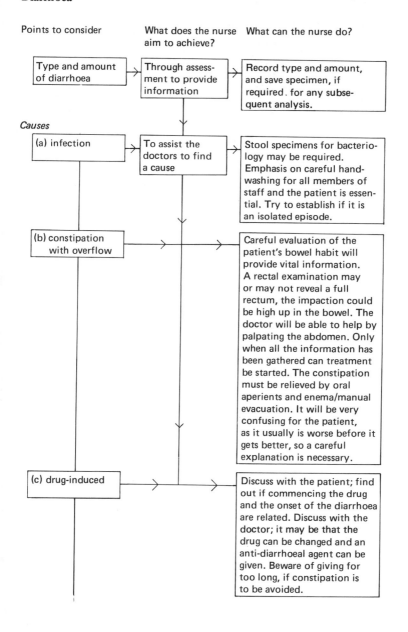

Points to consider | What does the nurse aim to achieve? | What can the nurse do?

Type and amount of diarrhoea → **Through assessment to provide information** → Record type and amount, and save specimen, if required. for any subsequent analysis.

Causes

(a) infection → **To assist the doctors to find a cause** → Stool specimens for bacteriology may be required. Emphasis on careful handwashing for all members of staff and the patient is essential. Try to establish if it is an isolated episode.

(b) constipation with overflow → Careful evaluation of the patient's bowel habit will provide vital information. A rectal examination may or may not reveal a full rectum, the impaction could be high up in the bowel. The doctor will be able to help by palpating the abdomen. Only when all the information has been gathered can treatment be started. The constipation must be relieved by oral aperients and enema/manual evacuation. It will be very confusing for the patient, as it usually is worse before it gets better, so a careful explanation is necessary.

(c) drug-induced → Discuss with the patient; find out if commencing the drug and the onset of the diarrhoea are related. Discuss with the doctor; it may be that the drug can be changed and an anti-diarrhoeal agent can be given. Beware of giving for too long, if constipation is to be avoided.

Diarrhoea *(contd)*

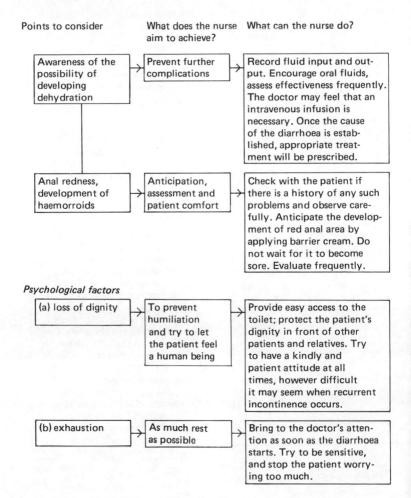

Points to consider	What does the nurse aim to achieve?	What can the nurse do?
Awareness of the possibility of developing dehydration	Prevent further complications	Record fluid input and output. Encourage oral fluids, assess effectiveness frequently. The doctor may feel that an intravenous infusion is necessary. Once the cause of the diarrhoea is established, appropriate treatment will be prescribed.
Anal redness, development of haemorroids	Anticipation, assessment and patient comfort	Check with the patient if there is a history of any such problems and observe carefully. Anticipate the development of red anal area by applying barrier cream. Do not wait for it to become sore. Evaluate frequently.

Psychological factors

(a) loss of dignity	To prevent humiliation and try to let the patient feel a human being	Provide easy access to the toilet; protect the patient's dignity in front of other patients and relatives. Try to have a kindly and patient attitude at all times, however difficult it may seem when recurrent incontinence occurs.
(b) exhaustion	As much rest as possible	Bring to the doctor's attention as soon as the diarrhoea starts. Try to be sensitive, and stop the patient worrying too much.

Dry Mouth

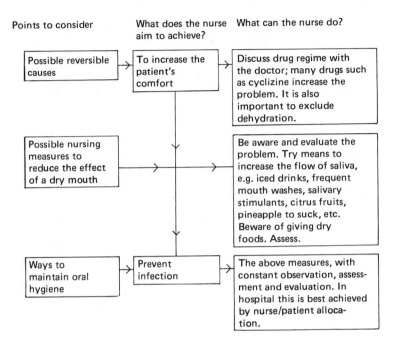

Points to consider	What does the nurse aim to achieve?	What can the nurse do?
Possible reversible causes	To increase the patient's comfort	Discuss drug regime with the doctor; many drugs such as cyclizine increase the problem. It is also important to exclude dehydration.
Possible nursing measures to reduce the effect of a dry mouth		Be aware and evaluate the problem. Try means to increase the flow of saliva, e.g. iced drinks, frequent mouth washes, salivary stimulants, citrus fruits, pineapple to suck, etc. Beware of giving dry foods. Assess.
Ways to maintain oral hygiene	Prevent infection	The above measures, with constant observation, assessment and evaluation. In hospital this is best achieved by nurse/patient allocation.

Dysphagia

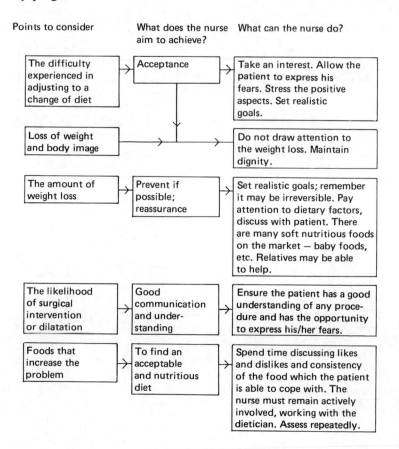

Points to consider	What does the nurse aim to achieve?	What can the nurse do?
The difficulty experienced in adjusting to a change of diet	Acceptance	Take an interest. Allow the patient to express his fears. Stress the positive aspects. Set realistic goals.
Loss of weight and body image		Do not draw attention to the weight loss. Maintain dignity.
The amount of weight loss	Prevent if possible; reassurance	Set realistic goals; remember it may be irreversible. Pay attention to dietary factors, discuss with patient. There are many soft nutritious foods on the market — baby foods, etc. Relatives may be able to help.
The likelihood of surgical intervention or dilatation	Good communication and understanding	Ensure the patient has a good understanding of any procedure and has the opportunity to express his/her fears.
Foods that increase the problem	To find an acceptable and nutritious diet	Spend time discussing likes and dislikes and consistency of the food which the patient is able to cope with. The nurse must remain actively involved, working with the dietician. Assess repeatedly.

Dyspnoea

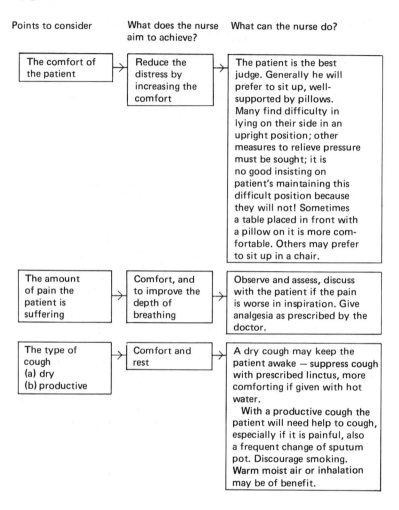

Points to consider	What does the nurse aim to achieve?	What can the nurse do?
The comfort of the patient	Reduce the distress by increasing the comfort	The patient is the best judge. Generally he will prefer to sit up, well-supported by pillows. Many find difficulty in lying on their side in an upright position; other measures to relieve pressure must be sought; it is no good insisting on patient's maintaining this difficult position because they will not! Sometimes a table placed in front with a pillow on it is more comfortable. Others may prefer to sit up in a chair.
The amount of pain the patient is suffering	Comfort, and to improve the depth of breathing	Observe and assess, discuss with the patient if the pain is worse in inspiration. Give analgesia as prescribed by the doctor.
The type of cough (a) dry (b) productive	Comfort and rest	A dry cough may keep the patient awake — suppress cough with prescribed linctus, more comforting if given with hot water. With a productive cough the patient will need help to cough, especially if it is painful, also a frequent change of sputum pot. Discourage smoking. Warm moist air or inhalation may be of benefit.

Dyspnoea *(contd)*

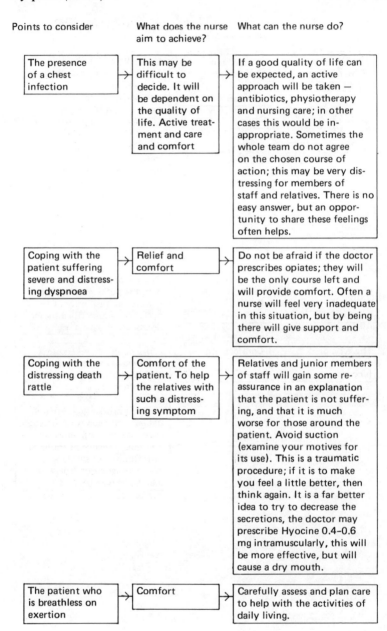

Points to consider	What does the nurse aim to achieve?	What can the nurse do?
The presence of a chest infection	This may be difficult to decide. It will be dependent on the quality of life. Active treatment and care and comfort	If a good quality of life can be expected, an active approach will be taken — antibiotics, physiotherapy and nursing care; in other cases this would be inappropriate. Sometimes the whole team do not agree on the chosen course of action; this may be very distressing for members of staff and relatives. There is no easy answer, but an opportunity to share these feelings often helps.
Coping with the patient suffering severe and distressing dyspnoea	Relief and comfort	Do not be afraid if the doctor prescribes opiates; they will be the only course left and will provide comfort. Often a nurse will feel very inadequate in this situation, but by being there will give support and comfort.
Coping with the distressing death rattle	Comfort of the patient. To help the relatives with such a distressing symptom	Relatives and junior members of staff will gain some reassurance in an explanation that the patient is not suffering, and that it is much worse for those around the patient. Avoid suction (examine your motives for its use). This is a traumatic procedure; if it is to make you feel a little better, then think again. It is a far better idea to try to decrease the secretions, the doctor may prescribe Hyocine 0.4–0.6 mg intramuscularly, this will be more effective, but will cause a dry mouth.
The patient who is breathless on exertion	Comfort	Carefully assess and plan care to help with the activities of daily living.

Dyspnoea *(contd)*

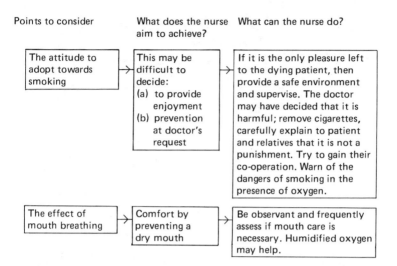

Points to consider	What does the nurse aim to achieve?	What can the nurse do?
The attitude to adopt towards smoking	This may be difficult to decide: (a) to provide enjoyment (b) prevention at doctor's request	If it is the only pleasure left to the dying patient, then provide a safe environment and supervise. The doctor may have decided that it is harmful; remove cigarettes, carefully explain to patient and relatives that it is not a punishment. Try to gain their co-operation. Warn of the dangers of smoking in the presence of oxygen.
The effect of mouth breathing	Comfort by preventing a dry mouth	Be observant and frequently assess if mouth care is necessary. Humidified oxygen may help.

Hiccups

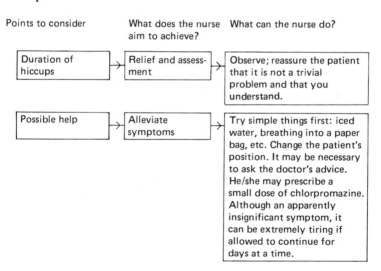

Points to consider	What does the nurse aim to achieve?	What can the nurse do?
Duration of hiccups	Relief and assessment	Observe; reassure the patient that it is not a trivial problem and that you understand.
Possible help	Alleviate symptoms	Try simple things first: iced water, breathing into a paper bag, etc. Change the patient's position. It may be necessary to ask the doctor's advice. He/she may prescribe a small dose of chlorpromazine. Although an apparently insignificant symptom, it can be extremely tiring if allowed to continue for days at a time.

Insomnia

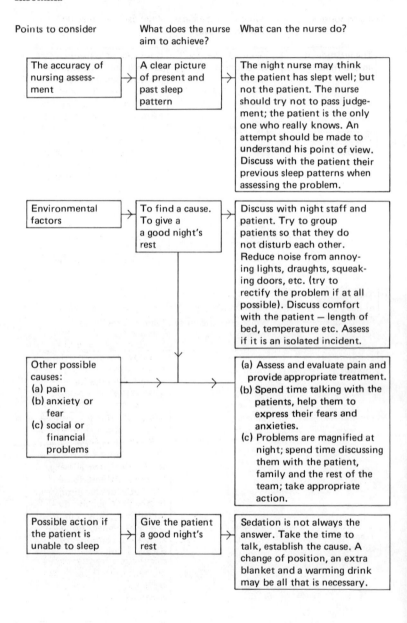

Points to consider	What does the nurse aim to achieve?	What can the nurse do?
The accuracy of nursing assessment	A clear picture of present and past sleep pattern	The night nurse may think the patient has slept well; but not the patient. The nurse should try not to pass judgement; the patient is the only one who really knows. An attempt should be made to understand his point of view. Discuss with the patient their previous sleep patterns when assessing the problem.
Environmental factors	To find a cause. To give a a good night's rest	Discuss with night staff and patient. Try to group patients so that they do not disturb each other. Reduce noise from annoying lights, draughts, squeaking doors, etc. (try to rectify the problem if at all possible). Discuss comfort with the patient — length of bed, temperature etc. Assess if it is an isolated incident.
Other possible causes: (a) pain (b) anxiety or fear (c) social or financial problems		(a) Assess and evaluate pain and provide appropriate treatment. (b) Spend time talking with the patients, help them to express their fears and anxieties. (c) Problems are magnified at night; spend time discussing them with the patient, family and the rest of the team; take appropriate action.
Possible action if the patient is unable to sleep	Give the patient a good night's rest	Sedation is not always the answer. Take the time to talk, establish the cause. A change of position, an extra blanket and a warming drink may be all that is necessary.

Intestinal Obstruction in the Terminal Stage

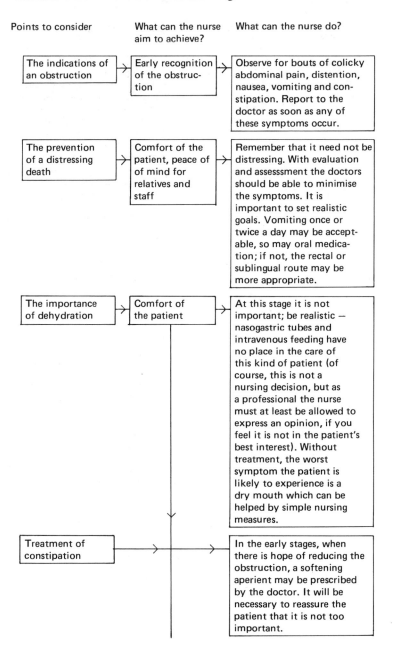

Points to consider	What can the nurse aim to achieve?	What can the nurse do?
The indications of an obstruction	Early recognition of the obstruction	Observe for bouts of colicky abdominal pain, distention, nausea, vomiting and constipation. Report to the doctor as soon as any of these symptoms occur.
The prevention of a distressing death	Comfort of the patient, peace of of mind for relatives and staff	Remember that it need not be distressing. With evaluation and assesssment the doctors should be able to minimise the symptoms. It is important to set realistic goals. Vomiting once or twice a day may be acceptable, so may oral medication; if not, the rectal or sublingual route may be more appropriate.
The importance of dehydration	Comfort of the patient	At this stage it is not important; be realistic — nasogastric tubes and intravenous feeding have no place in the care of this kind of patient (of course, this is not a nursing decision, but as a professional the nurse must at least be allowed to express an opinion, if you feel it is not in the patient's best interest). Without treatment, the worst symptom the patient is likely to experience is a dry mouth which can be helped by simple nursing measures.
Treatment of constipation		In the early stages, when there is hope of reducing the obstruction, a softening aperient may be prescribed by the doctor. It will be necessary to reassure the patient that it is not too important.

Intestinal Obstruction in the Terminal Stage *(contd)*

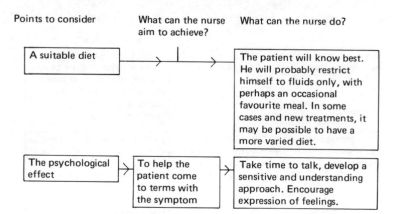

Points to consider	What can the nurse aim to achieve?	What can the nurse do?
A suitable diet		The patient will know best. He will probably restrict himself to fluids only, with perhaps an occasional favourite meal. In some cases and new treatments, it may be possible to have a more varied diet.
The psychological effect	To help the patient come to terms with the symptom	Take time to talk, develop a sensitive and understanding approach. Encourage expression of feelings.

Mood/Emotion

Points to consider	What does the nurse aim to achieve?	What can the nurse do?
The normal pattern for the patient	Assessment of how the patient usually appears, before passing an opinion on their mood	Talk to the family and friends. Try to discover if the patient's personality is normally intro-verted or extroverted, as this may influence the future care of the patient.
The degree of 'suffering' the patient is experiencing	To gain an understanding; reduce to a minimum	Alleviate as many physical factors as possible, such as pain, discomfort, social or financial problems. This will help to improve the overall morale, but the nurse's compassion, empathy and awareness may be the most important factor in reducing the 'suffering'.
The effect on the patient of the so-called 'conspiracy of silence'	For the patient to come to terms with the illness on whatever level he is able to cope with it	*Time* is the key word; time for a patient to discuss his fears and anxieties. The nurse should not be afraid of saying the 'wrong thing' or giving secrets away, the patient will pick up cues from what is not said anyway. The nurse must learn to develop the power of listen-ing, not to change the subject, or feel uncomfortable if silences develop. Eye contact and physical contact should be maintained. The patient probably does not want direct answers, but the oppor-tunity to talk. Always discuss with the rest of the team.
The effect of a change of dependency or image	To help the patient adjust to the situa-tion	The nurses must show he/she cares and is aware. The posi-tive aspects should be stressed, concentrating on those things the patient can do. Involve the patient and relatives in planning and implementing care.

Mood/Emotion *(contd)*

Points to consider	What does the nurse aim to achieve?	What can the nurse do?
The degree of mood swing and loss of memory, etc.	To help the patient through understanding	The patient may fear the changes in his mental state and believe he is going 'mad'; a simple explanation that this is not so may be necessary. The patient must know that the nurse understands.
External factors that may contribute to a change of mood: (a) social (b) marital	Improvement in patient's mood through understanding and help with problems	Constant awareness of potential problems. Develop a relationship where trust is of prime importance, involve the patient. Give patient and relatives the kind of environment in which they can explore their own relationships and feelings.
The spiritual aspect	An understanding of the spiritual side of the patient's life	It is a nursing responsibility to give spiritual help if it is required, even if it does not reflect his/her own beliefs. The patient may prefer to talk to a minister or a member of his own faith. It may be the patient's first interest in the spiritual side of his life and he may find it a great source of strength.

Nausea and Vomiting

Points to consider	What does the nurse aim to achieve?	What can the nurse do?

Contributing factors

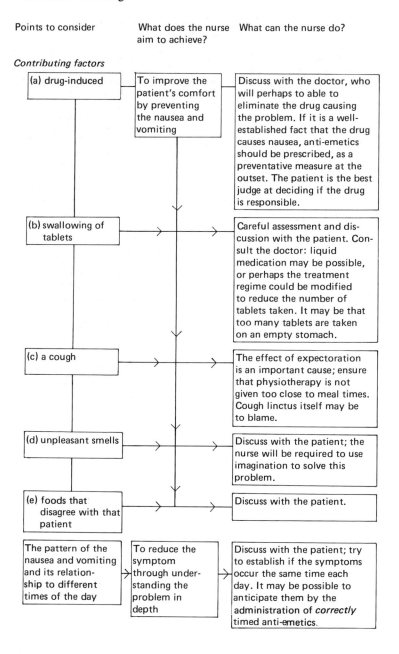

(a) drug-induced	To improve the patient's comfort by preventing the nausea and vomiting	Discuss with the doctor, who will perhaps to able to eliminate the drug causing the problem. If it is a well-established fact that the drug causes nausea, anti-emetics should be prescribed, as a preventative measure at the outset. The patient is the best judge at deciding if the drug is responsible.
(b) swallowing of tablets		Careful assessment and discussion with the patient. Consult the doctor: liquid medication may be possible, or perhaps the treatment regime could be modified to reduce the number of tablets taken. It may be that too many tablets are taken on an empty stomach.
(c) a cough		The effect of expectoration is an important cause; ensure that physiotherapy is not given too close to meal times. Cough linctus itself may be to blame.
(d) unpleasant smells		Discuss with the patient; the nurse will be required to use imagination to solve this problem.
(e) foods that disagree with that patient		Discuss with the patient.
The pattern of the nausea and vomiting and its relationship to different times of the day	To reduce the symptom through understanding the problem in depth	Discuss with the patient; try to establish if the symptoms occur the same time each day. It may be possible to anticipate them by the administration of *correctly* timed anti-emetics.

Nausea and Vomiting *(contd)*

Points to consider   What does the nurse   What can the nurse do?
                              aim to achieve?

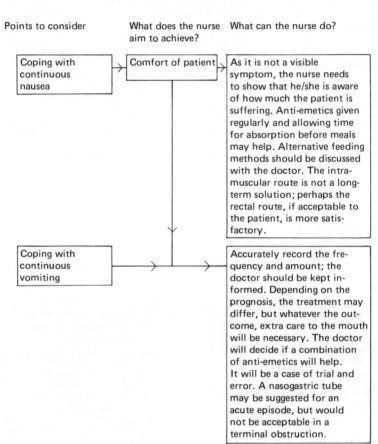

| Coping with continuous nausea | Comfort of patient | As it is not a visible symptom, the nurse needs to show that he/she is aware of how much the patient is suffering. Anti-emetics given regularly and allowing time for absorption before meals may help. Alternative feeding methods should be discussed with the doctor. The intramuscular route is not a long-term solution; perhaps the rectal route, if acceptable to the patient, is more satisfactory. |
| Coping with continuous vomiting | | Accurately record the frequency and amount; the doctor should be kept informed. Depending on the prognosis, the treatment may differ, but whatever the outcome, extra care to the mouth will be necessary. The doctor will decide if a combination of anti-emetics will help. It will be a case of trial and error. A nasogastric tube may be suggested for an acute episode, but would not be acceptable in a terminal obstruction. |

Pain

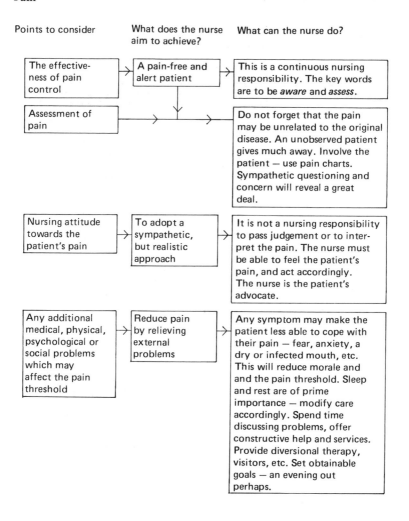

Points to consider	What does the nurse aim to achieve?	What can the nurse do?
The effectiveness of pain control	A pain-free and alert patient	This is a continuous nursing responsibility. The key words are to be *aware* and *assess*.
Assessment of pain		Do not forget that the pain may be unrelated to the original disease. An unobserved patient gives much away. Involve the patient — use pain charts. Sympathetic questioning and concern will reveal a great deal.
Nursing attitude towards the patient's pain	To adopt a sympathetic, but realistic approach	It is not a nursing responsibility to pass judgement or to interpret the pain. The nurse must be able to feel the patient's pain, and act accordingly. The nurse is the patient's advocate.
Any additional medical, physical, psychological or social problems which may affect the pain threshold	Reduce pain by relieving external problems	Any symptom may make the patient less able to cope with their pain — fear, anxiety, a dry or infected mouth, etc. This will reduce morale and and the pain threshold. Sleep and rest are of prime importance — modify care accordingly. Spend time discussing problems, offer constructive help and services. Provide diversional therapy, visitors, etc. Set obtainable goals — an evening out perhaps.

Pain *(contd)*

Points to consider	What does the nurse aim to achieve?	What can the nurse do?
The effectiveness of prescribed analgesia	To gain and maintain an adequate level of pain control, resulting in a pain-free and alert patient	Before dismissing the dose and type of analgesia, check that it has not been administered on a p.r.n. basis, or that a dose has not been missed. Establish the type of pain; exclude other causes. If the pain is mild, use diversional tactics — a cup of tea, provision of heat, a change of position, a cooling wash, a relaxing voice, an opportunity to talk is maybe all that is required. The doctor should be aware; if all this fails, the doctor may well have to review the analgesia.
Coping when the medical staff are unavailable or do not appreciate the problem	The best for the patient	Continue with simple measures. Persistent attempts must be made to contact the doctor, and the patient kept in touch. The nurse must believe in his/her own judgement and keep the patient's interest. It may be necessary to contact a senior doctor. The nurse must not give in; do not be afraid, time wasted may reduce the patient's faith and trust.

Sore Mouth

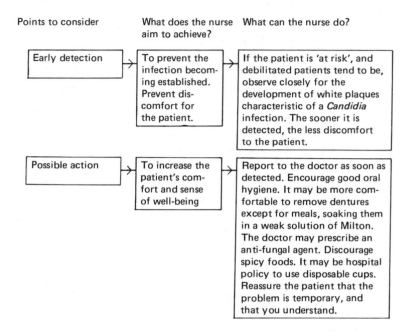

Points to consider	What does the nurse aim to achieve?	What can the nurse do?
Early detection	To prevent the infection becoming established. Prevent discomfort for the patient.	If the patient is 'at risk', and debilitated patients tend to be, observe closely for the development of white plaques characteristic of a *Candidia* infection. The sooner it is detected, the less discomfort to the patient.
Possible action	To increase the patient's comfort and sense of well-being	Report to the doctor as soon as detected. Encourage good oral hygiene. It may be more comfortable to remove dentures except for meals, soaking them in a weak solution of Milton. The doctor may prescribe an anti-fungal agent. Discourage spicy foods. It may be hospital policy to use disposable cups. Reassure the patient that the problem is temporary, and that you understand.

Bibliography

Baines, M. (1981) 'Drug control of common symptoms', *World Medicine*, 14 November

Janes, F. (1979) 'Constipation: keeping a true perspective', *Nursing Mirror*, 27 September, 149(14), supp. i–ii, iv–v, viii, x

Kubler-Ross, E. (1970) *On Death and Dying*, Tavistock Publications, London

Saunders, C.M. (ed.) (1978) *The Management of Terminal Disease*, Edward Arnold, London

Stedeford, A. (1980) 'Common psychological problems' in R.G. Twycross and V. Ventafridda (eds), *The Continuing Care of Terminal Cancer Patients*, Pergamon Press, Oxford

Twycross, R.G. and Ventafridda, V. (eds) (1980) *The Continuing Care of Terminal Cancer Patients*, Pergamon Press, Oxford

17 PSYCHO-SOCIAL ASPECTS OF CHRONIC DISABILITY

Elizabeth L. Cay

The practice of medicine has changed dramatically in the second half of the twentieth century. The virtual elimination of many previously fatal illnesses and improved living standards have resulted in an increasing proportion of the population surviving to reach the era of chronic degenerative disease: arthritis, ischaemic heart disease, peripheral vascular disease, strokes and chronic bronchitis. New techniques of medical care during the acute stage of illness have meant that more patients survive, but often with residual handicap and disability. Intensive care units, new methods of anaesthesia, assisted ventilation, resuscitation and surgery, together with the internal combustion engine which has changed our pattern of living dramatically, and the improvement in medical care means more accidents, but also more survivors. As a result of all these factors, the numbers of those with disability of all gradations of severity are increasing rapidly.

By far the greatest number of disabled persons are those who become ill. After years of normal living they have to learn, suddenly or gradually, to live with serious disability. Adjustment is a painful process and, as the natural course of disease progresses, they must keep pace with and change according to the change in physical state. At the same time, the individual must learn to adjust to profound social changes which may result from his illness. The attitudes of his family influence his ability to adjust successfully, and to a lesser extent those of his friends, workmates and employer. All will be affected by the attitude to disability prevalent in his culture.

Looking after the individual with chronic physical disease is a long-term commitment with its goal of 'caring' not 'curing', and requires the constant efforts of many people of differing professional skills. This is easy to state, but not nearly so easy to put into practice; it requires a change of attitude amongst staff whose training in all the modern technological advances has been directed towards curing the patient. It also needs the ability to stand back and withdraw services as the individual must be encouraged to be as independent as his disability will allow.

Psychological Reactions to Illness

Although for practical purposes it is convenient to talk about the psychological reactions to or sequelae of physical illness, it is important to remember that illness is a holistic concept and that the psychological aspects form an integral part of the disease process. They are still relatively neglected, but there is little doubt that they play an important part in influencing the course of an illness and the outcome of treatment. The intensity of psychological changes following illness forms a continuous spectrum, and there is no clear dividing line between normality and abnormality. Minor degrees of anxiety and depression are very common and are usually regarded as understandable and, given the circumstances, are not inappropriate. But if the emotional or behavioural changes themselves cause the patient significant distress or interfere with adjustment to the illness or orderly progression through a rehabilitation programme, they are considered to be pathological (Lloyd, 1977).

In response to illness, the individual brings various coping processes into action, the term 'coping' being used to describe various ways of dealing with threat (Lazarus, 1966). These coping processes may be adaptive or maladapative; they, therefore, can have a good or bad influence on prognosis. Patients free from major psychological conflict appraise their illness, seek medical advice and actively co-operate with treatment. Assuming that they are given good advice, this pattern of behaviour may be expected to allow them to adjust successfully. With persisting disability, the individual who cannot resume former activities looks for alternative sources of gratification. The illness in this case is regarded as a challenge to be overcome. Occasionally this may be so successful that the illness may lead to the development of intellectual and creative abilities that previously lay dormant. Music, art and literature can furnish many examples of individuals who have had such a positive result of illness (Eareckson, 1976).

Anxiety and depression are the most frequent reactions to physical illness. Although we have been aware of this at a clinical level for many years, it is only fairly recently that systematic efforts have been made to examine the extent of the problem. Groups of patients, including those with myocardial infarction (Stern, Pascale and McLoone, 1976), peptic ulcer (Small *et al.*, 1969), chronic intestinal disease (Philip and Cay, 1972), backache (Crown, 1980), on renal dialysis (Farmer, Snowden and Parsons, 1979) or admitted to a general hospital ward (Moffic and Paykel, 1975), have been studied. Although the results vary, depending on who is assessing the patients and the various methods to determine emotional upset which have been used, the striking feature to emerge is their similarity, rather than their difference.

It does seem possible to generalise the findings of these studies to all patients with chronic disease. In at least one-quarter of individuals with all kinds of handicap, emotional upset is severe enough to prevent successful adjustment. Severity of emotional disturbance is not necessarily related to severity of physical illness; those most severely disabled are not always those who are most disturbed (Cay *et al.*, 1972). Anxiety and depression is found in all age-groups and in patients from differing backgrounds. Women are more willing than men to admit that they are anxious or depressed (Billing *et al.*, 1980).

Clinical Manifestations

Although manifest anxiety does occur with restlessness, palpitations, sweating and insomnia, symptoms are often masked, making recognition difficult, unless those involved with the handicapped individual are alert to this. Anxiety can present with a rise in pulse rate or blood pressure, breathlessness, nausea and vomiting, diarrhoea or urinary frequency for which there is no clear physical explanation. Anxious patients may appear over-dependent, demanding immediate attention and care. Hostility may occur when various external sources, including the physician, are blamed for the illness and sensible medical advice is disregarded. Patients search frantically for a 'cause' of their illness, trying to alleviate its consequences. The depressed patient appears sad, disinterested and listless, is slow of speech and despondent about the future; he dwells on increasing dependence, inability to earn his living, sexual incompetence and premature death. On the other hand, he may seem to be merely hypochondriacal, excessively concerned with his symptoms, bodily function and medication. He may be considered the 'model' patient; quiet, well-behaved and easy to manage as, on the surface, he accepts increasing disability, treatment and advice without question. Such a maladaptive response may even lead to suicide, and there is now firm evidence on the association between physical illness and an increased risk of suicide (Reich and Kelly, 1976).

Anxiety may be difficult to identify, because patients consciously or unconsciously deny it. There has been considerable controversy in the role of denial in physical illness. Some authors feel that denial hinders adjustment, because it prevents the patient's objective assessment of the situation. This was supported by Ruskin's (1970) finding in patients after myocardial infarction that the aware and cautious patient improved most during follow-up, co-operated best with his medical advisers and returned to work readily. Other researchers have shown that denial, as a belief in the 'self' without disease, promotes rehabilitation. Hackett's group in Boston (1975) found that moderate denial was associated with decreased mortality and morbidity after infarction, and that it was the small proportion of minimal deniers who were likely to remain maladjusted. The results of a recent Swedish study suggest that the role of denial as an adequate defence mechanism may be culturally determined. Unlike the American patients, denial did not protect their post-infarct patients from anxiety and depression. Although no conclusions could be drawn from this study on the long-term consequences of denial, the Swedish research workers pointed out the marked differences between men and women in their psychological reactions to an infarction. Men were more likely to exhibit denial and reported fewer physical symptoms than women (Billing *et al.*, 1980).

Clinically, the patient who is denying the severity of his illness may appear elated and overactive and insist on continuing to work. This may be expressed in a more indirect fashion; the patient chooses to remain confused about his illness and to disregard its implications as much as possible.

Some defence patterns against anxiety are more successful than others in aiding psychological adjustment. A degree of dependence, rationalisation and identification with others with the same illness who have done well allow the patient to accept disability and cope successfully with its implications. Depression, excessive dependence, blaming others for the illness and identification with colleagues who have speedily become invalids decreases the likelihood of successful adjustment.

Factors which Influence Reaction to Disability

The reactions of an individual to chronic disability will depend on his previous psychological state and, in particular, on the methods of coping with stress developed over the years. Because the way in which stress is managed is closely bound up with the individual's personality traits, the patient's pre-morbid attitudes are important in influencing his response to illness. Patients with obsessional traits tend to find illness particularly stressful if there is doubt about the diagnosis, treatment or prognosis; they seek to set up well-defined guidelines and demand detailed explanations from those involved in their care. Those with narcissistic traits are likely to find illness stressful if there is a danger of disfiguration or loss of some highly esteemed bodily function. On the other hand, illness may be welcomed by inadequate, dependent personalities who are likely to be satisfied with the sick role (Mechanic, 1962).

The mental state and life experiences of the patient prior to and at the onset of the illness may be expected to influence the type of response. If the patient was already depressed previously, this emotional state may be expected to worsen. Women differ considerably from men in their psychological reactions to physical illness. There is some evidence that disabling disease proves more of a threat to men, whereas disfiguring illness is more stressful to women (Verwoerdt, 1972).

These personal attitudes are influenced by a number of environmental factors. Many studies have demonstrated the relation between illness behaviour and cultural background (Report of a Working Group, Warsaw, 1969). Compared to Irish and those of Anglo-Saxon origin, patients of Italian and Jewish extraction shared a tendency to earlier consultation for equivalent symptoms and to respond more emotionally to pain.

The more immediate social environment is important, because the emotional responses of close relatives, friends, workmates and employer influence the patient's own attitude. The whole family must adjust successfully to the new situation of illness; if they are experiencing serious problems in their personal life and social and economic difficulties, illness can provide a welcome escape and the patient role may be only reluctantly relinquished. A similar picture is seen if the possibility of litigation and compensation is a factor. On the other hand, illness is a threatening experience for the self-employed man or if promotion is likely to be deferred. The socio-economic situation prevailing in the country at the time of the individual's illness will affect family attitudes to the prospects of earning a living or accepting early retirement. Particularly stressful to the individual with severely incapacitating disability and to his family is the complexity of the social benefit situation in many countries. Bewildered, frightened and angry at the complicated bureaucratic system, many individuals do not get the benefits to which they are entitled (Blaxter, 1976).

The relationship between the patient and members of the therapeutic team has a profound effect on the way an individual reacts to illness. Hellerstein has demonstrated that anxious doctors have anxious patients (Hellerstein and Ford, 1957). Methods of treatment may provoke anxiety. A striking example of this has been shown in patients surviving cardiac arrest. Some years ago, the first reports on their quality of life were published (Druss and Kornfeld, 1967). The incidence of depression, nightmares and the level of chronic anxiety were high. The survivors complained of 'being different from other people'. These observations have not been substantiated in later studies, and there now seems to be little or no adverse psychological sequelae to cardiac arrest (Dobson *et al.,* 1971). The reason for this is most likely to be the way in which the patient learns about his arrest. In the beginning there was no uniform policy and often the wife or relative informed the patient, frequently in highly dramatic terms. Doctors and nurses, probably unsure of themselves, usually remained silent. Since the experience was unique to doctor and patient alike, distortion, exaggeration and misinformation accrued. Nowadays the patient is told of his arrest within 24 hours of the event, its routine nature is emphasised, and patient and family are informed that his future is not more gloomy because of it.

Effect of Psychological Factors on Outcome

Recognising that many patients with chronic illness are anxious or depressed is important if distress is to be relieved. It is also important because outcome of treatment depends as much on psychological as on physical factors. Upset patients have a poorer outcome following peptic ulcer surgery than those who are not disturbed (Small *et al.,* 1969); 75 per cent of those who react well to a myocardial infarction are working as hard as ever within four months, compared to only 20 per cent of depressed and anxious individuals, though they have not had more severe heart attacks (Cay, 1982). The survival rate over 3½ years of patients with chronic renal failure is better in those who are free of upset, have fewer physical symptoms, are able to return to work and who have wives who are coping well (Farmer *et al.,* 1979).

Acute onset of illness allows little time to adapt, but, although emotional disturbance often follows, if the physical disorder is of short duration there is usually associated resolution of upset. On the other hand, chronic illness allows the patient more time to adapt to his disability, but any related psychological disturbance is likely to persist in view of the implications of long-term handicap that the illness carries. Stern *et al.* (1976) reported that 73 per cent of those depressed immediately after infarction remained so throughout the follow-up, and in a similar group examined by Singh *et al.* (1970), 34 per cent of patients remained depressed or anxious for two years following an infarct.

Psychological Reactions of the Spouse

The spouse may, in some circumstances, be more distressed than the patient. During the acute illness, the wife's anxiety is often greater than her husband's (Cay, 1982). Later on, Ruskin (1970) found that neuroticism scores were higher for the patient than for the spouse, although the wife tended to be more realistic as her level of anxiety depended on the severity of her husband's illness. She may blame herself for her husband's illness and try to relieve her own anxiety by over-protecting the patient and encouraging him to become too dependent. She will have to cope with changes in roles within the family or the natural changes that occur as a result of illness. The lack of structure caused by increasing chronic disability in the lives of those accustomed to a busy existence results in boredom, irritability, frustration and loss of confidence with resultant strain between husband and wife. Mayou, in a study of wives of patients with infarction, found 42 per cent of wives depressed at two months, with 30 per cent still depressed at one year. Predictive factors for the wife's progress were her mental state, work satisfaction, marital satisfaction and a previous history of neurotic illness (Mayou, Foster and Williamson, 1978). Sexual problems, both physical and psychological, are frequent in disabled individuals (Stewart, 1974) and, not unexpectedly, their divorce rate is high. Personality changes in the patient, particularly if these result from brain damage, are often resented. The spouse may be more aware than the patient of the likely prognosis and be unable to face the prospect of dying and death.

Psychological Reactions of the Staff

Looking after the patient with chronic physical illness makes undoubted emotional demands on all those involved in his care, irrespective of the profession to which the individual belongs. This is particularly true if the patient is young; doctors, nurses and therapists identify with the patient and become sensitised to the tragic nature of the situation (Stedeford and Bloch, 1979). It is too easy to regard modern medical technology as able to prolong life indefinitely and staff may resent the patient who is obviously deteriorating physically while being maintained on regular renal dialysis. Similarly, they may become angered by the patient who does not conform to high standards of behaviour, particularly if they feel he is benefiting from expensive care which may not be readily available to all patients (De-Nour, 1968).

Members of the therapeutic team, aware of the distress of both patients and family, especially if they have been involved with them for a long time, may share the common fear and prejudice which surrounds emotional illness. They suspect that such obviously upset patients are more vulnerable and more difficult to understand than 'normal' patients, requiring specialised skills to handle this aspect of care. This attitude can obviously inhibit a spontaneous response by the staff, who may be quite capable of coping with the situation. There is evidence that the psychologist or liaison psychiatrist who is a member of the therapeutic team can act as educator, supervisor and supporter of his fellow team members. They become very competent at recognising and handling the more straightforward psychological problems associated with chronic disability, leaving the specially trained individual to deal with patients with complicated psychological difficulties (Stedeford and Bloch, 1979). This policy increases the chance that someone will be available to respond to the immediate psychological needs of patients, whether the psychologist or psychiatrist is there or not. The general level of psychological care is likely to improve, allowing the specialist to concentrate on the small proportion of patients whose problems clearly require his expertise. Also, he can play a valuable role in supporting colleagues when they are exposed to exceptional stress.

Such an approach is of value when patients are perceived to have problems in other areas, which are not traditionally part of medical care. Individuals with physical disability were not thought to have sexual desires or needs and, if in rare cases sexual difficulties were mentioned, doctors and nurses, largely ignorant of this field, tended to ignore this aspect and avoid discussion with the patient, dismissing sexual problems as being outside medical care. For example, the first mention in Western literature of sexual problems after myocardial infarction occurs in 1964, when Tuttle found that two-thirds of patients after an infarct reported a marked and lasting reduction in the frequency of intercourse, largely because of lack of information and fear (Tuttle, Cook and Fitch, 1964). Nowadays, with increasing knowledge of the physical requirements of sexual intercourse and the demonstration that it accounts for only a tiny proportion (0.6 per cent) of sudden deaths (Veno, 1963), doctors feel confident to discuss this topic with their patients. As a result, recent studies have shown that the great majority of post-infarct patients return to a normal and satisfactory sex life (Skelton and Dominian, 1973). The psychologist can help fellow members of the team to feel comfortable when discussing patients' sexual problems. They then feel confident to tackle those that arise, referring for specialist help only those with complicated difficulties.

Assessment of the Patient

It is important to stress that psychological assessment is part of total patient care and must be closely allied to an accurate assessment of physical state. The methods used will depend on the stage of illness. At each stage, the psychological assessment must take into account those factors within the patient which promote or hinder adaptation to disability and the factors in his environment which will influence this.

The physician has two aims in his assessment of the psychological state of the patient; diagnosis and prediction. Diagnosis of the individual's psychological reactions to the stress situation and the methods of defence which he mobilises to help him to cope with it allows the physician to predict how successful his patient will be in learning to live with disability. Using this information, he can then treat his patient effectively. It is important to see the spouse and close relatives separately; chronic illness puts a strain on any marriage, particularly one in which there are underlying problems. The spouse may need guidance and treatment.

Awareness by the physician that his patient is likely to be anxious or depressed and that he may have social problems is the first step in positive identification of these aspects of patient care. An attitude of encouragement by the doctor is essential. This is particularly important in patients who have shown evidence in the past of inability to cope with other stresses of adult life. Some indications of this are poor work records, previous psychiatric illness, alcoholism, excessive work activities, excessive invalidism after other illnesses, a poor marital relationship and pre-existing financial problems (Cay, 1982). The reasons why the patient is reacting badly are as important as the diagnosis of disturbance. They determine the method of treatment, which may be relatively simple — involving only minor adjustments at home or at work — or prolonged and difficult, if emotional disturbance is arising on the basis of pre-illness personality traits which may cause the individual to seek to prolong the invalid role.

Many methods have been used in research to estimate the level of anxiety, depression, denial, personality traits and motivation. Psychologists have used a combination of interviews, projective tests and questionnaires. Many of these are unsuitable for the non-psychologically trained physician to administer and interpret, and others, originally developed for neurotic patients, are not very relevant to patients with chronic physical disease. They reflect the need for maximum information and are therefore quite unsuited to routine clinical practice. Recently, much shorter questionnaires have come into use to estimate emotional disturbance in a 'normal' population. Philip (1981) has demonstrated that a self-administered questionnaire of emotional upset, taking 5-10 minutes to complete, is sufficiently accurate to be used to screen patients; 85 per cent of emotional disturbance estimated by a psychiatrist using an interview was detected by the test. A significant step forward in assessing emotional upset in routine clinical practice has been taken as a result of a recent study by DeBusk and his co-workers. They showed that a technician on the staff of the cardiology department, trained to use a standardised interview, was as accurate as a psychiatrist in detecting those patients requiring treatment for depression after a myocardial infarction (Taylor *et al.,* 1981).

Although such work is promising, for the physician faced with the task of assessing his patient, there is at present no one simple screening test. The clinical interview is, at the moment, the most reliable method to obtain the information that he needs. Psycho-social factors to be included in the interview are anxiety, depression, denial, work problems, family problems, sexual activity, problems involving leisure and social activities, financial difficulties and problems in complying with medical advice.

Management

Treatment of emotional distress in those with advanced disease can be summarised as awareness, education, continued support, co-ordination of care and practical help. Drug therapy is important, particularly to relieve pain, but it cannot replace these measures. Appreciation by staff that many of their patients will be anxious or depressed and encouraging them that such reactions are normal and to be expected do much to help and may decrease the need for tranquillisers and antidepressant medication. Patient behaviour reflects the attitudes of those involved in their care, and it is important to remember that time spent talking to patients is never time wasted. The great majority of patients with psycho-social problems can be treated by members of staff looking after their physical needs. Only a minority with severe disturbance or grave social problems will require specialist treatment – approximately 15–20 per cent of patients (Cay *et al.*, 1973; Stern *et al.*, 1976).

Patients who feel they are not being told enough about their illness are often suffering from a feeling of insecurity due, not to insufficient frankness about their exact diagnosis or their long-term prognosis, but to lack of sustained professional interest in their symptoms, lack of good care or lack of information about what is going on and what to expect in the immediate future. It is important always to have a plan and to tell the patient what it is. In the advanced case, if there is a reasonable chance of achieving one or more short-term objectives such as less pain, easier breathing or a better night's sleep, this should be explained to the patient in a suitably positive and optimistic way. It is very seldom that nothing can be done for the patient with advanced physical illness (Brewin, 1977).

Being a good listener need not necessarily take more than a few minutes. The main thing is to appear interested, not only in all current symptoms, but also in the patient as a person in his own right. If the patient is very disabled, this sort of respect for him with a brief word about his past life or his opinion about current happenings in the world, is especially important, as it counteracts the indignity that so often accompanies advanced disease and, combined with technical efficiency, helps to reassure him that he is in good hands. Unspoken communication may have a greater impact than words. The patient may quickly decide, sometimes from little more than a smile or the firm touch of a hand, that the person speaking to him wants to help, knows how to, and has at least some idea of how he feels. Busy members of staff have to try to appear relaxed, unhurried and above all not embarrassed or afraid and very willing to answer any questions. To deny the patient with advanced disease the humour, good fellowship and gossip that he would expect if he were fit, serves only to increase his sense of isolation. These various forms of basic background communication are very important, as the effect of what is said, or not said, about the diagnosis and prognosis may depend on them.

Education of the patient about his disease, like adjustment to it, is a gradual process with no one 'right' way to do it, as it depends on the relationship formed between the patient and his family and various members of staff. Most doctors will agree that they regard it as part of the art of being a good doctor that they do not hand out to every patient the same 'take it or leave it' policy when they communicate diagnosis and prognosis. They prefer to adapt, as best they can, to his personality and background and to what seems to be going on in his mind. This is not easy, however. It is impossible to read the patient's thoughts and, although the spouse or a close friend may be very helpful, quite often even in a close or happy marriage the marriage partner is as much in the dark as the doctor. Even the patient himself is sometimes not sure exactly what he fears, or what he already knows, or suspects, or wants to know, about the seriousness of his illness. Faced with these problems, it is all too easy to fall back on so many technical words and jargon that the claim to have 'told the patient' could equally well be described as 'not telling the patient'. The patient in fact often guides members of staff as to what they should say at any one time. Some vital clue is not the first question, but the second or indeed the absence of a second question. The attitude of the patient may at any time change completely, so that the doctor may be confronted by a situation quite different from the one he faced in the past. Communication of diagnosis and prognosis is not a dilemma faced once and then forgotten. It is a matter for continuous reassessment and sensitivity in changing circumstances.

Denial of the illness, a useful and perhaps essential protective mechanism, can be quite fragile and can be easily upset by a chance remark, an item in the newspaper or the death of another patient. It is important to recognise the extent to which the patient is using this. Sometimes he appears to 'know' and at others he does not. Perhaps when he is with one person he seems to know and with another he seems not to know. Perhaps he accepts deteriorating physical capacity, but still hopes for remission or possible recovery. He may show denial to such an extent that friends and relatives can scarcely credit it. They and the staff looking after him, perhaps unwilling to accept the concept of denial, may attribute such apparent lack of insight to stupidity or brain damage. Frank discussion of denial with relatives and other members of staff is necessary so that all are aware of and respect the patient's wishes (Brewin 1977).

Continual support with relief of pain may be necessary for a long time. Repeated assessment of needs has to be undertaken as changes in physical state occur. Drug therapy may be intermittently necessary to tide over crises and such care does not always end with the death of the patient, if his family still needs help.

Inevitably, the efforts of many individuals with differing skills may be required as the disease progresses. Few patients suffer a sharper drop in morale than those transferred from one doctor or medical team to another, who get the impression that little or no information has been passed on. Consistent, efficient and immediate inter-professional communication, so hard to achieve in practice, should not only be good, but be seen by the patient and family to be good, and they should be specifically reassured on this point.

Practical help, promptly available to deal with social problems as they arise, does much to relieve distress. Often only simple adjustments are necessary; day-centre attendance or holiday admission to give the family a break, putting relatives in touch with others facing similar problems or arranging for the care of the patient, if the relative becomes ill.

Although the actual organisation of services will vary from place to place, the general principles of management of psychological problems are the same. Whatever the outlook, the main aim is to maintain morale and to help the patient and his family to face the future with courage, equanimity and peace of mind. There is no set pattern to follow; it is necessary to assess as well as possible, with the help of relatives and friends, the immediate and late effects of what is said, to modify accordingly future policy in similar circumstances and to try to learn from mistakes, just as occurs in any other aspect of patient care.

This is not a new concept and Montaigne's words some 400 years ago are just as true of today: 'It is fear that I stand most in fear of. In sharpness it exceeds every other pain.'

References

Billing, E., Lindell, B., Sederholm, M. and Theorell, T. (1980) 'Denial, anxiety and depression following myocardial infarction', *Psychosomatics*, 21, 639–45
Blaxter, M. (1976) *The Meaning of Disability*, Heinemann, London
Brewin, T.B. (1977) 'The cancer patient: communication and morale', *British Medical Journal*, 2, 1623–7
Cay, E.L. (1982) 'Psychological problems in patients after a myocardial infarction', in J.J. Kellermann (ed.), *Advances in Cardiology*, Karger, Basel, Vol. 29, pp. 108–12
Cay, E.L., Vetter, N., Philip, A. and Dugard, P. (1972) 'Psychological status during recovery from an acute heart attack', *Journal of Psychosomatic*

Research, 16, 425–35

Cay, E.L., Vetter, N., Philip, A. and Dugard, P. (1973) 'Return to work after a heart attack', *Journal of Psychosomatic Research*, 17, 231–43

Crown, S. (1980) 'Psychosocial factors in low back pain', *Clinics in Rheumatic Diseases*, 6, 77–92

De-Nour, A.K. (1968) 'Emotional problems and reactions of the medical team in a chronic haemodialysis unit', *Lancet*, ii, 987–91

Dobson, M., Tattersfield, A.E., Adler, M.M. and McNicol, M.W. (1971) 'Attitudes and long term adjustment of patients surviving cardiac arrest', *British Medical Journal*, 3, 207–12

Druss, R.G. and Kornfeld, D.S. (1967) 'Survivors of cardiac arrest: a psychiatric study', *Journal of the American Medical Association*, 201, 291–6

Eareckson, J. (1976) *Joni*, Pickering and Inglis, London

Farmer, C.J., Snowden, S.A. and Parsons, V. (1979) 'The prevalence of psychiatric illness among patients on home dialysis', *Psychological Medicine*, 9, 509–14

Farmer, C.J., Bewick, M., Parsons, V. and Snowden, S. (1979) 'Survival on home haemodialysis; its relationship with physical symptomatology, psychosocial background and psychiatric morbidity', *Psychological Medicine*, 9, 515–23

Hackett, T.P. (1975) *Coronary care: patient psychology*, American Heart Association, New York

Hellerstein, H. and Ford, A. (1957) 'Rehabilitation of the cardiac patient', *Journal of the American Medical Association*, 164, 225–31

Lazarus, R.S. (1966) *Psychological Stress and the Coping Process*, McGraw-Hill, New York

Lloyd, G.G. (1977) 'Psychological reactions to physical illness', *British Journal of Hospital Medicine*, 18, 352–8

Mayou, R., Foster, A. and Williamson, B. (1978) 'The psychological and social effects of myocardial infarction in wives', *British Medical Journal*, 1, 699–701

Mechanic, D. (1962) 'The concept of illness behaviour', *Journal of Chronic Diseases*, 15, 189–94

Moffic, H.S. and Paykel, E.S. (1975) 'Depression in medical inpatients', *British Journal of Psychiatry*, 126, 346–53

Philip, A.E. (1982) 'Measuring the outcome of rehabilitation', in J.J. Kellermann (ed.), *Proceedings of 2nd International Congress in Cardiac Rehabilitation, Jerusalem, 1981*, Karger, Basel

Philip, A.E. and Cay, E.L. (1972) 'Psychiatric symptoms and personality traits in patients suffering from gastro-intestinal illness', *Journal of Psychosomatic Research*, 16, 47–51

Reich, P. and Kelly, M.J. (1976) 'Suicide attempts in hospitalized medical and surgical patients', *New England Journal of Medicine*, 294, 298–301

Report of a Working Group, Warsaw (1969) *Psychological Aspects of the Rehabilitation of Cardiovascular Patients*, WHO Regional Office for Europe, Copenhagen

Ruskin, H.D. (1970) 'MMPI: Comparison between patients with coronary heart disease and their spouses together with other demographic data', *Scandinavian Journal of Rehabilitation Medicine*, 2, 99–101

Singh, J., Singh, S., Singh, S., Singh, A. and Malhotra, R.P. (1970) 'Sex life and psychiatric problems after myocardial infarction', *Journal of the Association of Physicians of India*, 18, 503–7

Skelton, M. and Dominian, J. (1973) 'Psychological stress in wives of patients with myocardial infarction', *British Medical Journal*, 2, 101–3

Small, W.P., Cay, E.L., Bugard, P., Sircus, W., Falconer, C.W.A., Smith, A.N., McManus, J.P.A. and Sir John Bruce (1969) 'Peptic ulcer surgery: selection for operation by "earning" ', *Gut*, 10, 996–1003

Stedeford, A. and Bloch, S. (1979) 'The psychiatrist in the terminal care unit', *British Journal of Psychiatry*, 135, 1–6

Stern, M.J., Pascale, L. and McLoone, J.B. (1976) 'Psychological adaptations following an acute myocardial infarction', *Journal of Chronic Diseases*, 29, 513–28

Stewart, W.F.R. (1974) *Sex and the Physically Handicapped*, Monograph of the National Foundation for Research into Crippling Diseases, SPOD, London

Taylor, C.B., Debusk, R.F., Davidson, D.M., Houston, N. and Burnett, K. (1981) 'Optional methods for identifying depression following hospitalisation for myocardial infarction', *Journal of Chronic Diseases*, 34, 127–33

Tuttle, W.B., Cook, W.L. and Fitch, E. (1964) 'Sexual behaviour in post myocardial infarction patients', *American Journal of Cardiology*, 13, 140

Veno, M. (1963) 'The so-called coition death', *Japanese Journal of Legal Medicine*, 17, 333–40

Verwoerdt, A. (1972) 'Psychopathological responses to the stress of physical illness', in I.J. Lipowski (ed.), *Advances in Psychosomatic Medicine*, Vol. 8, Karger, Basel, pp. 119–40

18 BEREAVEMENT

Fiona Cathcart

Previous chapters have described the emotional stress of the patient and family approaching death. This chapter will explore some of the stress faced by the bereaved as they learn to live with their loss. It is divided into two sections; in the first, the psychological and practical difficulties encountered are described; and in the second, ways are suggested in which these difficulties may be alleviated.

Psychological Experiences and Practical Difficulties

Introduction

Birth and death are universal phenomena, but we forget how they can be viewed differently according to the time and place in which they occur. In some societies, it is considered highly irresponsible and anti-social to have more than one or, at most, two children. In other societies, producing many children, particularly sons, may be a source of public congratulation, and medals may be awarded to Mother Heroines. As attitudes to birth vary, so may attitudes to death. In twentieth-century western culture, life expectancy has increased (Figure 18.1). We expect our children to survive to adulthood and produce grandchildren. We expect our spouses to retire into a healthy old age with us. We would feel cheated by less, but only a hundred years ago this would have been an exceptional family pattern.

Was death less distressing to our ancestors, because it was more familiar? The experience of being a young widow with two or more children dead in infancy would have been common to other relatives and neighbours in the community. The sense of social isolation and stigma would have been less. There was more certainty of an after-life and reunion with the deceased. The financial consequences would have been severe for many working-class families losing either an adult or child wage-earner. The emotional impact was probably as great. Literature through the centuries describes the pain of bereavement as something we can recognise. Surviving correspondence reveals anxieties for the health of new nieces or grandchildren, which suggests that high infant mortality did not blunt family affections.

391

Figure 18.1: Expectation of life at different attained ages. England and Wales 1832-1972 (years)

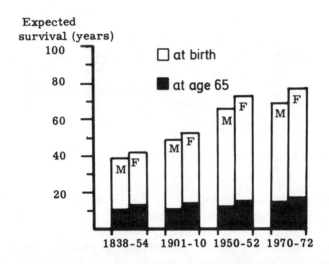

Source: Williamson, J. (1979) in D. Doyle (ed.), *Terminal Care*.

The analogy of physical pain may be useful. The pain of an abscess may be experienced more frequently by people in Third World countries with inadequate health services, but it cannot be considered as less painful even though the cultural expression of that pain may be different.

Children's Experience of Death

Death is rarely discussed openly with children and it is assumed that they are kept in blissful ignorance. 'If we don't talk about it, they won't know about it.' This protects the adult rather than the child. The child's understanding of death develops from an early age and is dependent, not only upon what it is told within its family, but also upon what it observes, learns from its peers and takes from television and fairy-tales. The age of the child determines its ability to form concepts about many aspects of its world, of which death is only one. Personal maturity, regardless of chronological age, will affect the depth of understanding.

Rutter (1966) compared children referred to a London child psychiatry department with children referred to paediatric and dental clinics. He found that more than twice as many children attending the psychiatric clinic had been bereaved by parental death compared with those attending a paediatric department. Five times as many psychiatrically disturbed children had been bereaved than had the children attending dental clinics. It should be noted that the majority of the children referred to the psychiatry department had *not* been bereaved, approximately eleven in twelve. Rutter suggested that the most vulnerable time was between three and four years of age. Referral was not within the first six months except for adolescent boys. The most likely time was some years later at puberty.

Pre-School-Age Children. In infancy, the child requires physical touch to develop fully, in addition to its more easily recognised needs of food, drink and warmth. Emotional deprivation alone is a cause of infants failing to thrive. The bereaved parent, who is absorbed in his or her own grief, may have little warmth left to comfort or amuse a fretful child.

Bowlby (1951) has stated that separation from the mother had severe and long-lasting effects. More recently, Rutter has argued that the outcome was variable and depended upon other factors such as the quality of the previous relationship and other care-takers being available for the child. The effect of leaving home to be fostered upon a rota of reluctant relatives is quite different from remaining at home with familiar friends and schoolmates and a popular gran or aunt moving in.

Toddlers appear to have a crude understanding of the concept of death. One active 2½-year-old was running round a room and stopped suddenly to flop on a cushion, shouting 'I'm dead'. He lay completely still for a few moments before jumping up to start another game. He had tried this role spontaneously, as he tried many others. The young child acts out life in games and may re-enact a funeral or accident with dolls or playmates. Dolls are buried in boxes in the sandpit. A car crash is re-enacted with toy cars. At this age, children will experiment with whatever is around them in an effort to understand how things work. They will see a dead cat by the roadside and ask what happened, what the cat felt, what it feels now and what will happen next. Similarly, when playing in the garden a child may cut a worm in two. It is interested to see both bits wriggle and may cut again or stamp on a part to see the effect. Insects may have wings or legs removed to see when they stop wriggling. This curiosity is as natural as the interest in blowing bubbles in juice or seeing how far he can throw something. The curiosity about death may be uncomfortable for an adult who has uncertainty about his own feelings about death. It causes anguish when the questions asked are about a dead friend or relative.

When talking about death with young children, it should be remembered that they have a limited attention span and are distractable. Conversation may switch from the dead person, a family pet, to other children passing by and back to death again. Taking it in stages may be a way of reducing anxiety, but it can also reflect the usual attention span of a young child and, as such, it is normal, if disconcerting for the adult.

The child of this age understands matters literally. If told that an angel has taken Daddy, he may become fearful of going to bed in case the angel comes and takes him too, when he would rather stay with Mummy, thank you. Fears of going out, crossing open spaces or sleeping with open windows have been observed in bereaved children. Cooper (1980) visited homes in which there had been a stillbirth and observed a larger proportion of siblings out of bed than might have been expected during an evening visit. She was uncertain whether it was the children's or parents' anxieties that kept them from their beds.

5 to 8-Year-Olds. The child's understanding is growing, but death is not yet seen as inevitable and irreversible. Death is visualised as a concrete figure like a skeleton or bogey man, rather than a biological decline. There is an assumption that if you are wary enough or get the right kind of attention, you may avoid it. This is important in helping us understand a child's distress. If Granny can be made better by being wrapped in warm blankets and given hot milk, why have we left her in that hole in the ground?

The child may become very obedient and quiet. Children learn that bad behaviour has unpleasant consequences, but that behaving well may win back a forfeited treat. The mother harassed by an unruly toddler during her morning chores may threaten not to visit Grandpa in the afternoon, because he would not want to see such a naughty boy. The child conforms and is rewarded by the planned visit (which probably would have taken place anyway!). It is not a large step for a young child to assume that if one is very good now, Grandpa will be available again for visits.

Adults may show similar behaviour. When a patient dies on a hospital ward, other patients may become markedly quieter and more compliant for a few hours. The subdued atmosphere may be explained as respect for the dead, but a more primitive need to pacify and perhaps avoid attracting Death's attention to oneself may play a part.

Nine Years and Older. The young person has a more adult understanding of death, but its takes place in the context of the strong emotional upheavals of adolescence. The youngster who had been challenging parents in the usual trials of strength finds him/herself in an empty field. Echoes of previous arguments return — 'You'll be the death of me' or 'Your father worries himself sick about you'. The young male is advised that he is the man of the family or the daughter may be told she has to mother the young ones and care for her father. The surviving parent may resent any increased show of authority by the youngster and oppose it as a threat to his/her own fragile strength.

Some parents use the teenager as a substitute for the dead partner. This way of coping may be effective until the teenager starts dating regularly or is offered further education or work away from home. Pincus (1976) describes families where a child has been used in this way.

The dead parent may be used to enforce the authority of the survivor for many years. The argument of 'You know your father/mother would not have liked it' may silence a disagreement, but causes guilt and resentment, particularly if the teenager suspects the deceased parent would not have objected.

Children's Practical Difficulties

Psychological Deprivation. There is the grief for the dead parent with the anger, anxiety and depression that this entails. In addition to the loss of a loved person, the child has lost an important model for its own future development. We establish our future relationships using our past experiences with others, particularly parents; for bereaved children, these experiences are diminished.

One common reaction to bereavement is loss of affection a feeling of coldness and loss of warmth to those around. The young widow may be able to wash and dress her children, but has no wish to cuddle them or play. This initial coldness can be intensely distressing for both parent and child at a time when they have an increased need for physical contact. Fortunately, it is almost always temporary. It is difficult to meet somebody else's emotional needs when there is nobody to meet one's own.

Financial Deprivation. One-parent families are poorer and this financial loss affects both widows and widowers. A mother may be obliged to return to work at a time when her resources for learning new skills and forming new relationships are low. A father is obliged to pay for childcare and household services that he may have taken for granted until this time. Where the financial difficulties are severe, the family may be dispersed among relatives or a desperate parent may consider rapid, premature remarriage to provide another parent for the children.

At a simpler level, money can provide some comforts. One widow who feels unable to sit in the house a moment longer can put her children in the car and drive across town to visit a friend. The cost of bus fares would make this prohibitive for another mother, even if she could manage the three small children, a pushchair and the change of buses. The guilt of always having to say 'No' to treats adds to feelings of depression and anxiety.

Social Deprivation. Financial difficulties may curtail the family's social activities. Membership of clubs, visits to swimming baths or school trips are no longer possible. The child feels different from other children and may be viewed as an object of curiosity by them. The surviving parent experiences tiredness as part of the grief reaction, but also feels exhausted by the loss of a practical helper. The effort of trying to be both mother and father leaves little energy to play games or listen to chatter. In this way, the child loses a part of its surviving parent too.

The child's adjustment to the loss will be determined to a large extent by the adaptation of the surviving parent. The effects of bereavement on an adult will now be explored.

Adult Experience of Bereavement

It is arbitrary to divide child/adult reactions to bereavement. The reaction may be expressed more nakedly in the child, but both may experience emotional and physical distress. Similarly, the distinction between the physical and psychological experience of grief is of limited value, as is the debate as to whether bereavement is an 'illness' or not.

Bereavement has both components, but the emphasis may centre upon one or the other, depending upon the individual's personality, sex and age.

There are varying theories about what happens during resolution of grief. Freud described it as needing to decathect or detach one's energy from an object/person in whom there was great investment, hypercathesis. Bowlby (1961a) described it in terms of animal behaviour, the pining search of an animal who has lost its mate, Parkes (1972) sees it as altering one's inner model of the world so that it accords with the changed reality of living without the loved one.

Physical Effects of Bereavement. There is evidence that bereavement can have major effects on physical health. Young, Benjamin and Wallis (1963) examined the deaths of 4486 men over the age of 54 years, who had been widowed during a two-month period. They found a large increase in deaths among the widowers during the first six months of bereavement. The mortality rate was 40 per cent higher than expected, based on figures for married men in the same age-group. This was extended by a later study (Parkes, Benjamin and Fitzgerald, 1969), which indicated that the greatest proportional increase in deaths was from heart disease.

Rees and Lutkins (1967) examined the effects of bereavement upon the parent, child and siblings as well as the spouse of the dead person. They surveyed over 900 close relatives of 371 people who died during the period 1960-5 in a small Welsh community. The survey revealed that nearly 5 per cent of the relatives died during the first year, compared with less than 1 per cent of a non-bereaved group living in the same area and matched for age and class ($p < 0.001$).This effect was more noticeable in male than female relatives ($p < 0.005$). The effect was least where the death had occurred at home, greater where it occurred in hospital, and greatest elsewhere and — presumably — was unexpected, such as at the roadside, pond or golf course.

Maddison and Walker (1967) and Maddison and Viola (1968) studied the subjective impact on physical well-being using self-report. They surveyed two groups of widows in the year following bereavement. In one group of American widows of men aged 45-60 years, over 20 per cent indicated that they believed themselves to have sustained a marked health deterioration. In a larger group of Australian widows whose husbands had died before reaching 45 years of age, 33 per cent indicated poorer health. Although it is tempting to conclude from this that bereavement is more difficult for the young widow, it should be remembered that this is a cross-cultural study. Each country would have had different social and financial supports for its widows. In addition, the respondents to the questionnaire were a self-selected group in that only 50 per cent of those approached returned completed questionnaires.

Parkes (1964b) examined the GP consultation rate of 44 widows eighteen months before their bereavement and during the following eighteen-month period. The rate rose significantly from an average of 2.2 visits per patient for each six-month period prior to bereavement, to an average of 3.6 during the first six months post-bereavement, and remaining high during the next twelve months. There was a 200 per cent increase in consultation for psychological symptoms in widows under the age of 65 ($p < 0.001$). There was a slight but insignificant increase in consultations for psychological symptoms in older widows. In addition, there was a significant increase in consultations for physical symptoms.

Psychological Aspects of Bereavement. It is appropriate at this point to examine in more detail the psychological aspects of grief work. (The bereaved person will be referred to as female for convenience.) It is usual to present this as a sequence of stages which the person is required to work through: that is, shock, denial, physical distress, guilt and idealisation, depression and anxiety, and finally resolution. This can be misleading and is simplistic. In general terms, some aspects may be more common earlier than later. There is no clear time-scale, rather, a jumbled series of phases. It may be more helpful to think of the bereavement process as a spiral rather than a linear sequence. The person may experience the same emotion again at a later time, but with a different intensity and understanding. It is with these reservations that the process of grief will be discussed. The widow may feel that she has accepted the death and is resigned to the loss. The sight of a familiar car stopping at the door creates a sudden surge of hope which is dashed and causes her to question if she had accepted anything as real. This can be a devastating blow to the confidence which had been regained. She may need reassurance that she is not back at the beginning.

Shock/Numbness

Frequently, the news of the death is experienced as a sudden physical blow that takes the breath away. The person may ward it off by physically striking the person who tells them. This sudden violence can be as alarming and unexpected to the bereaved person as it is to the carer on the receiving end. It adds to the guilt experienced by both parties, even though the reason is understandable. More commonly, the person appears outwardly composed and can act as an automaton. This disassociation may help for a brief period while certain practical tasks are done, but it usually lasts only minutes or hours.

Lindemann (1944) described waves of distress which sweep over the person, lasting 20 minutes to one hour. Intense pangs of grief are experienced as a feeling of tightness in the throat with the sensation of gasping and shortage of breath. There may be heavy sighing or gulping, dry sobs.

Denial

Denial softens the blow: full realisation comes by degrees, as we are more able to cope with it. The bereaved person continues many of the daily rituals such as setting an extra place at the table or preparing a meal for a certain time. These may have become meaningless to the outside world, but they maintain a comforting security. Parkes (1972) describes us as having an inner model of the world which is now faulty. We search to replace the loss. A person of the same physique nearby can cause an overwhelming desire to touch.

The smell of the person's possessions, ironing shirts for the last time, can cause an intense desire for their physical presence. The person may regress and sleep with a garment for a while as a child sleeps with a comforter. Less commonly, the need for physical touch and search for the dead person may lead the bereaved person to act out sexually and start an affair or behave promiscuously. This causes more problems if it comes to the attention of the extended family, and is likely to result in withdrawal of support.

Seeing a person in similar clothing may cause the bereaved person to think momentarily 'There's Dad'. Mistaking an object or person who is present for something else is called an illusion. A hallucination is the sensation of seeing something in the absence of any physical stimulus. Hypnagogic hallucinations have been described. These are experienced when the person is in a semi-sleeping state and believes that the dead person is standing by the bed or lying next to them. This is more common in the initial stages, but similar sensations may recur years later at a significant time for the surviving relative. One young woman whose mother had died years before felt her physical presence on her wedding day. As she dressed for the ceremony and moved from room to room, she had a strong sensation that her mother had only just left that room and she had missed seeing her by seconds. She had not experienced this before, but found it consoling to feel she had shared this major event in her life with her mother.

Frequently the presence, whether seen or only felt, is considered a positive experience, but it may be viewed negatively and seen as confirmation by the bereaved person or their family that he/she has broken down under the strain and is becoming insane. It may be a frightening experience which is not confided to anyone, particularly for a controlled person whose concentration and memory have become unreliable and who is subjected to strong emotional distress. It is helpful to be reassured that it is as much a part of grieving as tears and that it is not an uncommon experience.

One young woman complained of insomnia. She was afraid to sleep with the lights off and slept regularly in her child's room. On questioning, she revealed she was frightened of ghosts. This was explored further and she stated that she was fearful of her father's ghost. It was apparent that this fear was balanced by an equally strong longing to see him again. The woman had left home in disgrace as a pregnant teenager. Subsequently, she had returned, but by this time her father was dead. She had not had the opportunity to be reconciled to him. Interestingly, her child's imaginary playmate was an old man with many of the habits of the grandfather she had never met. The deceased man was being kept alive at a number of levels within this family.

If the loss is acknowledged in waking life, the gap may be filled in dreams for some bereaved people. Sometimes the dream may be so clearly wish-fulfilment that awakening to the reality leaves the person more bitterly aware of the loss. A woman died unexpectedly after surgery. Her daughter recounted a vivid dream in which she had gone to the ward as usual at visiting time to be greeted by the ward sister saying 'Oh, Miss S, we're so sorry we made a mistake. It was not your mother who died but somebody else's.' Another bereaved daughter recalled a dream in which she was sitting with her sisters and mother looking at family photos developed since her mother's death. They were chatting and she had laughed and said 'Isn't it funny? We all thought you were dead and here you are.'

The person may avoid the pain by avoiding people who would discuss it, avoiding the possessions or music preferred by the dead person. If a favourite tune is one the radio, it is switched off. It is hard to maintain this avoidance in the face of incoming letters of condolence, religious ceremonies and visits from the dead person's relatives, friends and colleagues. It is more appropriate if the person can allow herself to be overcome by the distress at the time of the bereavement, because at that time social support is mobilised. If the person fights against it and is overcome weeks afterwards, it is harder to find the necessary support. By that time, workmates expect one to be functioning efficiently again, relatives have dispersed and friends and neighbours are less likely to visit.

Physical Distress

Some of the immediate sensations were described earlier. In addition, there may be gastrointestinal upsets. The person may lose appetite and complain that everything tastes like sawdust. If the bereaved person is living alone, particularly on a reduced income, there can be malnutrition. There are complaints of muscular weakness. The bereaved person will complain of a lack of energy and feeling weighed down. The person who enjoyed garden work or carried heavy shopping finds it a struggle; 'Everything I lift seems so heavy.' Parkes (1964b) noted a trend for the newly bereaved to complain more of muscle and joint conditions.

In contrast to the lethargy is the restless agitation experienced by others. The person may seem to be keeping themselves busy, but little purposeful activity is completed. A wardrobe is half-emptied to pack clothes for charity, but clothes are left strewn around as the person remembers people who should be contacted. Half-written letters are left as the person reflects that the dead person would be upset by the state of the garden. Gardening tools are left as yet another task is seized upon, only to be abandoned in its turn. This exhausting treadmill parallels the difficulties of planning and executing purposeful behaviour as the cognitive processes are strained. Despite exhaustion, frequently there is insomnia for which the person may seek help from their general practitioner.

Guilt and Idealisation

As the dead person is idealised, the survivor feels he/she is responsible in some way for the death, was not worthy of the love or did not work hard enough for the dead partner's happiness. The mother of a stillborn child blames her diet or activities during pregnancy. A wife may blame herself for not encouraging her husband to stop smoking, exercise more or go to the doctor sooner. Previous events are scrutinised for some clue that could have made the death avoidable. The bereaved person reproaches him/herself for quarrelling when it would have been easy to agree, for not wanting to visit a particular place, take a foreign holiday or sometimes not wanting to make love.

Although these differences are part of any relationship, the counsellor should not reassure too readily. When a spouse says: 'I was not
the wife/husband I should have been', encourage further explanation. It
may be that the person is testing the listener out before confiding an
ongoing affair or previous marital indiscretion. If there has been too
ready an answer of 'No wife could have done more for him; you were
devoted', it leaves the person with little chance of dealing with such
problems.

An anticipated death does provide some opportunity of expiating
real or imagined wrongs. This is one reason for discussing the diagnosis
in terminal illness. It is helpful for the mother or spouse to be involved
with the care, particularly routine physical tasks. When the terminal
phase of the illness is prolonged, the person needs careful support so
that she is able to maintain her input without becoming exhausted
and resentful about this. It will help her subsequent readjustment if
she can keep some outside contacts or activities. Support can come
from the ward sister or community nurse who 'gives permission' for the
person to take time off.

Anger

When denial has lessened and the fact of the death becomes more real,
anyone or anything may be blamed in an effort to give meaning to the
death. The family doctor may be blamed for not diagnosing the illness
sooner; the hospital doctor may be blamed as the final care-taker whose
care has failed. Technology which is poorly understood may be held
responsible for the death. A man in terminal renal failure received
peritoneal dialysis. His immigrant relatives, who had poor command of
English, attributed his subsequent death to 'having his insides washed
out with cold water'. Poor communication in hospitals can be the cause
of added distress. A woman grieving at the anniversary of a miscarriage,
wept angrily when describing the nursing staff whom she had overheard 'discussing my abortion'. She had left the hospital shortly after
without speaking of this to anyone. It was some time afterwards,
during the course of crying for this child she had lost, that the misunderstanding of the jargon came to light and the pain that it had
caused.

Where there is no specific focus for the anger, it may be experienced as an unreasonable but persistent irritability towards neighbours,
colleagues and friends. This hostility can deprive the bereaved person
of those who would give support. When attempts to help are sharply
rebuffed, the offers stop. This may be forgotten in future months and

the survivors may complain that nobody visited them when their partner died, forgetting how uncomfortable they had made visitors.

Resentment is a common reaction to loss. A woman with a mastectomy can find herself walking down the street hating other two-breasted women. A woman who has had a stillbirth or cot death may experience bitter resentment towards pregnant women, 'I know something that will wipe the smile of her face.' The world seems full of contented couples or secure families and the bereaved person feels unfairly singled out.

The anger may be directed at the dead person and appear selfish. 'How could he leave me at a time like this, when the children are so helpless/so demanding/have left home and we should be enjoying our retirement?' Where the marriage has been disappointing, there is resentment for the wasted years.

Anger can be a positive force, which drives us to change an intolerable situation to one of greater satisfaction. When the anger produces no change, helplessness replaces it.

Depression and Anxiety

Depression is the aspect of grief which we can most readily accept. The loss of a person who fulfilled many roles — companion, protector and lover — whose life has become part of our own daily routines, leaves the bereaved person feeling naked and vulnerable. Panic may set in at the prospect of performing routine but unfamiliar tasks such as dealing with tax, buying children's clothes or remembering family birthdays.

Socialising for the first time as a single person can mean entering rooms of strangers alone, going to and leaving parties by oneself and being excluded from some invitations. If the widow does find the courage to attend a party where there is dancing, she may become self-consciously aware that some woman always sits out so that she has a partner. Invitations accepted freely once are rejected because 'I don't want anyone feeling sorry for me'.

Relationships with the opposite sex become fraught. Sexual manners have changed in the last twenty years and mutual misunderstandings can increase anxieties and withdrawal. Help offered and accepted in good faith may become the topic of neighbourhood or family gossip and lead to further bitterness.

Alternatively, fear at the prospect of being alone may cause a hasty remarriage. One woman, on her way to her mother's funeral, was informed by a neighbour: 'By the way, dear, I think you should know that your father's just proposed to me.' Another woman's father invited a stranger to live with him within weeks of the mother's death. She dreamed that she was kneeling, trying to wrap her mother's corpse in a winding sheet, but that the father and the new woman kept stepping back and forth over the body, preventing her from doing this. It seemed that concern about the new relationship was interfering with her grief work.

When counselling the bereaved person's anxiety, it is important to assess how independent the person was before being bereaved. The support appropriate for somebody who coped well previously but is temporarily helpless is different from that required for sombody who has never mastered basic living or social skills.

Resolution/Reinvestment

Finally, it is hoped that the energy invested in the dead person is released for other relationships and activities. The dead person is not forgotten, but the death is accepted and the intensity and frequency of the emotional reaction is diminished. How long does a 'normal' grief reaction last? Clayton argued that this had been overestimated, as early work had been based upon traumatic death and atypical populations (Clayton, Desmarais and Winokur, 1968). She suggested that by four months over 80 per cent of bereaved relatives had improved. Although the most intense pangs of grief may have diminished by then, most workers would suggest that it is a year before the major impact has passed. This would be in keeping with the research cited earlier (Parkes, 1964 and 1972; Rees and Lutkins, 1967). During that year, the person has many experiences to face for the first time alone, for example, the first birthday, the first Christmas, the first Mother's Day and planning for the holiday.

Some dependent individuals seem to find their identity through their partner after death as they had during life. This has been the norm in some cultures and may not be a problem. It can create difficulties in a social group of widows, where one feels ready to establish new relationships with the opposite sex, but is subjected to criticism, explicit or implicit, from other members of the group who feel threatened. A support group can act destructively by colluding in not facing reality, and the counsellors or group leaders involved need to be aware of this.

Ways in which Difficulties Relating to Bereavement may be Alleviated

Some of the practical questions for those working with the bereaved are:

1. Who is most likely to have problems?
2. What can be done to help?
3. Is bereavement counselling effective?

Who is Most Likely to have Problems?

Individuals will react in a characteristic way to a new stress. The person whose preferred way of coping with a problem was anxiety or anger with others will tend to use this mechanism when faced with the stress of bereavement also. There is general agreement in the literature that the person who continues to avoid emotional expression of grief is likely to experience chronic grief. Where the family inhibits emotional expression, or where the person avoids it through attempting to become immersed in work or other activity, then that person is more likely to experience a delayed grief reaction.

Certain psychological factors are reported regularly as indicating the vulnerable person (see Table 18.1).

Table 18.1: Risk factors for bereaved adults

Perceived lack of support
Pre-existing marital stress
Nature of death: for example, suicide, protracted terminal illness *or* very sudden death
Young age (below 45 years)
Additional stress around the time of bereavement: for example, moving house, illness
Earlier unresolved bereavement

Parkes suggested that the factors listed in Table 18.2 indicated that a person was at high risk for experiencing health problems subsequently. It is known that among the factors which differentiate those who kill themselves by suicide from those who make suicidal gestures are: living alone, having other physical illness and being male. More widowers than widows remarry, but it was noted earlier that as a group their mortality increases. The profile of a vulnerable person might be a retired man, housebound with bronchitis or arthritis, with no family nearby. At the other end of the scale of those most at risk is the widow

Table 18.2: Risk factors for bereaved adults subsequently to experience
health problems

Lack of supportive family
Clinging to the patient before death
Angry, self-reproachful behaviour
Young age
Low socio-economic status
'Intuitive' guess by nursing staff

---

in her late twenties or early thirties, with three or four young children,
who has no work outside the home and is of low social class.

What Can Be Done to Help?

Financial Support. In the United Kingdom, the current death grant is
£30 (September 1982), but the cost of a modest funeral is approximately £350-400. The widow's allowance is £41.40 for the first 26
weeks, followed by a widow's pension of £29.60, the latter figure
varying accordingly to the age of the widow and the number of
dependent children. Further details of statutory benefits in the United
Kingdom can be found in leaflet NI 51 from the Department of Health
and Social Security and 'What to do after a Death', from the Scottish
Home and Health Department. Costs of funerals vary enormously in
different countries, and in many little, if any, financial support is
available.

Some registered charities and trusts provide single cash grants or
support with children's schooling. Sources of possible help are listed in
the *Directory of Trusts*, which is available in the public library. The
professional body or trade union to which the person belonged may be
able to help. There are a number of organisations to help ex-service
personnel or their dependants.

A further source of help might be a local voluntary group such as the
Rotarians or the Round Table. The bereaved family may have no link
with such a group themselves, but the professionals involved with the
family, such as the general practitioner or child's teacher, may be able
to make approaches on their behalf. Large nationalised industries (such
as the Gas Board and Electricity Board in the UK) are usually willing
to accept deferred payment of bills in these circumstances. The local
branch of the Cruse Organisation, or similar bereavement support
organisation, should have a committee member who can advise upon
financial problems.

The house, savings or bank account is often in one name only. This custom is becoming less common, but it is an added strain to the new widow to find that she has no direct access to the family income. When this happens, most bank managers will be helpful and, if desired, a solicitor could make the necessary approaches on behalf of the widow.

When the death is anticipated, it is appropriate for somebody involved with the family either personally or professionally to raise this matter. It is a consolation for the dying person if these matters are openly discussed, so that he/she knows that the family will be taken care of in their coming absence.

Finally, a note of caution. If goods arrive COD cash-on-delivery, or workmen turn up claiming that they have been booked by the dead person to do decorating, renovation or so on, this should be refused. The query should be passed on to a relative or family friend who can ascertain if this is genuine. It is unfortunate that occasionally the bereaved are preyed upon in this way.

Physical Support. The family doctor is consulted more frequently (Parkes, 1964). In a busy surgery, minor symptoms may be overlooked. The family's own GP may be aware of the situation, but a locum or another partner may not. Physical symptoms which resemble the dead person's terminal illness are of major importance to the bereaved person, but their significance may be overlooked. The bereaved spouse may not present him/herself, but bring children to the surgery with more than the usual number of coughs or colds.

It would be helpful if the family's case notes could be tagged for the first twelve months after a death has occurred. For a family doctor in the United Kingdom with 2500 patients, there are likely to be approximately 40 deaths per year, so this would not place an undue burden on the practice administration. The Royal College of General Practitioners has long recommended tagging of notes for all patients thought to be at risk of suicide.

The role of medication in bereavement is controversial. Parkes noted an increase in sedative consumption in the first six months after bereavement. General practitioners may feel pressured into prescribing psychotropic drugs such as antidepressants. There is an expectation that 'help' comes as a prescription, and the bereaved may feel they have wasted the doctor's time until they have been seen to be 'ill' enough to justify tablets. Receiving medication can be seen as confirming one's distress and being identified as somebody who needs additional help at this time. The pressure for prescribing may come from neither the family doctor nor the bereaved person, but from the family. The doctor may be cornered in the hall on a home visit or in the surgery by a married daughter, who demands something for her mother who 'can't cope since Dad died and is crying all the time'. The additional but unspoken message is 'and that makes me want to cry'.

Physical health may deteriorate through self-neglect. Loss of appetite, lack of interest in cooking, forgetfulness and possible shortage of money might cause dietary deficiencies. It can be a help if another relative or neighbour could visit and bring a pre-cooked meal. If this is unacceptable, perhaps visits could coincide with mealtimes when the visitor just happens to have groceries with them. Eating meals alone is a reminder of the lost company. The loss of appetite and physical symptoms described earlier may deter the person from a full meal, but a light snack might meet with less resistance.

Community nursing staff may be able to monitor the well-being of the family. A home visit may reveal a concealed difficulty, for example, the smell of alcohol at unlikely times during the day. It has been observed that the use of tobacco and alcohol rises after bereavement (Parkes, 1972).

It may be difficult for health service staff to offer support when they or colleagues are held responsible, either explicitly or implicitly, for the death. In this situation, the person should seek support from a colleague, but maintain contact with the bereaved so that they can continue to ventilate their distress.

Social Support. Gorer (1965) has described the change in mourning rituals in our own society during the last few decades. It is important that the loss should be acknowledged in the social network, even if there is not formal mourning. Neighbours or colleagues who write or visit confirm that the dead person was worth grieving for and that the distress is appreciated. This may have little apparent impact at the time, but the number of letters received can be a source of consolation to the person who re-reads them subsequently. It was commented earlier that the social acknowledgement encourages the bereaved person to grieve. If friends can take over some of the practical tasks, this permits the bereaved person to spend time talking about what has happened with others. Some cultures encourage the members of the community to sit with the bereaved and discuss the dead person; the Irish 'wake' and the Jewish period of 'Shiva' can be used for this.

A number of organisations can offer impartial advice and information, for example, in the United Kingdom Cruse, CAB and Gingerbread. There are many organisations which might be of use. At first, the person may want no personal contact, but would accept a more distant link such as the Cruse newsletter. Some community groups may offer help with household tasks such as decorating or gardening. Others can offer company through trips to local theatres, cinemas or hold coffee mornings or lunch clubs. Some bereaved persons feel able to socialise initially only with somebody who has shared the same experience. Others feel stigmatised by this and would prefer a wider social grouping. The bereaved person may need to be encouraged to experiment with a few, probably in the company of a friend, before finding a compatible group.

It should be remembered that not everybody is a joiner of clubs, bereaved or non-bereaved. It may be that in pushing the bereaved into a group, we are doing more to assuage our own feelings than theirs.

Religious Support. This is dealt with fully in Chapter 19, so will not be discussed here. The growth of secular organisations such as Cruse and the National Society of Compassionate Friends may be answering the needs of those who do not have a religious group. Also, some apparently devout people do not find consolation in their religion. They seem to have used it as an insurance policy which, if practised regularly, will prevent any distressing event befalling them. They feel cheated when this does not happen.

Counselling Support.
Befriending: Many people do work through their grief with families and friends. The disintegration of close communities and the scattering of families, which is a relatively new development, takes away the traditional supports. In the nuclear family we ask a very small number of people to fulfil our emotional needs in a way that perhaps 20 people would have done only two generations or so ago. When the demand is that they should support us through an event that has been devastating for them too, they may fail. An outsider who is able to listen without becoming distressed may be needed. Non-directive counselling, based on Carl Rogers' work (1951) is one method of counselling. The aim of this approach would be to facilitate emotional expression by reflection without analysing or interrogating.

Alternatively, the counsellor may be more directive and invite the person to explore other aspects of their grief by suggestion; for example, where the bereaved person has spoken at length and in glowing terms only about her dead partner, 'You've told me what a good father Mac was when the boys were young. What about when they became teen-agers?' 'You've told me how hard Jimmy worked for the family. How were things when he was tired?' The widow who describes her husband as a cheerful optimist, who never thought about the future, may be beginning to feel that if he had, she would not a facing so many diffi-culties.

The phrase 'Never speak ill of the dead' suggests both a courtesy and a fear of being overheard by them. In some cultures, it is customary to fire arrows in the air to chase away vengeful spirits. In our culture a final volley of shots is fired over a military grave. One group of Maoris do this formally. The community gathers for a farewell over the grave and praises the dead person. This is followed by a period of abusing the deceased. It is important to review both the positive *and* the negative aspects of a relationship.

Professional Support: Professional support is available from a number of sources, but the help available tends to depend upon the skill/ interest of the particular individual, rather than their membership of a specific discipline. The family doctor may choose to provide this sup-port himself or may refer the person to a nurse, clinical psychologist, psychiatrist or social worker.

Studies on the treatment of pathological grief reactions have been published in recent years (Volkan, 1970; Raphael, 1975; Ramsay, 1977; Hodgkinson, 1980). One recent approach suggests that morbid grief should be viewed as a phobia in which the bereaved person avoids dealing with the distress. Treatment consists of confronting the person with photographs, objects, associations and memories, and repeating this exposure until the anxiety and avoidance associated with the situa-tion are no longer present. It can be a gruelling experience for both therapist and patient. A study by Mawson *et al.* (1981) reported that patients receiving this type of guided mourning showed more improve-ment on a number of measures than a controlled group who were asked to, and advised on how to, avoid their distress.

When assessment reveals that the person had limited abilities, such as deficient social skills, before the death, help may be required in learning them. Role-playing and the setting of weekly goals may be helpful. Behavioural techniques can be used with other therapies to help the person adapt to the new situation.

Is It Effective? Raphael reported a significant difference between supported and unsupported groups. The Mawson study, cited above, indicates a positive outcome following structured therapy. Parkes (1980) suggested that the risk for the high-risk group was reduced to about that of the low-risk group following counselling by a volunteer service. He concluded that 'professional services and professionally supported voluntary and self-help services are capable of reducing the risk of psychiatric and psychosomatic disorders resulting from bereavement.'

Summary

1. For many people, bereavement is both a physical and psychological stress that has demonstrable effects for at least a year afterwards.
2. Practical help is available from both professional and voluntary agencies. There are a number of very useful leaflets which could be given routinely to a bereaved household. The bereaved spouse may not read them at the time, but they can be helpful to other members of the family or consulted at a later date.
3. Articles describing the processes of grief and bereavement are more common. Controlled research is recent, but scanty. Priorities for research should clarify which individuals require what kind of help, when this can best be given and for how long.
4. Staff working with bereaved people need support. Often it is assumed that health professionals are exposed to death so often that they can deal with it easily. Many professionals have little formal teaching in dealing with distressed relatives and even less teaching in dealing with their own distress.
5. Discussion of sex was considered taboo, but now we accept sex education in schools. Death and dying could be part of the curriculum also. Children are aware of death from an early age. It would be useful to provide an opportunity to discuss it openly with them, rather than ignore it. Books and films are available as teaching aids.
6. Death is one of the traumas we face through being human. As with other difficulties, one may learn from it and gain self-awareness and strength, or one may reject it, becoming embittered and fail to grow. Support can be offered through the pain, but the individual needs to accept the challenge.

Useful Contacts and Reading for Bereaved People

United Kingdom

Cruse. The National Organisation for the Widowed and their Children, 126 Sheen Road, Richmond, Surrey. Cruse offers counselling, practical advice, social activities, a monthly newsletter and other literature.

The Stillbirth and Perinatal Death Association: 15a Christchurch Hill, London NW3
1JY. Scottish Contact: c/o Scottish Health Education Group, Woodburn
House, Canaan Lane, Edinburgh. The association is a source of counselling and
literature, such as the booklet *The Loss of Your Baby.*

The Foundation for the Study of Infant Deaths: 5th floor, 4/5 Grosvenor Place,
London SW14 7HD. This organisation has some excellent leaflets for bereaved
parents and the professionals caring for them, including *Information for
Parents following the Sudden and Unexpected Death of their Baby*; *Your Next
Child*; *Checklist for GPs.*

Society for Compassionate Friends: National Secretary, 25 Kingsdown Parade,
Bristol BS6 5UE.

United Kingdom Publications

1. *What to do after a Death . . . Practical Advice for Times of Bereavement.* This
   booklet covers the practical details of the funeral, legal aspects and finances.
   It is available from the Citizens' Advice Bureau.
2. *What to do when someone dies,* Consumers' Association.
3. *Widows Guidance about NI Contributions and Benefits,* NI 51 from the
   Department of Health and Social Security and the Scottish Home and Health
   Department.
4. Judith Viorst (1981) *The Tenth Good Thing about Barney,* Collins, London.
   This is a study of a boy who has a cat that dies. It is suitable for 3 to 6-year-
   olds.
5. Jean Richardson (1979) *A Death in the Family,* Lion Publishing, London. A
   short book offering practical advice and support from a Christian viewpoint.
6. Sarah Morris (1971) *Grief and how to live with it,* Published by Allen and
   Unwin, London.

American Contacts

1. Theo Inc., 11609 Frankstown Road, Pittsburgh, Pennsylvania 15235.
2. The Nairn Conference, 109 North Dearborn Street, Chicago, Illinois 60602.
3. Post Cana, Family Life Movement, 1721 Rhode Island Avenue, NW, Washington DC 20006.
4. Parents without Partners, 80 Fifth Avenue, New York City, New York.

References

Bowlby, J. (1951) *Maternal Care and Mental Health*, WHO monograph 2, Geneva, p. 9

Bowlby, J. (1961a) 'Processes of mourning', *International Journal of Psycho-
analysis,* 44, 317

Clayton, P., Desmarais, L. and Winokur, G. (1968) 'A study of normal bereavement', *American Journal of Psychiatry,* 125, 168

Cooper, J.D. (1980) 'Parental reactions to stillbirth', *British Journal of Social
Work,* 10, 55–69

Gorer, G. (1965) *Death, Grief and Mourning,* Cresset Press, London

Hodgkinson, P. (1980) 'Treating abnormal grief in the bereaved', *Nursing Times,*
17 January, pp. 126–8

Lindemann, E. (1944) 'Symptomatology and management of acute grief',
American Journal of Psychiatry, 101, 141–8

Maddison, D.C. and Viola, A. (1968) 'The health of widows in the year following
bereavement', *Journal of Psychosomatic Research,* 12, 297

Maddison, D.C. and Walker, W.L. (1967) 'Factors affecting the outcome of
conjugal bereavement', *British Journal of Psychiatry,* 113, 1057, 37

Mawson, D., Marks, I., Ramm, L. and Stern, R.A. (1981) 'Guided mourning for morbid grief: a controlled study', *British Journal of Psychiatry*, 138, 185–93

Parkes, C.M. (1964) 'The effects of bereavement on physical and mental health: a study of case records of widows', *British Medical Journal*, 2, 274

Parkes, C.M. (1972) *Bereavement Studies of Grief in Adult Life*, Tavistock Publications, London

Parkes, C.M. (1980) 'Bereavement counselling: does it work?', *British Medical Journal*, 5 July, p. 3–7

Parkes, C.M., Benjamin, B. and Fitzgerald, R.G. (1969) 'Broken heart: a statistical study of increased mortality among widowers', *British Medical Journal*, 7, 741

Pincus, I. (1976) *Death in the Family*, Faber and Faber, London

Ramsay, R.W. (1977) 'Behavioural approaches to bereavement', *Behaviour Research and Therapy*, 15, 131–7

Raphael, B. (1975) 'Counselling and loss: counselling following a disaster', *Mental Health Australia*, 1, 118

Raphael, B. and Maddison, D.C. (1976) 'The care of bereaved adults', in Oscar W. Hill (ed.), *Modern Trends in Psychosomatic Medicine*, Vol. 3, Butterworths, London

Rees, W.D. and Lutkins, S.G. (1967) 'Mortality of bereavement', *British Medical Journal*, 4, 13

Rogers, C.R. (1951) *Client-centred Therapy*, Houghton Mifflin, New York

Rutter, M. (1966) *Children of Sick Parents: An Environmental and Psychiatric Study*, Oxford University Press, Oxford

Volkan, B. (1970) 'Typical findings in pathological grief', *Psychiatry Quarterly*, 44, 231

Young, M., Benjamin, B. and Wallis, C. (1963) 'Mortality of widowers', *Lancet*, ii, 454

Further Reading

Antony, S. (1940) *The Child's Discovery of Death*, Routledge and Kegan Paul, London

Bourne, S. (1968) 'The psychological effects of stillbirth on women and their doctors', *Journal of the Royal College of General Practitioners*, 16, 103–12

Burton, L. (1974) *Care of the Child Facing Death*, Routledge and Kegan Paul, London

Foster, S. (1981) 'Explaining death to children', *British Medical Journal*, 14 February, 540–2

Glick, I., Weiss, R. and Parkes, C.M. (1974) *The First Year of Bereavement*, Wiley, New York

Harari, E. (1981) 'Pathological grief in doctors' wives', *British Medical Journal*, 3 January, 33–4

Keddie, K.M.G. (1977) 'Pathological mourning after the death of a domestic pet', *British Journal of Psychiatry*, 131, 21–5

Kennel, J.H., Slyter, H. and Klaus, M.H. (1970) 'The mourning response of parents to the death of a newborn infant', *New England Journal of Medicine*, 283, 344

Lewis, E. (1976) 'The management of stillbirth: coping with an unreality', *Lancet*, ii, 619–20

Lewis, E. and Page, A. (1976) 'Family reactions to child bereavement', *Proceedings of the Royal Society of Medicine*, 69, 835–8

Maddison, D.C. (1968) 'The relevance of conjugal bereavement for preventive psychiatry', *British Journal of Medical Psychology*, 42, 223

Martin, I. (1980) 'Many unhappy returns', *Nursing Times*, 24 July, pp. 1319–20

Strachan, J. (1981) 'Mentally handicapped adults and bereavement', *Appendix to Journal of the British Institute of Mental Handicap*, 9, (1), 20–1

Yorkstone, P. (1981) 'Dealing with the disadvantaged', *British Medical Journal*, 11 April, 282, 1224–5

PASTORAL CARE

Derek Murray and David Lyall

Some Clinical Vignettes

Mr A. was a recently retired married man with a bronchial carcinoma who was admitted to a hospice in a terminal condition. His wife and family were active in the local church, but he 'had always been too busy for that'. Now, however, he began to express anger with God for allowing vandals to be healthy, while he − a good, respectable tenant − was dying. In further conversation, he admitted to feeling deeply guilty about his neglect of religious observance and his refusal to accompany his wife to church.

Mrs B. was a married woman in her fifties. Although not a member of any church, she had her own very particular and individualistic religious views derived from a variety of sources. These she had inculcated into her family, though her husband was quite outside this part of her life. Now that he had been admitted to a hospice with terminal cancer, she was very afraid of the God with whom she had threatened her children. She seemed to have no conception of forgiveness and divine love. God seemed to her to be a capricious tyrant, but she showed few signs of guilt.

Miss C. was a 65-year-old spinster with strong evangelical convictions. On admission to a hospice with terminal cancer, she professed inability to believe that she could be dying, as her friends and her pastor were praying for her. She would not discuss spiritual problems except with her own minister, although she preached at the staff. She exhibited strong symptoms of denial and fear, and her strict propositional faith seemed to give her little comfort. Her 'hope of heaven' only made her miserable.

Mrs D. was a 60-year-old married woman admitted to a radiotherapy unit to have her radiotherapy treatment for carcinoma of the uterus. During her first and subsequent admissions to the hospital to receive palliative treatment for metastatic growths, a strong pastoral relationship developed with the hospital chaplain. During one visit she spoke with great hesitation of her belief that the cancer has been 'caused' by her marital infidelity 35 years previously, while her husband had been at sea during the war. 'I think God must be punishing me for my wickedness,' she said.

Mr E. was a 40-year-old married man with a young family, admitted to a neurological ward with a degenerative disease of the nervous system. When visiting the ward, the chaplain introduced himself to the patient, who could hear but had lost the power of speech. The patient communicated by laboriously pointing to the letters of the alphabet on a card specially printed for the purpose. Very early in this 'conversation' Mr E. pointed to the letters 'w-h-y-d-o-e-s-g-o-d-a-l-l-o-w . . .' and burst into tears.

Staff Nurse F., a 45-year-old widow, had returned to nursing when her two teenage children had become less dependent on her. She was an experienced, competent nurse who was particularly good at supporting the student nurses when there was a crisis in the ward. One day when she was in charge of the ward, there were three deaths. After seeing off the last group of relatives, the chaplain returned to the ward to find Nurse F. in the duty room looking unusually distressed. She began to tell her story. The previous night she had found out that her father had been diagnosed as having a malignant growth . . .

Introduction

These brief case studies illustrate the truth that in seeking to alleviate the sufferings of the seriously ill, the task is far more complex than the relief of physical symptoms. The subject of every set of case notes is a human being, with his own distinctive network of relationships and his own modes of thinking and feeling. His outlook on life is peculiarly his, with deep roots in his past, though possibly distorted by present physical pain and emotional turmoil. Some of his thinking may be irrational, but have its own inner logic. He may or may not think of himself as a religious person, though he will have his own creed, and this is important to him as he tries to find some meaning in the strange and sometimes frightening events at the centre of which he finds himself. If he is a religious person, he may find that previously-held beliefs raise questions rather than provide answers. Even if he is not an active member of a church, there may be many non-medical questions that he wishes to explore.

The purpose of this chapter is twofold: (a) to help doctors, nurses, and other paramedical staff gain some understanding of the spiritual issues which may arise in the care of patients who are seriously ill and who are unlikely to get better; and (b) to communicate some under-standing of the help that can be offered by chaplains and visiting clergy.

Not infrequently, it is medical and nursing staff who first encounter problems which may broadly be defined as spiritual. This is so for a variety of reasons. For one thing, it is they who are most intimately involved with the patient. It is the doctor on his rounds who is deemed to have the answers to the most urgent questions. 'Can you give me something to alleviate my pain/sickness/diarrhoea?' 'I am going to get better, aren't I doctor?' The simple (or not so simple) medical questions sometimes lead to deeper ones. 'What could possibly have caused this illness?' 'Why should this happen to me?' And it is the nurse who, help-ing the sick person in the most intimate of bodily functions, or bringing the cup of tea during the long hours of a sleepless night, is there when the deepest questions are most near the surface of consciousness.

Nevertheless, the visit of a minister or priest – be it the hospital chaplain or the patient's own clergyman – can also have the effect of provoking the patient into exploring some of the more profound issues integral to a serious illness. Ministers are regular visitors to hospital wards and to sick people in their own homes. A minister will almost certainly visit a sick member of his congregation, if aware of the situa-tion. Further, every hospice or NHS hospital has its own officially appointed chaplains of the main Christian or Jewish traditions, who may be either full-time (as in the case of the large teaching hospitals) or part-time. Ministers and chaplains will expect to be actively involved in the support of seriously ill patients and their families. This is part of their traditional ministry of pastoral case. This chapter will attempt to set out what this ministry may involve, not only in order that hospital staff may have some understanding of what the minister is trying to achieve and so make more appropriate use of him, but also so that these same staff may respond more effectively to the pastoral crises in which they themselves will inevitably find themselves involved. One must, however, dispose of one or two misconceptions concerning the nature of pastoral care.

What Pastoral Care is Not

Pastoral Care is not Evangelism

Some medical staff may hesitate to involve a minister in the care of a seriously ill patient, because of a previous negative experience where a patient was 'upset' by an over-enthusiastic minister, whose main aim seemed to be to preach at the patient and achieve some kind of death-bed conversion. Undoubtedly such instances do exist, but they do not constitute good pastoral care. The good pastor starts from where the patient is, allows him to talk or be silent and does not attempt to impose his own theological views upon the patient. As one contemporary writer puts it: 'The task of the pastor is not to give the patient religious words – it is that of helping him get behind his words to their truth' (Wise, 1980). This does not mean that the pastor comes to the patient unaware of his own attitudes – rather the opposite, for the pastor certainly must be in touch with his own faith (and doubt!). But it does mean that the pastor must realise that his own religious formulations may not be appropriate for that particular patient at that particular time, that he must walk with and support the patient as he explores his own way forward.

There is nevertheless a paradox here, for it may well turn out that there is nothing so profoundly evangelical as sensitive pastoral care, that the acceptance and understanding offered in the pastoral relationship may come to symbolise for the patient that deeper acceptance and understanding which Christians call the love of God.

Pastoral Care is not Social Work

To disclaim an identification of pastoral care with evangelism is to highlight another misunderstanding which frequently exists concerning the nature of pastoral care; namely, that the minister has nothing to offer which a social worker cannot give more competently. To deny this is not to denigrate for one moment the professional skills of the social worker, which are described in Chapter 20. There are admittedly occasions when, from the outside, there appears to be little difference between the kind of supportive relationships offered by the two professions. Indeed, whether it be the minister or the social worker who is primarily involved with a given patient or his family may depend upon the accidents of availability or personality. Nevertheless, although there may be a 'grey area' in the interdisciplinary boundaries, the tasks and methods of social work and pastoral work are different. It is too facile to say that whereas the social worker is mainly concerned with 'practical matters', the minister must deal with 'spiritual issues', for both are involved in the support of the person. It is the task of the remainder of this chapter to set out the most important features of the pastoral care of the seriously ill.

Pastoral Care: A Working Definition

What, then is pastoral care? *At its most basic, pastoral care is an active and purposeful concern for people within the context of ultimate meaning and value.* Others might wish to be much more specific in their definition. It is hoped, however, that this rather general definition might be broad enough to encompass the varieties of both individual religious experience and of denominational practice. Nevertheless some quite definite consequences follow from such an approach.

First, the fact that this definition contains no mention of clergy implies that pastoral care is part of the task of all who have professional concern for the person being cared for. The doctor, the nurse, the social worker must be concerned with the whole person, not simply with drugs or dressings or sickness benefit as the case may be.

Second, to speak of 'people' rather than 'patients' is to be conscious that pastoral care is more than a one-to-one relationship in which a professional does something to or for a patient. Both the patient and the professional are parts of interlocking systems. The patient is a member of a family and of a community, the professional is a member of a team and often of the same community as the patient. Frequently these systems overlap and impinge upon one another.

Third, to speak of an active and purposeful concern is to imply that in the exercise of pastoral care one must assess a situation and, on the basis of experience and/or knowledge, decide whether or not to intervene in it. If a decision is taken to intervene, one must decide in what manner, realising all the time that one's judgement may be wrong and need revision in the light of fresh information or changing circumstances.

Finally, to declare that the context of pastoral care is that of ultimate meaning and values is to begin to define its boundaries and subject matter. Clebzch and Jackle (1967), historians of the development of pastoral care, express this point thus: 'Pastoral care calls forth questions and issues of deepest meaning and highest concern for it is exercised at a depth where the meaning of life is involved on the part of the helper as well as on the part of the helped.'

It is not, of course, implied that all who either seek or receive pastoral care are active church members, for though there may be a decline in institutional religion, there are few among the seriously ill or among those involved with them who are unaware of 'issues of deepest meaning and highest concern', although these issues may not be expressed in religious language. This means that pastoral care must be exercised with the greatest sensitivity to the beliefs and value systems of the person being cared for. What is critical and central to pastoral care is its freedom to respond in a manner which is appropriate to the expressed or perceived needs of the other person. This freedom may involve a simple sharing of the Christian message, or it may involve a sensitive reticence. For some, care will be expressed in very traditional Christian ways, involving a conversation about the deepest things of the Faith and ending with Scripture reading and prayer. For others, for example, Roman Catholic or Anglican patients, the receiving of Holy Communion will be of the highest pastoral significance. And there are many people who are helped by unobtrusive befriending over a period of time.

What is important is that pastoral care should be a free response to the needs of the cared for, and not the consequence of some inner compulsion and need on the part of the carer.

Some Spiritual Questions

Illness and the loss of one's normal health and ability to cope with life inevitably cause anxieties. The prospect of going to hospital for an operation, of being off work for a time, or of being diminished in some way changes one's perspective on life, at least for a time. The knowledge that a limit has been set to one's lifespan, when that knowledge has been truly absorbed, makes a person more than ordinarily anxious, and raises a number of particular questions. The form that the questions and anxieties take is widely varied and only a few of them can be dealt with here, to illustrate the theme.

The contemporary theologian Paul Tillich distinguishes three types of anxiety of the human spirit, and these give us a useful framework for our comments. The first of the three main types which he describes is the anxiety of fate and death, the absolute threat to man's very being. The second is the anxiety of emptiness and meaninglessness, questioning the worth and value of life; the third is the anxiety of guilt and condemnation, when man both wants to know the reason for his suffering, and tries to take the blame for it himself.

The first type of suffering is present in some form in almost every patient, although often not overtly. It is probably true that the majority of patients fear the dying process more than they fear death, and they can be to some extent reassured by a sensitive explanation of of what they may expect to undergo, by symptom control, by a warm and accepting environment, and by consequent growing confidence in the medical and nursing staff. But those who cannot face the reality of death, who have no hope of another life, and who are vexed or angry at having to let go, face other challenges. Such patients may be reluctant to believe that they are dying, and some will practise denial with great skill. Others may succumb to terror. The objective of good pastoral care will be to help the patient to come to an affirmation of the worth of his own life. It may be that at this point the faith of the carer will be most put to the test.

The second type, the anxiety of meaninglessness, presents itself in a variety of ways. 'Why has this happened to me, of all people?' 'How can God, if He loves me, let this happen to me?' The despair at the heart of these questions must not be underestimated. When life is suddenly or slowly to be cut short, it is not surprising that the patient should be bewildered, ready to put the blame on God, and to call into question the more comfortable aspects of his religion which have sufficed him up to this time. The problem of apparently unnecessary and unproductive suffering is not to be solved by a few easy words at the bedside, but will be eased by acknowledging the patient's anxieties, and by 'sitting where he sits'. From time to time, a patient will be met who appreciates the concept of God's identification with human suffering through Christ, and some patients will find meaning in their own suffering by meditating on this. Most, however, must be helped to climb out of the 'slough of despond', less by the offering of theological concepts than by the carer's evident concern and sharing of their own mystification.

Another form of this second anxiety is a nagging doubt concerning life after death. The Christian patient, taught to believe in the resurrection and accepting this as part of his faith, finds when faced with the prospect of his own death that this part of his faith is less easy to hold. Human parting, the sense of loss in leaving behind a younger member of the family, the break-up of close relationships prompt speculations about reunion in another life. The carer can try to build on the expressed beliefs of the patient, urging him to explore them, and to hold on to what has been a comforting faith. It is important to be gentle in correcting views which may seem to us to be ill-founded, for clumsiness in asserting our ideas could knock away yet another of the props that make life bearable.

The anxiety of guilt and condemnation is widespread and also takes many forms. It may be asked: 'How could God love a failure like me?' or 'Is it not too late to return to God, or be reconciled with the Church?' or the patient might well catalogue all the things that make him regretful and ashamed, and conclude that he is outside God's mercy. This guilt may be projected on another — a member of the family, or the doctor, or the minister, or God. Personal inadequacy to face death is seen to arise from upbringing, or an early experience, or the general unfairness of things. That guilt is endemic to humanity, and that self-condemnation is a saddening and often unnecessarily depressing emotion are commonplaces that the carer can use to reassure the patient that he is not abnormal if he feels such guilt. It is much harder to relieve guilt, even with those who believe in the saving work of Christ. It is necessary to lay emphasis on the unconditional love of God, who welcomes His children home, and who finds His people even in their guilt. This is not direct evangelism, but comfort and reassurance. All those who contemplate their death with any self-awareness ask questions. Those which are practical may have a positive and clear answer, but those which are connected with the great themes of philosophy and theology, those which concern meaning and worth, do not have easy solutions, and part of the work of the carer is to ask himself over and over again just these questions, and to walk with the dying in their search for light.

The Pastoral Response

Ministers in wards seem difficult to place. They do not come with medicines or injections, they do not produce forms to be filled, they can be ignored and they go away, they appear to have an endless capacity for small talk, and only occasionally do they do 'religious' things such as conducting services or praying at the bedside. Sometimes they are not immediately identifiable as clergy, some are women, and not all wear the clerical collar. Members of religious orders appear and add to the confusing picture. Yet patients are remarkably tolerant and accepting, and soon 'place' the chaplain or visiting minister, drawing on their previous experience of clergy and the church. What does the minister have to offer? First, he can bring pastoral conversation. Occasionally, he may be able to start immediately speaking about God, but usually he has to get to know the patient as a person, to ask about family and home and career, and to build up a picture of the individual, so that a right approach to a pastoral relationships can be discovered. Quite trivial conversation may lead to an exploration of the deepest issues, when confidence has been established, and quite profound insights can be given and gained through growing friendship. Not only the minister, but all concerned in care must at least try to have time for confidence-building conversation.

At the right time the word of faith may be spoken. Of course, not only clergy may read the Bible and pray with patients, but they, so obviously representing the Church, will have the most opportunity to do so. The reading of familiar scripture, such as the 23rd Psalm, John 14, Romans 8 or 1, Corinthians 13, can mean a great deal, even to the very ill patient who has previously shown an understanding of and a need for such directly spiritual help. Prayers, read or extempore, according to circumstances and tradition, bring great strength, especially to the patient who finds himself, to his alarm, no longer able to pray himself. For privacy, and to avoid embarrassment in what for many is a most private transaction, screens or curtains can usually be drawn, but it must be remembered that screens and curtains are not walls.

Physical contact is important in prayer and pastoral conversation. It is very comforting to the patient to be touched on the brow or for the hand to be held in friendship, acceptance and solidarity. The 'laying on of hands' is not just an ancient eastern rite. It is a recognition of a universal human need to be close to others. Above all, the carer must never appear to withdraw, in dignity or in revulsion.

Sacramental ministry, which consists in different traditions of confession, absolution, anointing and communion, is in essence a specialised form of pastoral conversation, linked with specific meaningful Christian rites. Most Christians, accustomed to the sacramental ministry of their churches and, in illness, feeling isolated from their fellow believers, greatly value sacramental acts; the familiar form and words of the ritual enable those who are very ill, or somewhat confused and forgetful, to share in the worship of the church and to recall familiar responses and feelings of comfort and strength.

A separate chapel, set aside for worship and quiet, is a most important part of any institution caring for the very ill. Although it may not be possible for more than a minority of patients to make use of it, its existence is a symbol of Christian presence in the building. Regular services, even if sparsely attended, are an opportunity for some to continue a lifetime's practice, and for others to make a return to religious observance in a less embarrassing way than would be possible elsewhere. The programme for worship will be adaptable, and the chapel will be open to all, but it has been wisely stated that such chapels are areas of ecumenical co-operation, not ecumenical experiment.

Telling the Truth

Not infrequently, it is within the context of a relationship of trust that the patient will begin to explore the nature of his illness. He may want to know what the various tests have revealed and what the probable outcome of his illness will be, although these issues may be raised obliquely rather than in a direct manner. Fortunately the days are rapidly passing when attempts are made to fob off an inquisitive patient with 'fairy tales'. Having said that, the trend towards more open communication with patients raises incredibly complex questions. How much should the patient be told at a particular time? Who should do the telling? There are no easy answers in this area, and the following suggestions are made tentatively with an awareness that the realities of a given situation will frequently inhibit their application.

The patient should not be told lies. There is only one version of the truth, whereas untruth may take many forms and a patient will soon detect when different members of staff are telling him different tales. Whatever confidence has been built up will soon be destroyed. This does not mean that the patient must be told the whole truth all at once. Indeed, to ask: 'What should the patient be told?' is frequently to pose the wrong question. Far more relevant is the question: 'What does the patient really want or need to know?' Although the conspiracy-of-silence approach is tending to disappear, there is the opposite danger that the patient may be burdened with more information than he can handle at a given moment in time. A gentle exploration of what the patient understands about his illness will frequently facilitate a sensitive communication of that degree of knowledge which the patient wants and can cope with.

Ideally, important information should be communicated by a doctor who already has a good relationship with the patient. There are no such things as 'simple facts'; once a patient has begun to assimilate the reality of a poor prognosis, there are always questions which he will wish to ask and can only properly be answered by a doctor. 'How long do I have?' 'Will I suffer pain?' The fear of the process of dying is nearly always greater than the fear of death itself, and it is normally a medically qualified person who will be in the best position to give whatever reassurance is possible. When the question of time-scale is raised, it is better not to be too specific (who does know anyway?). It is not unknown for patients who have been given a rough estimate of how long they have to live to receive this as a definite 'sentence', with disastrous results. Neither is it unknown for patients to be fit and well long after their 'sentence' has expired!

Having said that ideally it is the doctor who should communicate a bad prognosis, if this has to be done, it is often others, especially nursing staff, who are faced with the awkward questions. Hopefully there will be enough mutual trust within the ward team to allow nurses, particularly trained staff, to be honest with patients without necessarily telling the whole truth.

All members of the caring team should be aware of what the patient has been told, and ideally the patient should be aware that the others know. This will greatly enhance the support for the patient. Not that all members of the team will seek an opportunity to discuss the patient's prognosis with him, for each patient will select his own confidants with whom to discuss his innermost thoughts. What is important is that the rest of the team should be sensitive to the emotional and spiritual needs of the one who is most deeply involved with the patient (be that the consultant or the tea lady).

As far as specifically pastoral care is concerned, the starting-point must be the patient's understanding of his illness. The pastor (and everyone else) must not fall into the trap of assuming that the patient has 'taken in' all he has been told. Sometimes there is a wide gap between what is said and what is heard. The minister or priest must not give the impression of knowing much more than the patient, for to exercise a ministry of pastoral care is to stay with the patient where he is, and to be led by him into those highways and byways of the spiritual pilgrimage which the patient himself wishes to explore.

The Pastoral Care System

Although there is a one-to-one relationship at the heart of good pastoral caring, it is obvious that there are many people involved in the care of one patient, and that the carers and the patient are part of their own networks of support and help. Relatives will normally be visiting the patient, and their distress can be as real as, and more open than, that of the patient himself. They may be in a position to help or to question the carers. The medical, nursing and ancillary staff are all at different times and in different ways affected by the presence of the very sick patient, and will relate to him in various ways. Often the patient will belong to some club or association and, in particular, a fairly high proportion will have a church connection, so that the system of support includes the minister, and the people of the church.

Usually, the chaplain, with the agreement of the patient, will tell the patient's minister of the situation, and try to make the minister's visiting as well-informed as possible. Many clergy find it helpful to talk to one of their own number who is outside normal parish responsibility, who can give advice on his approach to the patient, and who can introduce him to ward staff. In the case of the seriously ill, ministers may feel both more involved and less adequate, and they will need the active co-operation of other staff.

Patients choose their confidants carefully, and may very well ask the deepest questions when the minister is absent. Professional boundaries may easily be crossed in pastoral caring, and the ordained clergy have no monopoly of skill in this field. What they do have is, in many cases, a wider knowledge of the patient as he was before he was ill, and of his family connections and background, so that a more comprehensive understanding of the likely reactions and anticipations of the patient can be given to other carers. It is important to see the seriously ill patient in the context of his family and his interests, his personal history and his faith. By this he is 'placed' as a human being.

All those who care for the seriously ill are potentially in a vulnerable state. However strong one's faith, or disbelief, there are poignant questions of human worth, of loss and justice and values being raised, and the strain of such exposure to questioning can be considerable. There has been some interesting research carried out recently on the phenomenon of 'burn-out', which has been shown to affect carers at all levels and is now being better understood. The chaplain must try to support other staff, for no one can undertake such stressful work in isolation, and he must be aware of his own liability to strain and need for support. The care of the carers is a serious problem. Support system's, formal or informal, must exist in the hospital, and will include the chaplains.

The argument so far has tried to hold together two concepts which may at first sight appear contradictory. On the one hand, it has been argued that pastoral care is not the task of the minister and priest alone, but of all who have a responsibility for the welfare of the patient. On the other hand, there has been a recognition that the relationship between the patient and his minister or priest has a peculiar significance in the pastoral care of the patient. This apparent contradiction may be resolved somewhat when it is realised, as indicated above, that pastoral care of the patient is seldom carried out in isolation from the network of caring relationships, at the centre of which is the patient. This is particularly the case with officially appointed chaplains. Whereas the relationship of a visiting minister with the staff will be limited by the time of a patient's stay, the relationship between the chaplain and the other members of staff is ongoing, possibly over a period of years, with a common concern with the care of many patients. This shared concern should provide the context for the development of close working relationships based on growing mutual confidence and support between chaplains and other members of staff.

Officially appointed chaplains will on occasion, as time permits, be participants in ward and team meetings, and will be involved in the continuing discussion regarding patient care. They will observe the same protocols of professional confidentiality as the other members of the team, being party to such information about patients and their families as is necessary to provide good patient care, and sharing with the team whatever can be shared without transgressing the boundaries of pastoral confidentiality. There has been discussion in the past as to whether chaplains should have access to case notes and other, similar material. Although theoretically there is no reason why a chaplain who is a member of staff should not be treated in the same way as other members of staff directly involved in patient care, in a sense the issue is an academic one, for a chaplain who enjoys good relationships with the staff has no need of such a facility (a quick word with Sister is far more informative!). A visiting minister is, however, in a different position and theoretically at least no confidential information should be divulged without the permission of the patient. In practice, what is disclosed will depend on the relationship established with the staff, and though this relationship may be of brief duration, it can be of crucial importance on the support of the patient. Good pastoral care can be said to be highly dependent on a good relationship between clergy and staff, with openness of communication and an appreciation of one another's professional roles and personal qualities.

Non-Christian Religions

The foregoing description of the pastoral care of the seriously ill has been written from a Christian perspective. It could not be otherwise, when both authors belong to churches with roots in the Reformation. Increasingly, however, society is becoming more diverse in the cultural backgrounds of its citizens, especially in urban areas, where large numbers of immigrants have made new homes. Many have come from countries where the missionary outreach of the nineteenth century has led to the establishment of indigenous Christian churches. There are, however, many newcomers whose backgrounds lie in the Muslim, Hindu, Sikh or other faiths, and who continue to practise their religion or at least be influenced by its customs. Such men and women will form an increasing proportion of the hospital population as they grow older and become part of that age-group which makes most use of the health services. To care for them adequately will demand some attempt at understanding their various attitudes to illness and suffering, and their customs relating to death and dying. A helpful summary of these is to be found in Peter Speck's book, *Loss and Grief in Medicine.*

Although the Christian minister may have something to offer people of other religions, this will be offered (at least initially, as in most pastoral relationships) through listening and befriending, rather than in any attempt at proselytising. A hospital chaplain will be aware of the different religious resources in his community and will know how to contact the representatives of the various religious groupings, where this is the wish of the patient or his family. 'Issues of deepest meaning and highest concern' belong to the human race and not to any one segment of it. Effective pastoral care respects the integrity of the person being cared for, and ultimately maintains its own integrity through a non-intrusive concern for those who may not share its own Christian presuppositions.

References

Clebzch, W.A. and Jackle, C.R. (1967) *Pastoral Care in Historical Perspective*, Harper Torchbooks, New York
Wise, K. (1980) *Pastoral Psychotherapy*, Jason Aaronson, New York

Bibliography

Autton, N. (1966) *The Pastoral Care of the Dying*, SPCK, London
Badham, P. (1976) *Christian Beliefs about Life after Death*, SPCK, London
Campbell, A.V. (1979) 'Meaning of death and ministry to the dying', in D. Doyle (ed.), *Terminal Care*, Churchill Livingstone, Edinburgh
Campbell, A.V. (1981) *Rediscovering Pastoral Care*, Darton, Longman and Todd, London
Edelwick, J. (1980) *Burnout: Stages of Disillusionment in the Helping Professions*, Human Sciences Press, New York
Faber, H. (1971) *Pastoral Care in the Modern Hospital*, SCM, London
Hinton, J. (1972) *Dying*, Penguin Books, Harmondsworth
Kubler-Ross, E. (1970) *On Death and Dying*, Tavistock Publications, London
Lamerton, R. (1980) *Care of the Dying*, Penguin Books, Harmondsworth
Speck, P. (1978) *Loss and Grief in Medicine*, Ballière Tindall, London
Thompson, I. (1979) *Dilemmas of Dying*, University Press, Edinburgh

20 PALLIATIVE CARE AND SOCIAL WORK
Audrey Boyle

In this chapter I shall consider the concept of social work in the health field relative to palliative care, where social work practitioners collaborate with the patient and his family, with multi-professional staff within the hospital and with agencies outside the hospital, to offer palliation or alleviation of the stress of intractable conditions to the patient and his family. Models of practice will refer to my present work in a department of neurology and a respiratory diseases unit.

Background

Social work has been in hospitals since 1895, when the first hospital almoner was appointed at the Royal Free Hospital in London. In 1905, Richard Cabot (1973) was working at the Massachusetts General Hospital in Boston, and in 1915 he was writing that 'team work of doctor and social worker is called for, and the professionals are beginning to hear the call'. He saw clinical social work as a major link between medical and environmental resources.

In the early days, as social work spread in hospitals, the professional status of the hospital social worker became well established, forming its own professional organisation and curricula of education and practice. The late 1930s saw the evolvement of the clinical social work concept of case work as the main function of the hospital social work department.

As social work services were accepted as adjuncts of hospital care in the 1940s and 1950s, there were shifting emphases for social work thinking, from discharge-planning primarily to treatment-orientated services. Today, the profession appears to be returning to its early roots by reaffirming the generic elements of social work practice which preclude separating the delivery of concrete services from clinical services and community organisation.

428

Clinical Social Work: The Case-work Concept

As we see that social work is a continuing and developing practice directly involved in hospital and health care, it is important to set forth its responsibilities in the health field, remembering that social work in hospital is in a secondary setting, that is, the patient enters the hospital for medical treatment and care. In our work with patients, we are aware of the many broad dimensions of the service, the many professions involved, the nature of illness and the impact of illness on the patient and his family; the need to make plans supportively, often in limited time, and to integrate personal, emotional and material resources for the patient's well-being. Of particular importance is the working relationship between the patient and social worker, which enables the patient to work positively with his illness or disability in order to obtain optimum function.

Decisions and judgements may have to be made which the social worker draws from knowledge, values and experiences, and from self-awareness, often in situations of uncertainty. The social worker makes priorities in the working situation to achieve effectiveness. The emphasis is on setting and achieving desired goals, and being able to evaluate outcomes based on an assessment of inner and outer resources which either exist or can be developed (Caroff, 1981).

Area of Work: The Health Field/the Hospital

As clinical social workers employed, and accountable, in the demanding health field and concerned with the needs of our patients, we see that good health is what we all wish for and disease is a hazard and problem which affects all of our society. Where there are severe forms of illness and physical handicap, or frailty in ageing, social and emotional stress can be burdensome and barely tolerable, or intolerable.

The goal of medicine is to effect a cure in illness and to return the patient well to his home and family and independent social function. Where there is no cure and the problem of illness continues, there are negative implications for the patient and his family and also for the professional staff, who may feel helpless and to have failed — the phenomenon of 'burn-out' being a known hazard in professional health care.

In addition to the emotional stresses of severe and lengthy illness and ageing, the socio-economic costs can be high for the patient and his family, and also for society because of loss of social function — for example, dependency and absence from work can have socio-economic repercussions. As research continues in medical science and produces new levels of treatment, and as we become an ageing society, and as those with severe physical handicap live longer, the responsibilities for social work and the implications for society become greater.

Cost-effectiveness in social work planning in the health field, a topical theme, has always been present, if latent. Although careful social work planning may also be cost effective to the health service and of course is important, it should not be the major priority in social work thinking and, in fact, social work planning may involve added hospital cost if it is felt, for example, that the premature and unprepared return home of a patient could be detrimental to that patient.

The Hospital Setting

Psycho-social Transition and Supportive Social Work Intervention

The basic tenet − 'start where the patient is and move with him' − is important as the crisis of illness and admission to hospital affect the individual patient and his family, and as he moves from the assumptions of past experience to the confrontation of a new experience (Garnett, 1972). Severe illness and physical handicap and the need for medical care as seen in neurological and respiratory units present many problems for the patient and his family: physical and economic disruption, anxiety, waiting for the diagnosis, fear of injections, sickness in radiotherapy, threat to body image (the loss of hair), confirmation of a routine of drug therapy in chronic illness, the poor prognosis. Uncertainty is a stressful factor as the individual wonders: 'What is wrong with me? Will I be disabled?' Self-blame is distressing as the patient says: 'What have I done to deserve this?'

Any illness is threatening, and fear and anxiety are expected reactions, as is regression, the fear of dependency and reactive depression. Some patients may be able to express themselves freely, whereas others deny symptoms and reject the nature of their illness. It is important that the social worker, in an equal, non-paternalistic partnership and in a professionally permissive and non-judgemental way, understands these responses. In counselling, she will need to understand the sadness of the lonely widower with respiratory failure, still grieving his lost marriage partner; the elderly lady with pneumonia, disorientated and depressed in a new environment; the vulnerable loneliness of the single man with cor pulmonale; the young teacher with multiple sclerosis, unable to return to her job and harassed by business matters; and the elderly man with Parkinson's disease, worried about his frail wife at home on her own.

While the social worker assesses and evaluates the at-risk situation and sets goals for purposeful intervention, it is important that the family is included in this planning. It may be that much social work activity is with the family, as the individual may be too ill to share. Tripartite meetings with the relative, the doctor and the social worker may be arranged to interpret medical information and clarify any confusion the relative may have. This may be very important, especially where the relative has denied and rejected the initial diagnosis. The family and the individual, are entitled to full information, participation, frank discussion and self determination.

Reactions by the family to social work counselling are of utmost importance and are integrated into the total outcome. In addition to the emotions already described, aggression and hostility may be expressed by the family consequential to guilt feelings, if the relative rejects the possibility of any responsibility, or regrets previous attitudes to the patient.

Practical problems of admission to hospital for the patient and his family combine with these emotional responses, as the patient needs help with the ongoing functions of daily living — the care of the children of the divorced mother admitted with malignancy, the anxiety of the elderly lady with pneumonia whose pet animal has been left on its own, and the everyday multitudinous worries that occur. The social worker will attempt to enhance the interaction between the person and his environment.

Counselling, emotional support and practical activity by the social worker permit the understanding of the total situation of the whole person and his family on his admission to hospital.

Visiting the Hospital

Visiting presents mixed emotions and problems, and the hospital social worker may be involved in assisting with financial difficulties caused by the high cost and inconvenience of travel to specialist units. Travel may be difficult for an elderly spouse. Separation from children can be distressing for the patient and child, and it is important to support in this area if necessary.

Where the patient is isolated, a visit from a voluntary source may be welcomed, peer-group visitors being usually more compatible, though not necessarily so. Self-help groups, university students and church groups are usually ready to help. Visiting by volunteers when the patient returns home should be considered, if the person is likely to be isolated, as visitors sometimes tend to drop away when the patient returns home.

Financial help for temporary accommodation, for example, can be obtained by the social worker, for example, if the relative of a terminally ill patient lives at a considerable distance from the hospital.

The Patient and the Ward Community

On coming into the hospital ward, the patient visited by his family and friends, usually at set times, begins to form new social attachments to his fellow patients. New positive supportive relationships may be formed which can help to reduce elements of fear and anxiety in the sharing of experiences and the demonstration of mutual comfort. The social worker may observe and participate in these informal groups and will come to know patients who are readmitted to hospital, for example, to the respiratory unit where there are acute episodes of complicated chronic chest disease, and where the security of the ward is welcomed. Patients will inform each other of financial resources and services and ask the social worker for details, and perhaps advise the social worker of new information, which can be shared. On return home, contact may be maintained between patients. Where a patient, newly admitted, is distressed by seeing very ill patients, the social worker, along with her professional colleagues, will try to be supportive.

An example of a spontaneous and informal group that occurred with a patient, ward sister and social worker is illustrated to show the beneficial effect of a small group discussion. The patient is very disabled with multiple sclerosis and confined to bed. She regretted Christmas ceiling decorations being taken down as they had provided a source of interest (the ceiling was her main focus of attention). In discussion, the idea of suspended mobiles was conceived by the patient and supported by the ward sister. The social worker approached the art college and a local school, and imaginative mobiles are now being produced for the ward. Our patient, deprived physically but not intellectually, had her self-esteem reinforced by making a valuable contribution to the ward, and two groups of young people and professional staff had further insight into the needs of others.

Social work practice in offering palliative care to the very ill and physically handicapped person is primarily with the patient and his family in the time available. However, professional social workers also have been practising group work in hospitals for many years, especially in the area of psychiatry and of long-term physical handicap, and beneficial results have been demonstrated in patient intercommunication and in the creation of greater staff awareness.

The Patient and the Multidisciplinary Team

Requests for social worker intervention in patient care, i.e. 'referrals', are made in various ways, from the patient, his family and friends, fellow patients or many outside agencies. Another source of referral, to effect maximum awareness of need, is the use of the multidisciplinary team meetings, the 'social meeting', where specialist knowledge is communicated, contributed and collated confidentially, assessment made and treatment formulated, geared to the care of the most vulnerable patients and the protection from risk of their quality of life. The group can be structured variously and many meetings of disciplines occur spontaneously with differing membership. Non-availability of social worker staff and other reasons may preclude regular meetings. However, a useful group may be composed of the medical and nursing staff, the physiotherapist, the occupational therapist, social worker and a liaising hospital health visitor. The meeting can be held weekly at a set time, day and place. Valuable additional information may be presented, for example, by a speech therapist, psychiatrist or geriatrician, and hospital chaplain.

The social worker, invested with the authority of the hospital by the patient, is readily accepted by him. The social worker has a dual role to the hospital and to the patient. In her role with the patient, she may act as advocate to intervene on the patient's behalf and to put forward his needs as he sees them and as understood by the social worker. In her role with the hospital, the social worker will normally follow the ward culture, for example, in the decision, or not, to tell the patient of a terminal diagnosis, but may wish to supplement and influence with knowledge obtained from the family, for example, by making aware the total needs of the family group.

In stressful ward situations, where there are many very ill and dying patients and staff anxiety is high, the multidisciplinary group meeting may be useful in meeting team needs by permitting the ventilation of stress, and by providing mutual support and understanding.

Planning for Discharge Home

The multidisciplinary team is part of a process that continues from the time the patient enters hospital. In this section, we shall look at social management and palliative care, by illustration. Areas of care may be classified as medical, social, economic, functional or psychological, but the borderlines may be blurred, overlap and interact. First, we can look at the needs of the elderly and the frail elderly on returning home.

The Respiratory Unit

As the frail elderly comprise a large number of those who are admitted and discharged from hospital and from the respiratory unit, they require careful team assessment. The elderly lady admitted with pneumonia may, for example, minimise her difficulties and be over-reassuring in her anxiety to be at home again. She may be unrealistic and over-demanding of her family. Mental attitudes may show depression, withdrawal and self-neglect, and behavioural problems may take the form of nocturnal ambulance or memory loss or incontinence. Assessment by the social worker of total patient needs and adequacy of support from family, friends and neighbours is essential. Rejection of responsibility by the family and possible aggressive behaviour to the team may reflect past difficult family relationships. The possibility of reactive physical or emotional abuse, so called 'battering' is not to be missed. Before final discharge from hospital, the team may suggest a trial visit home for the afternoon with the occupational therapist and social worker, to assess patient function and capability.

While the patient is alone, or where support for the family is required, the social worker can initiate the home-help service through the home-care team. Each new referral is visited by a home-care supervisor and an assessment made of the elderly person's needs. A home help usually assists in the mornings and the length of time spent depends on need and availability of resources. Meals on wheels can also be requested by the social worker through the home-care team; meals may be provided from one to five days each week. The patient is reviewed at home by the home-care team at regular intervals. There are private domestic and are private domestic and nursing agencies in the city.

Where recommended by the team and the consultant in geriatric care, the elderly person may attend a geriatric day hospital or a psychogeriatric day hospital, transport being provided by ambulance. Days of attendance vary, but are usually one to three days each week.

Lunch clubs, run by a church group or voluntary organisation, are enjoyable, for as well as offering a meal, they provide a useful meeting place. Day centres, run by voluntary organisations, offer opportunities for retired people to enjoy recreational activities in a friendly atmosphere, and also may offer chiropody, hairdressing and bus outings. The policy is geared to encourage and support the frail elderly to live in their own homes for as long as possible.

Sheltered housing, with special facilities and a warden service, can make a very real contribution to the quality of life for elderly people, and it is much sought after where existing accommodation is inconvenient or isolated. Housing associations and the local authority housing department operate sheltered housing schemes, but waiting lists can be very lengthy, unfortunately. The social worker and doctor can support by writing to the agencies concerned. The social worker can advise and initiate application for residential care in a local authority home; the procedure for selection is by a panel method. Registered voluntary homes may also be a source of help, with financial supplementation for accommodation requiring approval by the regional social work department. The local authority homes may also provide short-term holiday periods for the elderly, to give relatives a rest, where a little more care is needed, but there is pressure for accommodation especially in summer. Holidays can be offered by voluntary organisations, for example, through the central offices of a church, but usually the older person requires to be more active.

The Neurological Unit

I shall try not to repeat provisions already mentioned, but which may be equally applicable in this illustration. Sometimes the team may feel that return home is not desirable, for example, in the situation where a young woman, severely affected by multiple sclerosis, was also isolated at home from her peer group. It was felt that the health of her older parents was at risk, and there was some evidence of disturbed behaviour. Team support was offered to the patient and her parents, and by supportive help, the transition to long-term care in a young chronic sick unit was made less difficult; flexible arrangements were made for visits home for weekends or longer periods.

The pattern, however, in a busy neurological unit is for investigation, assessment, treatment planning and return home in a limited time, which reflects case management. Needs are identified quickly, with continuing care being planned in the home situation.

The social worker meeting a patient who has been confronted with the diagnosis of multiple sclerosis will not remain neutral, but will try to understand the stress of loss, and be aware of the need to support and enable the person who may feel stigmatised by physical impairment, and who may feel his self-esteem and dignity threatened. The belief of Mike Oliver (1981) is very relevant:

In working with disabled people, the social worker's task can be changed from helping an individual to adjust to personal disaster to enabling him to locate the personal, social, economic and psychological resources to live life to the full. This not only enhances the quality of life for the individual but will add considerably to the personal and professional satisfaction of the social worker involved.

The potential of people under stress is not to be underestimated, and team support may help in the growth and emergence of this potential. The term 'sufferer' is frequently used, and I wonder if we cannot simply talk of 'people'.

The team enlists the support of the family as carers in discharge-planning, but the full implication of looking after someone with a very severe disability, where the patterns of life-style are altered, is seen in the long term. The social worker must be concerned for and work with the elderly widowed mother, whose daughter has cerebral atrophy and epilepsy; the married woman, in a reversal of role situation, whose husband is severely disabled with multiple sclerosis, sexually impotent, and sees her marriage at breaking-point; the husband who works all day and has little sleep at nights looking after his disabled wife; the elderly parents of the mute son affected by excessive drink and drug addiction and referred for psychiatric care; the children of the severely disabled mother excluded by the bonding of parents; and the family in fear of congenital handicap.

If the health of the carer is to be safeguarded, we must be aware of the sheer physical hard work and emotional strain in caring. Carers need break periods to give them a release from attending. The social worker may be involved in counselling the patient, if need be to encourage him to see that a holiday would be helpful. Carers need information about resources, agencies and groups, and how to take up all appropriate benefits, and carers can be helped by social work counselling and understanding of their needs. Unless carers' needs, physically and emotionally, are given importance, there is danger of their breakdown under stress.

The Terminal Phase

For a proportion of those patients who go home, there can be no further medical treatment. For some, chemotherapy or surgical procedures will enhance the quality of life, at least for a time, but for others there will be no 'cure'. A proportion of those returning home will know that life is nearing the end, whereas others may believe there is to be betterment. There is a differing awareness of knowledge.

The team has a shared realisation of approaching death and is prepared, sharing an anticipatory grieving process, perhaps unthought out and unstructured. When the patient is at home, the relative may not have this opportunity to grieve openly in anticipation of loss for fear of distressing the patient. Where there are children in the family, the social worker may intervene with the team to consider the implication of loss for them. Children are very aware and the apparently sudden death, for example, of a loved father, who has always been at home, sitting in the chair for months perhaps, can shock and distress them, and they may not understand why he has left them.

In Britain, the health visitor, who is a valued member of the team, both as a counsellor and a trained nurse with specialised additional qualifications, has constant contact with the team, the social worker and, very importantly, the general practitioner. The relationship between the health visitor (in the UK) and the social worker is important; each complements the other, with the social worker being geared to support emotionally and practically.

The social worker with the team will have an expectation that there will be supportive care from families, but will be aware of the size of the family and the age, for example, of the widow living on her own, who is particularly vulnerable, relying on relatives, friends and neighbours to help. The burden of care for these older carers might be too great, especially where personal care, perhaps unpleasant and distressing, is overwhelming. Where there is a recognised inability to manage, because of apprehension or the scale of the task, the team may have to come to the decision that returning home is not possible and alternative care is needed. Where this happens, the social worker may be involved in planning arrangements with the relatives and must take care to reduce any feelings of guilt the relatives may have and support them in the decision that has been made, reinforcing the work and support they have already given.

When the patient returns home, caring and supporting services will be mobilised, and support from the primary care team enlisted. The social worker involved in obtaining help can seek financial aid from voluntary funds, for example, to install a telephone, provide a portable oxygen cylinder or by providing voluntary transport. Appropriate statutory benefits will be sought. The social worker will be aware of her anxiety and vulnerability in stressful situations and guard against using practical activity to screen her awareness of the emotions and spiritual needs of the patient and his family.

At all times in a counselling role, the social worker values and accepts the lifetime experience of the patient, valuing his vulnerability, his humour and his dignity. She will be aware that he may be in pain and physically uncomfortable. The terminal condition may go along with other conditions, for example, a drink problem may have been present for many years. The concern will be to help with total needs. The social worker will also be very aware of the multi-problems already existing within the family, and of the family response to the stress of the terminal phase of illness of a loved person, for example, a child may stress-react by truanting from school, or by petty thieving. There can also be a multi-physical condition causing multi-problem reactions, where, for example, the mother with terminal cancer has a mentally retarded daughter, who had grand mal epilepsy, and is cared for by a frail father.

Terminal illness presents with fear and uncertainty for the patient and his family. As we have seen, there may be a wall of silence around the patient lest he be distressed, even though the patient knows what is wrong, but it may be that this is how the stressful situation is handled. Others may value the breaking-down of a barrier of pretence and denial of communication. The ward culture is followed, but the social worker may intervene to influence from her knowledge of the patient and his family. A minister of faith will very often support and help the dying person and respond to the patient's beliefs and needs irrespective of creeds.

The hospital, with its caring team and, very importantly, the auxiliary and nursing team, come to know that patient over months of out-patient attendance and community care, and will continue to look after him if he returns to hospital to die and will grieve his loss.

Reflecting the growing interest in the care of the dying is the increasing establishment of palliative-care units, hospices and Macmillan Continuing Care Units, set up by religious and voluntary organisations and offering important areas of care for patients with incurable disease. The patients are referred to such centres by the primary care of hospital team. Nursing and medical staff from the hospice visit the patient and his family and enable the family to continue longer in their care.

When death occurs, the reaction of the family or friends is of shock and numbness, even when death is expected. In her relationship with the bereaved, the social worker will be aware of responses, of seeing or hearing the dead person. The social worker in a counselling role, a helping role, will offer the bereaved person the opportunity to talk through, perhaps many times, the accounts of illness and death, and by listening carefully, will hope to alleviate distress. Many feelings are expressed by the bereaved person, perhaps anger and guilt, for example, where the bereaved left the person for an hour or two to sleep and the person died on their own. Anger may be the reaction of being left alone to cope and assume unknown responsibility. Counselling in bereavement, devoid of platitudes, is the prerogative of all who may have been connected with the dying person. While we speak of the burden of stress and highlight the areas of need, the social worker will understand that dying is part of living and can be an experience that can bring people more closely together − the quality of death, and of dying, being respected, as is the quality of living. Death, when it comes, will be for the bereaved a physical loss, but also perhaps a source of spiritual gain and development.

Social Work Departments (in Scotland)

As a social worker working within a medical setting, it would be inappropriate for me to interpret the role of the community social worker. I know it is insufficient to say that without their co-operation and support the care of the patient would be seriously hampered. Liaison at times, by the case–conference method, is established with social workers in community offices.

Where there are workers with a special remit in the care of the elderly and the physically handicapped, a close sense of liaison may be established, and is of especial importance in these areas of long-term case management with the physically handicapped person. The visiting of patients may be made in either direction, with the hospital social worker visiting the patient at home, and the community social worker, a valuable support service, visiting her 'client' in hospital. Confidentiality, which is of prime importance at all times in all areas of social work, is respected.

Voluntary Associations and Funds

Long-established voluntary organisations have been very frequently the forerunner to statutory social work provision. The work of voluntary organisations and their funds add greatly to hospital social work capability, not only their financial provisions, but the visiting, the holidays, the counselling services, all areas of work which supplement and complement hospital and statutory social work provision.

Physically and Mentally Orientated Self-help Groups

The hospital social worker is frequently involved in communicating with self-help groups, These groups are voluntarily organised and cover a very wide range of age, disability and social functions. Some groups solely provide information and education. Others provide holidays and social clubs and visiting at home or in hospital; others act as pressure groups. Patrick Phelan (1981), who writes on social work, looking back at attitudes to disabled people and the International Year of Disabled People 1981, writes: 'The way in which International Years focus a spotlight of concern on a particular group of citizens and their sectional requirements can and does serve to highlight deficiencies in our knowledge, gaps in our understanding, loopholes in our provision and shortcomings in our caring.' The need for integration and the non-segregation of sections of society is a goal to be strived for.

Anticipatory Care – Prevention and Education

Social workers have always been interested in the concept of prevention to discover whether social worker intervention could be pushed back to an earlier stage, before stress begins. There are many areas of need for social work anticipatory care, for example, with the frail elderly, where research into need led to the setting-up of a network of community carers. Registers of people at risk could be extended to the bereaved and the isolated, but fundamental areas of confidentiality and privacy could be vulnerable. The hospital social worker is concerned to educate and to be involved in the community resources. She can draw attention to areas of need for older people and of needs relevant to the young chronically sick people. However, the resources of 'the community' will always fall short of expectation, demand and perceived need.

Conclusion

The social worker involved and in communication with the caring teams, with people – within and without the hospital – is concerned to help and to relieve stress for those who are very ill or physically impaired. In turn, the social worker gains strength from the warmth and personal qualities of the patients and the families she meets.

Agency	Worker	Service
Local government		
Social work department in area offices Citizens' Rights offices	Social Worker Occupational Therapist Home-care Team Residential/Day Care Team	Case management Aids to daily living, possum, ramps, cass alarm, etc. Home helps, Meals on Wheels, incontinent laundry service Residential home (Part IV), day centre for physically handicapped, adult training centres, supported accommodation Bus pass for elderly/disabled, parking disc for disabled, holidays, recreation
Education	Careers Officer	Employment, vocational guidance
Housing	Welfare Visitors Homeless Team	Housing applications/transfers Sheltered housing, Rent/rebate section Housing information service including housing associations
Central government		
Manpower Services Commision Job Centres (Employment Service Agency)	Disablement Resettlement Officer (DRO)	Register of Employment for Disabled Employment Rehabilitation Centre (ERC)
Department of Health and Social Security	Visitors Counter Officer Catalogue and Leaflets from: Government Buildings, Honeypot Lane, Stanmore, Middlesex or	National insurance benefits, FIS, mobility, attendance, invalid care, etc.
Supplementary Benefits Section		Supplementary allowance heating/diet, special single payment
War Pensions Welfare	Local DHSS offices	Welfare to pensioners
National Health Service		
Primary Care Team	General Practitioner, Health Visitor, Community Nurses	Appropriate services

Agency	Worker	Service
Lothian Health Board NHS Community Health Service	Community Health Specialist Chiropodist, Dietician, Speech Therapist, Physiotherapist Occupational Therapist, Special Care Nursing, Social Worker	Nursing aid centres (temporary-loan wheelchairs/commode) Vehicle for the disabled centre (wheelchairs) Hospital loans (including Edinburgh Simpson bed)
Young Chronic Sick Units Geriatric/Psycho Geriatric Rehabilitation	Medical Staff	Day hospital
Voluntary Associations and Funds Self-help groups — Epilepsy, Parkinson's, Multiple Sclerosis Muscular Dystrophy, Arthritis Care, Red Cross, WRVS, Chest, Heart & Stroke — see Directories	Workers attached to Associations and self-help societies	Variable Research Social activities Holidays Fund-raising/allocation Pressure

References

Cabot, R. (1973) *Social Services and the Art of Healing*, Classics Series, Washington DC National Association of Social Workers, Washington DC, reprint of 1915 edition

Caroff, P. (1981) *Clinical Social Work and Health Care*; and 'Clinical social work and health care practice', *Journal for National Association of Social Workers*, 6 (4), 69-73

Garnett, A. (1972) *Interviewing: Its Principles and Methods*, Family Association of America, New York

Oliver, M. (1981) 'Physical disability – society's handicap', *Community Care*, October, Sutton, Surrey, pp. 18-19

Phelan, P. (1981) 'Social work today', *Aiming at Integration in the IYDP*, vol. 12, no. 18, p. 13

21

COMMUNICATION

Ivan Lichter

Introduction

To be successful palliative care must provide comfort for the body, the mind and the soul. It is evident that psycho-social and spiritual problems require interpersonal communication. It is sometimes forgotten that even physical comfort is dependent on good communication; we can only be aware of the patient's needs if we give him of our time, if we relate to him, and engender in him the confidence to unburden himself of his anxieties. Even the limited aim of physical comfort cannot be achieved if the emotions are in turmoil. Symptom control can only be achieved, in fact symptoms may sometimes be avoided, if, by communication, sources of emotional and spiritual distress are identified and relieved. Nor will medication be fully effective unless symptoms are explained and therapies detailed, involving the patient, in so far as possible, in decision-making.

When an illness is serious, anxiety and stress for the patient and for the family are inevitable. A major cause of anxiety is a prevailing uncertainty about what is happening, what can be expected and what needs to be done. Lack of information, withdrawal from open discussion, discomfort in confronting an unhappy situation, and reservations about revealing feelings, all promote stress and induce tension, fear and anxiety. These are formidable barriers to communication which may prevent the patient from comprehending, remembering or even hearing. The health-care team, in particular the doctor, must give the necessary information about the illness and the measures for support that will be provided. The commitment to such support should be the message that remains with the patient, not merely the disclosure of diagnosis. If this does not come across, then the discussion may have increased his distress rather than lessened it. For relief of anxiety we must diminish uncertainty, give the patient the confidence of our continuing care and concern and of our ability to provide relief that may be needed. The manner in which information is imparted may be more important than the words.

We must also promote healthy communication on a cognitive and an emotional level within the family. In these ways much of the distress of serious illness can be avoided. Communication between the patient, between doctor and family, and between members of the health-care team are vital components of total care. It is particularly important when the patient cannot expect cure.

The Message

The belief that frank communication should be a feature of all our dealings with patients and their families is now more generally accepted, particularly in serious illness and especially in cancer. Experience suggests that this should begin when the diagnosis is first made and that it should not be left until the terminal stage of illness. If communication is delayed, the significant benefits of earlier sharing will be lost — in making the most of the life that remains and in achieving what Francis Bacon called 'A fair and easy passage'.

What is it that we should communicate? We want to communicate our concern and our support for the patient. We need to give information about his illness and his condition. We want to tell him what we shall be doing for his relief and comfort. We want him to know that we understand how he feels, we understand his loss, his grief, his sadness; that we know something of his needs, and we know something of what to do to help. We want him to know that he will be respected as an individual, and he will be able to make his own decisions regarding his care. We want him to know that we shall be available to listen to what he wants to say, to allow expression of his fears and anxieties, and to help resolve them. We want him to know that we shall answer his questions openly and honestly. We want to tell him about our continuing support — our commitment to him; that we shall stand by him and provide relief and comfort.

Non-verbal Communication

There is much we can *say* to make these communications, but for the most part, and most believably, it is what we feel and do that will transmit the message. This is the only communication that will carry real conviction. Our unconscious behaviour, the minute, barely perceptible, non-verbal ways in which we unknowingly communicate, convey the message. So, ultimately, the message is not in what we say, not even in what we do, but in how we feel. This cannot readily be disguised. If we do not really care, the patient will know; if we are uncomfortable with death, he will sense it; if we would rather be spared the discomfort of talking about terminal illness, he will be aware of it.

When two people come together, it is inevitable that they will communicate something to one another. Even if we do not speak, messages pass between us. By our looks, expressions and body movements, each will tell the other something, even if it is only 'I do not want to talk'. We show how we feel mainly by our facial expressions and movements. Any strong emotion will automatically show itself, even though we may not be aware of the signals that we are sending. These non-verbal signals and this 'silent' language are more important in an encounter than words. If the body language is at variance with the verbal communication, the contents of the verbal message will be largely discounted. Even though we may deliberately aim to deceive, the withholding of information is not easy. Without being aware of it, we emit non-verbal signals of our deception.

In a paradoxical way, words themselves may constitute non-verbal signals. Idle chat can be a means of enjoying a relationship; the message gets across. And in sorrow, although the talk may be about the weather and other trivia when the main concern lies quite elsewhere, it may be a way of communicating a bond.

In the light of these observations, we can no longer believe that telling is done only in words, or that we can avoid telling by silence, evasions, half-truths or outright lies. When the doctor talks to the patient about his illness, the information that the latter gleans will be more than that contained in the doctor's words; non-verbal behaviour will convey not only the diagnosis, but how he is preparing to handle the situation.

Do We Tell?

Studies have shown that most dying people are aware that they are dying. It is not only the way they themselves feel that gives them this information. They will not miss the whispers outside the door, the look of anxiety and stress in the eyes of relatives, the changed attitude of friends, the halting conversations, the hollow cheerfulness, the lack of touching and intimacy. We may think that our pretence has not been detected, but this is because, though found out, our lies have not been challenged, since it is more comfortable to go along with the deception. So it is not a question of deciding whether or not to tell — we cannot help telling; we read one another. We observe the patient, but at the same time *he* is making a psychological assessment of *us*. Patients are often more perceptive than we are — they recognise our needs and our fears, and will do nothing to upset the relationship. It is not just we who communicate with the patient. We must be aware of his communications — whether made verbally or non-verbally. Communicating requires that we respond, relate and interact with patients. It involves also responding to our own feelings and sometimes to our own fears. In our fear, it is usually we ourselves who create the barrier to communication.

Entering discussion on whether or not to tell patients that they have a serious illness is to immerse oneself in a cauldron of controversy. We can bypass the contentious question — 'Is there a moral obligation to reveal one's findings to the patient?' — and pose another question: 'Is it in the patient's best interest to know the truth?'

The Response to Disclosure

The first concern expressed is that the truth may harm the patient. When one decides against telling, one must accept — and weigh against each other not only the benefits believed to stem from this negative decision, but also the disadvantages of the positive decision not to tell — the harm that may be inflicted. The ill-effects that may result from evasion and dishonesty and the isolation attending non-communication are well enough documented. A negative approach aimed at doing the least harm may add considerably to the patient's distress. The manner in which communication is handled when the patient first consults his doctor with disturbing symptoms may determine, to a large extent, his future emotional status and his ability to function to the best of his capacity.

Yet the patient may find it difficult to get honest answers. The usual claim is that we shall decide for each patient whether he really wants to know and can 'take' it. The usual decision is that the patient should not be told — because he might become depressed, 'give up' or even commit suicide. These responses to disclosure anticipate a single permanent impact on the patient — that he will either 'be brave', 'plan for the future', 'go to pieces', 'become depressed'. In fact, disclosure sets off a response process through which the patient passes, and each stage can be modified by appropriate forms of interaction. The dynamic response process may at one time or another include denial, anger, anxiety, depression or acceptance, and the response may be modified by the patient's personality and resources, the manner of telling and staff-patient interaction. Moreover the response may stop at any stage and change direction. Basing a decision on a single probable impact is to focus on only one stage of the response process.

There are times in a terminal illness when patients feel depressed or show anxiety. This is frequently due to some specific worry or, even more commonly, an isolated distressing event or episode. Discussion often brings to light the immediate cause of the present mood and it can be worked through there and then.

When to Tell

It is commonly accepted that a decision on whether to tell or not must be made for each individual patient. We then face a difficulty — how to recognise those individuals who should be told and those who should not. One view is that those who want to know will ask. Those who adopt this approach seldom seem to encounter anybody who wants to know. This may be because the patients are not really given the opportunity to ask, or the necessary support to be able to handle it.

Many believe that people often do want to know — in their own good time — and that there is no real problem about identifying these people. They take the view that providing an opportunity for unburdening and a sensitive approach will allow the person to talk when he is ready; that in fact little telling is needed — he wants to talk, not listen. There is reason to believe that the patient's need for communication depends in large degree on the stage of the illness. It is necessary to differentiate between the need to give information in the earlier stages of the illness and its desirability in terminal illness. When people are dying, there is less often a need to communicate diagnosis and prognosis; at that stage they usually know what they need to know; what they require is understanding and support, and sometimes an opportunity to unburden. However, even at this time people may be bewildered as to what is happening, and show by their demeanour and even by their questions that much still needs to be resolved. Yet there is sometimes a tendency to wait for more clearly defined openings or for time to establish rapport or for the patient to 'settle down'. If this is done, the opportunity to communicate may be lost. The person who has met with evasion or equivocation has been failed — he will not try again. He will withdraw, and the conclusion may then be reached that he 'did not really want to know'.

It is necessary to consider an earlier stage, when the person may be uncertain about the nature of his illness. There are very few people who, even at the time of their first symptoms, are not concerned deep down that the illness may be serious. They may put their lung cancer down to a chill, dust or other environmental cause; they may say that they have no idea as to the nature of their illness. But beneath it all, closer questioning will reveal fear — they have already thought the worst. Despite all protestations and appearances that the person is not worried about the possibility of cancer and therefore that it might be better to keep it from him — he is worrying about it. On fuller discussion, he will admit it. Keeping him in ignorance will not remove his anxiety — not unless he is told an outright lie, which must be sufficiently convincing to remove his deep-seated anxiety. Nothing will do this, short of assuring him that he has not got cancer, and this assurance cannot be sustained for long.

What Don't Patients Ask?

We must remember, too, that the person is sometimes not sure of what he already knows or suspects or wants to know about the seriousness of his condition or what exactly it is that he fears. Despite the commonly held belief that 'the patient will talk when he is ready', without a direct approach, many patients never bring themselves to ask questions, although they may well wish to discuss their problems, and would do so if given some assistance. These patients make no overtures to us, show no inclination to discuss matters relating to their illness, despite our availability to listen and to answer questions.

There may be a number of reasons why no communication takes place. The patient may not be sure what questions are permissible. He may have difficulty in wording his question, or he may be unable to formulate questions to express his unease and distress. Frequently the patient will wait for us to talk — 'The doctor will tell me what I ought to know.' So he waits for us to initiate dialogue, while we wait for him.

Sometimes the patient remains silent because the behaviour of those about him has brain-washed him into thinking that 'he will not be able to take it'. Our attitudes towards cancer and death persuade him that the burden of knowledge will be intolerable. On occasion he says nothing, just because, when an alternative is available, it is often easier to do nothing than to take action — especially when the task is so formidable.

If these reasons sound less than convincing, it may be because we tend to project our own responses onto others. We are accustomed to talking with people, we are in the habit of questioning, we are used to taking the initiative. Many patients have a very different background. They are unused to expressing their thoughts or to posing questions.

The Distress of Uncertainty

There are times when we have to do more than wait for patients to ask their questions; when making opportunities for communication is not enough; when one has to take the initiative; when one must comment, invite, suggest, explore, set up talking positions, even ask the questions. The patient may not even realise that it is the uncertainty that is causing his distress — that it is the uncertainty he wants removed. But the relief is obvious, when communication has finally been established. People fear the unknown much more than the truth about their illness, however serious it may be.

The anxiety produced by uncertainty may only be dispelled by frank disclosure. Patients often say that once they have been 'told' about their illness they stop worrying. They then know what to expect. They sometimes say that they are almost relieved when they know the worst. They feel calmer and are better able to co-operate in their management. 'Telling' removes the uncertainty of the situation and often brings peace of mind.

Not everybody responds in this way. The initial response may be shock, tears, sadness, especially in younger subjects whose life expectations have been dashed. But one is impressed by how well people cope with the news of serious illness — how they face this crisis with strength and courage and often with equanimity. And such a response is quite common, even in patients whose previous history might lead one to expect otherwise.

Our main objective is to maintain morale and help the patient to achieve peace of mind, but not in a shortsighted way by evasions or concealment which will increase difficulties later.

What is the Truth?

To given honest answers we must distinguish between making a true statement and telling the truth. We must distinguish between accuracy (as far as we know it) and veracity — that is, telling the truth honestly — not withholding or changing or obscuring a part of what we believe to be true. One may say to a patient: 'You have a blocked bronchus.' The statement is true, but is it the truth? The test is, was the statement intended to deceive? Was it hoped that the patient would not interpret it as a diagnosis of cancer? Circumlocutions and evasions are likely to leave the patient in a state of uncertainty that provokes anxiety. Sooner or later the real truth will become apparent, and if we have been less than frank with the patient in the past, where does he then turn for the truth in which he can believe?

We must, however, be careful that the meanings that we give to words are the same as those put on them by the patient. A blunt statement of a diagnosis of cancer may to the patient mean a prolonged illness with a painful degrading death. We must determine the perceived meaning and implications of the disease for the patient and his family, so that not just the words we use are true, but that the message received is accurate.

It is sometimes said that we are not vouchsafed to know the truth. Indeed, we are only talking about telling the truth as we know it, or believe it to be. That is all the patient asks of us. He does not expect us to be omniscient, but he does expect us to be truthworthy and he places his trust in us to tell to the best of our ability what we believe to be true. He asks no more — and no less. We may confess ignorance about certain aspects of the disease or a degree of uncertainty. This is also part of the truth as we know it, and it should be conveyed to the patient, but always with a commitment to the patient of continuing care and support.

Truth is not necessarily an end in itself, and it is not suggested that we aim at truth as a moral objective. Truth is advocated as being in the patient's best interests. The aim of honesty is to avoid uncertainty, to establish and to maintain a trust the patient can rely upon, to promote a belief in what is disclosed so that there is no room for unrealistic fancies — which may be more disturbing than the truth.

The alternative is not to tell. This can only mean verbal telling — it is impossible not to give away information by non-verbal signals. Even silence may be eloquent. It tells the patient: 'Your illness is grim — too grim to talk about.' It also tells him: 'I don't think you are strong enough to take it.' The result is fear, loss of self-esteem and depression.

If we do not tell, it is not just the diagnosis we have withheld. We have not told the patient that we understand his illness, understand how he feels; we have not told him that we shall support him and that we shall keep him comfortable — this, at a time when he is dependent upon the emotional support of others. It is when the prognosis is bad that there is a need to belong — to family, friends, people.

Do Patients Want to Know?

There is often concern that patients will not be able to tolerate the knowledge that they have a serious illness. This may well be so if the information is given from the foot of the bed during a ward round, and without taking time to find out about the patient's fears and anxieties, and without emphasising the care and support that will be provided. If the information is given in an atmosphere of trust and confidence, allowing time for the patient to formulate his anxieties and receive assurance, then experience is that patients show remarkable strength.

We have extended a study of 300 patients admitted to an acute surgical ward where there is frank communication with patients in the context of a supportive staff environment, to determine attitudes to disclosure of diagnosis and prognosis. The findings were as follows.

> Only 1 per cent of all patients (cancer and non-cancer) did not approve that information regarding their illness was made known to them.
> Only 3 per cent of non-cancer patients would prefer not to have the information made known to them if they had cancer.
> Less than 3 per cent would not wish to be told if they had a terminal illness, and all but 3 per cent would wish to be told as soon as possible.

The findings tend to show that very few people say that they do not want to know about their illness when caring support is available. The study also demonstrated that those with cancer have already found out that with the support provided they can cope. It is probable that people who say they do not want to know about serious illnesses are often afraid that they will not be able to handle it.

We must examine the situation of the patient who says he would rather not have been told what is wrong with him. It is necessary to consider the effects of the two alternatives: telling and not telling. What the patient is saying is that the knowledge that he has cancer is distressing to him. In the first place, it is unlikely that he really had no suspicions about the diagnosis. He does not realise that continuing uncertainty causes more anxiety and inhibits effective functioning. he knows how he feels now, but not how he would have felt if kept in ignorance. He does not know the consequences of failure of communication. But it is known that these can be disastrous. He may feel, 'If I had not been told, I would not have known, and I would have been unworried'. But the alternatives are not distressing knowledge or comfortable ignorance. It is almost inevitable that sooner or later the evidence that he has cancer will crowd in upon him.

Those who are not 'ready to hear', who cannot cope with the information, will not be harmed. They will find a way to handle this information. Denial is a frequently used coping mechanism. Often it is a temporary measure. The information given to the patient is stored and available to him to be processed at any time when he is ready into more constructive coping behaviours.

Maintaining Hope

There is concern that telling a patient he has cancer will break morale and destroy all hope. The hope that is denied is unrealistic hope of cure, a hope that cannot be sustained. But in our last days we have other important hopes; hope that we shall be cared for by people who understand our illness, are honest with us, and on whom we can rely; hope that we shall be able to share our fears and anxieties with those caring for us, and our feelings with those dear to us; hope that we shall not experience pain and distress; hope that we shall not suffer isolation, and that those on whom we depend will stand by us and be with us; finally, hope for a 'safe passage'. These are realistic hopes, vital to the patient with a limited life expectancy. They are denied to him when he is kept in the dark about his condition.

Helplessness

A major factor responsible for distress in terminal illness is a feeling of helplessness. The terminally ill patient has to contend not only with a threatening disease, but also with impairment of his personal significance. In hospital he is subjected to impersonal routines and placed in a dependent, powerless situation. Even more importantly, when there is failure to communicate diagnosis and prognosis, the patient cannot be involved in vital decisions in his life, and in his dying. When a person has no control over the ordering of his living, when he has no power over those elements of his life that relieve suffering or bring gratification, he will come to feel helpless and hopeless. There is experimental evidence to show that learned helplessness leads to emotional disturbance, depression and anxiety. This is accompanied by loss of appetite and weight, and by social deficiency. When these manifestations are observed in the seriously ill or dying person, one should consider the contribution that helplessness, resulting from lack of communication, may have made to the patient's condition.

Support Systems

The dying person may be anxious and afraid. How he copes — whether he breaks down or bears up — depends upon the availability of adequate support systems. He needs an ego support system and an external support system. The external support is relatively easy to supply; it largely involves people, services and care of his environment. To bolster internal strength, the patient needs, not hollow pretences and empty assurances; rather, he needs to be able to command information about his illness and to maintain some control of his life. Once he loses this, he has little significance as an individual, he is no longer a person, he is already socially dead; he loses his self-esteem and with it his inner strength.

Touch

Dying people are isolated not only mentally and emotionally, but physically. People withdraw, no longer touch them, and this is true even of relatives. The kiss on the lips becomes a peck on the forehead, then the light touch on the arm, then the wave from the door. When the doctor visits, he stands at the foot of the bed, Touch is a form of communication; moreover people *need* physical contact. Tender loving physiotherapy (TLP) (see Figure 21.1) often alleviates discomfort and

Figure 21.1: Communicating — tender loving physiotherapy

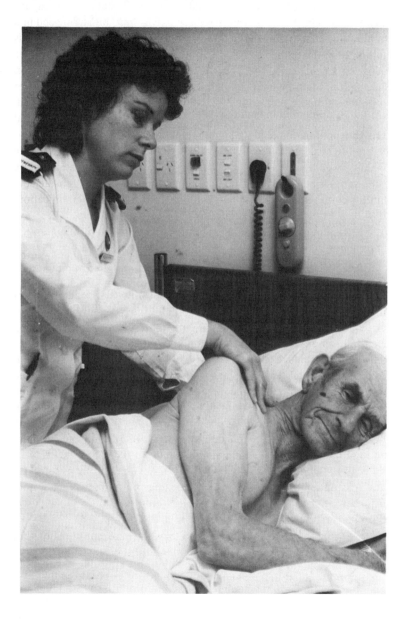

is always soothing – a back rub, neck stroking, gentle massage of muscles, or kneading of the shoulders. It also meets the need for physical human contact, what has been called 'skin hunger' (common to all mammals). This type of touch comfort should be prescribed just as one may order medication. It has an additional benefit; when the patient is receiving no other form of treatment, the physiotherapy given demonstrates that he is still being treated and is still important.

The Human Relationship

Finally, we should remember that communication is a basic human need and, as such, an essential requirement of patient care. Ordinarily, human beings spend a great part of their waking hours communicating. If we are deprived of communication, we cannot continue to function in a normal human way, we cannot maintain identity and role. Thus we should not deny the seriously ill patient the good fellowship, humour and idle chat that he could expect if he were well; to do so serves only to increase his sense of isolation.

Those who suffer lasting ill effects are the patients who have been left in doubt about diagnosis and prognosis, and the help and support they can expect. Uncertainty is more difficult to bear than the painful truth: it engenders anxiety, which increases the suffering of pain and other symptoms. Explanation, the security of a supportive relationship, the freedom to unburden fears, all the assurances and reassurances of communication can sometimes prevent the intractable pain that is often the lot of the rejected, isolated dying patient. It may also do much to prevent depression and to reduce confusion in the terminal stages of illness. This is the remarkable spin-off from a relationship of honesty, and the confidence it engenders. Intractable pain is seldom experienced by patients who are not afraid, anxious or demoralised by uncertainty and loss of self-esteem. It is rare indeed that routine medication does not suffice. Antidepressants are used only infrequently and the resources of the pain clinic are seldom needed. Terminal confusion is unusual. But all these problems occur when communication with patients has been poor.

Barriers to Communication

In numerous studies, the findings have shown that patients say they want to know if they have a serious illness, especially cancer; yet doctors frequently insist that patients seldom ask. If patients do not ask, even though they want to know, we need to postulate possible reasons. It may be that:

patients are not given the opportunity to ask;
attitudes discourage asking, with consequent fear of alienating the doctor;
they believe that the doctor will tell them what they 'ought to know';
the general climate of opinion transmitted to patients persuades them that they cannot cope with such information.

Communication between Professional Attendants

It is important that all health-care personnel involved in the care of the patient be aware of what he knows about his condition and what has been said to him about his illness. As far as possible they should also have an insight into his feelings about his situation. The latter may be made apparent by his comments to staff. At St Christopher's Hospice all significant conversations that throw light on the patient's understanding and feelings about his condition are recorded so that those caring for him can respond appropriately, answer questions and communicate constructively. Although the patient may well choose to unburden himself to a particular person, or to hint that further discussion might be welcome, that person may not be the one who is best able to provide the answers the patient seeks.

A great deal of information about the patient and his family is shared at ward rounds and at combined multidisciplinary meetings, where input from many sources serves to complete a picture that will enable all members of the health-care team to be better acquainted with the background, resources and needs of the patient and family, enabling them to respond with understanding.

Not all information comes from formal interviews, nor even from informal discussions with the patient about his illness. It is often while practical care and nursing are being given that the patient is likely to reveal his worries and anxieties. Much has been learned about a patient's feelings while a nurse has been scrubbing his back or during a gentle massage by a physiotherapist.

Communication within the hospice unit creates no difficulties where the team approach is fundamental and well understood. Greater difficulties arise in passing on information between health-care institutions and services. A study at St Christopher's Hospice regarding staff communication showed that patients receive most of the information about their illness from a member of the hospital staff rather than from their own family doctors, but that hospital doctors do not include in their discharge summaries a statement of what the patient has been told about his illness. General practitioners largely failed to discover how much patients knew about their malignancies and were therefore unlikely to be able to deal effectively with any resulting mental distress. In serious and terminal illness, what has been said to the patient about his condition, and his response to this, is at least as important a part of the medical record as an account of his physical symptoms.

Communication with Family

The hospice philosophy considers the patient *and* his family as the unit of care. This is a recognition of the impact on the patient of the family's response to the illness, and also that of the patient's illness on the family and on all those within his orbit. The patient cannot be at peace if family members are tense and anxious. He must feel isolated if those about him are trying to deny his condition and are maintaining a deliberate silence. When deceit leads to mistrust, he must bear his burden alone. Families who do not talk together are liable to grow apart. The failure to communicate may be evidence of denial, or of a genuine, if mistaken, desire to try to shield the family member from a distressing situation. It is the function of those caring for the patient to ensure that the importance of sharing information and giving support by communicating freely is not only accepted by the family, but practised.

    To achieve these objectives, it is necessary first to talk alone with the patient so that he has the opportunity of unburdening matters that he may not wish to discuss with his family, and to have a similar talk with family members alone. The next step is to bring patient and family together when some of the same ground is covered, so that each member is then fully aware that what has been discussed is common knowledge among them. Problems can be identified, fears allayed and realistic expectations determined. Even more importantly, dialogue begins at that meeting, facilitating what might otherwise be difficult for the family themselves to initiate. Once begun in this way, communication can proceed free of the barriers of uncertainty as to what is known or of the fear of the consequences of open discussion. The family can be assured that patients with terminal cancer are least anxious and depressed when communication is frank and when they are given answers to their questions. This is the response to those who ask that patients not be told about their illness. For the family, communication can bring about reconciliation when relationships have been poor, and can change tension and anxiety into peaceful acceptance.

Our other responsibility is for the well-being of the family who bear the brunt of terminal illness. They suffer the same emotional and spiritual distress as the patient and frequently have social and financial burdens to bear. The stress on the family is often greater than on the patient and may be particularly damaging when the decision has been taken to try to 'protect' the patient by discouraging talk about his illness. When they nurse the patient at home, family members may be subject to severe physical distress and to great anxiety, resulting from fear as to what is going to happen and concern regarding their ability to cope.

The family requires information. They need to know about the patient's condition, about the significance of his symptoms, about his medications and about the likely course of the illness. They must know whom to contact when worried and they need to be assured that help, and if necessary admission to an in-patient unit, will be rapidly available. They want to know when death is imminent and how to manage.

Particular attention should be given to children, who are commonly 'protected' from the realities of serious illness. Great harm can result from such exclusion; participation benefits the child, especially in the long term, and also the patient.

When the family breaks down, the patient can no longer remain at home. An understanding of the family's needs, and the giving of necessary support, may enable the patient to be nursed at home for long periods.

After the patient's death, the family must live on. Support at this time can prevent pathological bereavement and its associated morbidity and mortality. Experience shows that providing support for the family during the patient's illness, allowing them to ventilate their feelings and share these with the patient, encouraging them to assist with the care of the patient, and helping them work through their preparatory grief reduce stress and give them strength and peace in their bereavement. Communication becomes true preventive medicine.

Communication is Therapy

Ultimately the needs of the dying person are no different from those of anybody else. There is need to feel needed, for self-esteem and dignity, for love and for communication. Communication should at all times be conducted in an atmosphere of trust and honesty — otherwise the patient is shackled in chains of uncertainty and anxiety. When death can no longer be denied, the aim is to help the patient live the remainder of his life as fully as possible. To live effectively requires good communication. There is much we can and should say to help the dying patient. But more important than the words is the communication that we make. Our attitudes and feelings will affect this communication. Words cannot be spoken without our colouring what is said. We cannot separate ourselves from the communication — we are part of the message.

This will affect not only the patient's emotional comfort, but his physical comfort as well. It will determine to a large degree his perception of pain and other symptoms — in other words, it will influence the suffering he experiences. Many of the most pressing problems of the seriously ill patient and of his family relate to a breakdown in communication; difficulties are erased when the relationship has been frank and honest. For the person who is ill, communication is not a bonus handed out with therapy; it is therapy.

Recommended Reading

Wass, H. (ed.) (1979) *Dying: Facing the Facts*, McGraw-Hill, New York
Weisman, A. (1979) *Coping with Cancer*, McGraw-Hill, New York

22

ETHICAL ISSUES IN PALLIATIVE CARE

Ian Thompson

Homo sum: humani nil a me alienum puto. (I am a man, and reckon nothing human alien to me.)

Terence (*c.* 195-159 BC), *Heauton Timoroumenos*, 25

Introductory: The Ethics of Palliative Care

The ethics of terminal care are founded upon the ethical principles which govern our everyday relationships with other people and are *ultimately* no different from the ethics of ordinary life. However, there is an immediate difficulty here, in that we tend to regard death as an extraordinary event, requiring extraordinary measures and extraordinary ethical responses. Why is this the case?

In the first instance, there *is* something extraordinary about death. Whereas dying is an event in life, death is not. Dying is an experience, death represents the end of experience as we know it. Because death represents the unknown, and in human terms the unknowable, we all tend to shun death, to be afraid of death. The Great Religions do not make light of death and recognise that the *timor mortis* (or what Tillich calls the anxiety of fate and death) is a universal part of human experience (Tillich, 1952). The hope of life beyond the grave is based on faith grounded in a variety of metaphysical beliefs, and while some have this faith, others do not. Some face death with equanimity, others do not. We all instinctively want to live and resist dying — even if we ultimately accept it with resignation. So it is not surprising that men and women facing death make extraordinary efforts to keep death at bay. Caring professionals and families may make heroic sacrifices, and go to extraordinary lengths, in the attempt to save lives. Patients may make extraordinary demands for every effort to be made and every latest miracle cure to be tried, or they may paradoxically ask for all treatment to be stopped and even request euthanasia.

Then, too, the circumstances of death in contemporary society make it appear that there is something special about ethical issues in terminal care. Death in contemporary society has been characterised as having

461

been *privatised, institutionalised* and *medicalised* (Aries, 1976; Boyd, 1977; Choron, 1973; Illich, 1975). Death is less of a social event for two reasons: first, because urbanisation and industrialisation have tended to isolate the nuclear family from its traditional community supports and the extended family; and second, because changes in the pattern of mortality mean that less young people die and most dying is done by the elderly. These changes are quite recent. Only thirty years ago less than 40 per cent of deaths occurred in hospital; now 66 per cent do (and as many as 75 per cent in some areas) (Cartwright *et al.*, 1973). Man in urban and industrial society has in general a greater dependence on institutions and professional services to provide for his needs, and this is particularly true of his needs for health care. Because most dying is done by the elderly, this means that their deaths tend to be hidden from the rest of society. The elderly live in relative social isolation at the periphery of modern society. They have, as a result, greater dependence on institutions and professionals to care for their needs — particularly when they are dying. (Among the growing number of the very old, their immediate surviving relatives may be too old and enfeebled themselves to be able to provide any support.) The current generation of the elderly also belongs to a generation with greatly raised expectations of the power of medicine to provide miraculous cures. As a result, doctors and nurses are both obliged and expected to care for the dying and to preside over the last rites. This medicalisation of death is partly the result of demographic changes and partly the expectations which medicine itself has created. It is not surprising therefore that health professionals are being obliged to examine the ethical basis of their clinical practice in terminal care, or that their moral attitudes and ethical decisions are being brought under public scrutiny, in the courts, the press and on television.

Thirdly, it can be argued that just as the breakdown of Victorian sexual taboos was followed by a period of voyeuristic interest in sex in literature, films and the media, so too in the past decade, with the development of the hospice movement, advances in death technology and a breakdown in social taboos on the discussion of death and bereavement, we are witnessing at present a preoccupation with death in modern society. In terms of interest in literature, films and the media there has been an explosion of material devoted to exploring death and dying, and there is a risk that some of this is essentially voyeuristic in nature — a tendency encouraged by our ignorance of death and lack of social experience in handling death and bereavement. With death in the family becoming more rare, the privatisation, institutionalisation and medicalisation of death encourage what may be a morbid preoccupation with the subject. There is a risk that this kind of interest may skew our understanding of ethical issues in terminal care, investing them with an exaggerated subjective significance or melodramatic importance encouraged by the media.

It is important therefore that any discussion of the ethics of terminal care should be placed in the context of an understanding of the ethical principles underlying ordinary relationships between people in everyday life as well as in professional relationships and institutions. In this book, a number of ethical issues have been raised in the course of discussing the general principles of terminal care as well as detailed cases and practicalities. In general, these centre on the following issues: the respective rights and responsibilities of professionals and their clients/patients, the ethics of intervention (including decisions to change from therapeutic measures to palliative ones, regarding truth-telling and the limits of pain control), the rights of the dying (including the issue of euthanasia), issues relating to conflicting attitudes and values of different caring professionals and families, and issues relating to the limits of professional responsibility. Central to all these issues are three key questions: How do we protect and enhance the autonomy of patients? How do we interpret the rights of patients and duties of professionals in the context of their full communication with one another? How do we understand the limits within which professional responsibility is to be exercised? It is to these questions that we shall turn, after making some necessary preliminary ethical distinctions.

The Ethics of Different Situations are Different

When a patient approaches a doctor or nurse and asks for help, the circumstances in which the approach is made profoundly affect the way in which the respective rights and duties of the parties involved are interpreted. If the patient approaches the health professional independently in the consulting room or invites the professional to attend him at home, that is quite different from the situation where the patient finds himself in hospital having been referred there by his doctor, or where the patient is bed-bound and dying and decisions have to made between continued hospital treatment, hospice care or discharging the patient home.

The status of the patient affects the way his rights are understood (and respected). Where the patient is lucid and ambulant and approaches the health services on his own initiative, he is in the strongest position to assert his rights and he can vote with his feet if he does not like the treatment he receives. Although in principle the situation appears the same when a patient is admitted to hospital (in that the patient, or his relative, has to sign his admission form and consent to treatment, and retains the right to discharge himself), in practice his status is changed. On entry, the patient surrenders some of his rights (for example, to privacy) and professionals acquire both responsibility for him and greater power over him within the institution. In the extreme situation where the patient is unconscious, mentally disordered or a dependent infant, the professional acquires virtually total control over the patient's life and responsibility for his well-being.

It has been suggested by William May (1975) that it is useful to distinguish between at least three different kinds of ethical relationships between health professionals and their clients; namely, *code, contract* and *covenant*. The first is perhaps the most traditional, the ethics have been based on the situation where the patient is wholly dependent on the professional for care and treatment (classically where in a medical emergency the patient is comatose, insane or a child incompetent to give consent). The ethics of such a relationship are governed by the assumption of the helplessness or dependence of the patient and the need for the professional to exercise beneficent paternalism in protecting the patients' interests. The limits of such professional responsibility have been defined by professional *codes* of practice and usually supervised by professional associations.

In the situation where the patient approaches the health professional actively soliciting help, where the parties meet on terms of relative equality and negotiate terms of co-operation (and perhaps payment), then it is more appropriate to speak of a *contract* — whether this is a formal contract or an implicit understanding. Such a model is particularly suitable to a system of health care based on fee-for-service, where consumers and providers enter into explicit legal commitments. However, the contract model has a general value in emphasising the autonomy of the contracting parties and their respective rights and duties — even if the relationship is inherently unequal, in terms of the need of the patient and the power of the professional controlling medical resources.

In the case of the dying patient, there is a need for a different model which is more flexible and takes account of the shift in the balance of rights and responsibilities from the original situation, where the patient has a right to expect investigations and therapeutic treatment, to one where palliative care is appropriate. When the patient reaches the point where he is recognised to be dying and the medical team are powerless to do more than offer symptom control it is arguable that the terms of the original contract have to be renegotiated, and that the patient acquires an enhanced right to be consulted about decisions relating to his care and management. Because the presuppositions of the original contract change as hope of cure fades, and there is a need for a more flexible contract based on care and mutual trust and fidelity, it is suggested that the term *'covenant'* might be more appropriate. Explicit recognition of this changed ethical situation may not only help to clear the air and facilitate decision-making, but, in giving greater emphasis to the autonomy of the dying patient and releasing the doctor and nurses from inappropriate obligations, it creates a new atmosphere of freedom, in which the parties involved can be responsive to the changing needs and demands of the situation.

The Rights of Patients and Responsibilities of Professionals

While we may argue about rights — about whether they are inalienable and based on our intrinsic nature as persons, or whether they are socially acquired and sanctioned by convention — it is a matter of fact that certain general rights of patients are recognised in our society and are given both the sanction of morality and the law. However, rights can never be unconditional and absolute, for people do not exist in isolation and their rights may conflict. If we recognise that people have rights, then by the same token we accept that they impose certain duties or obligations on us. If I claim certain rights, I am seeking to impose certain obligations on others. This is why society does not readily recognise a right to abortion or a right to die. If these were recognised rights, then others would have a duty to enable women to terminate their pregnancies on demand, or members of society would be obliged to assist those who wish to die either to commit suicide or kill them. We consider that it would be morally offensive to oblige others to assist with such actions, if it is against their conscience.

In Britain, the current legal position is that the Abortion Act permits the termination of pregnancy under specified conditions, but it is merely an enabling Act exempting those from prosecution who procure or assist with abortions under the prescribed conditions, but not obliging anyone actually to assist. The Suicide Act, likewise, allows individuals who attempt suicide immunity from prosecution, but does not create a 'right to die'. On the contrary, the Homicide Act still makes it clear that to assist someone to commit suicide is a criminal offence. In part, at least, the debate about abortion and euthanasia is about the degree of discretion which can be allowed to professionals in decisions relating to the termination of pregnancy or the ending of life, and how much weight to give the autonomy of patients requesting help. However, there is no moral consensus which would currently recognise either abortion or euthanasia as rights of individuals, because they appear to conflict so fundamentally with the moral rights of other individuals. Even those rights which are recognised are not unconditional, because the rights of others may have to be taken into account. Nevertheless, when we speak of rights, it is another way of emphasising the corresponding duties of others, particularly professionals in the context of health care.

When a patient approaches a doctor (or another caring professional) for help and treatment, the law and morality recognise that a contract is established, whether it is explicit or implicit, in terms of which certain expectations are created relating to reciprocal rights and responsibilities of the contracting parties. In the context of health care, the most fundamental of these are: (a) the right to know, (b) the right to privacy, and (c) the right to treatment (Thompson, 1979).

When a patient entrusts himself into the care of a doctor or nurse, the professional acquires the right to examine the patient. This examination may include taking a medical, psychiatric and social history, physical examination, tests and investigations, psychological tests, psychiatric interview, social enquiry. In return for the trust whereby the patient exposes himself to intimate physical, mental and social examination, the patient is entitled to be adequately informed about his condition and its proposed management. He has a *right to know* relevant details concerning his diagnosis, prognosis and treatment. Obviously the patient's rights are not absolute, and the carer may have to exercise discretion about when and how much is told – in terms of his wider knowledge and responsibility for the patient. In fact, like all rights, their bearers may not wish to exercise or claim their rights, and patients may also be said to have a right not to know!

In general, patients only approach their doctors or other professionals for help when they are extremely vulnerable and acting under the duress of pain, disease, fear or distress. In addition to their physical vulnerability, they make themselves psychologically vulnerable by exposing themselves to intimate personal examination. By placing himself in the professional's care, for example, the patient gives the doctor or nurse the right to touch, examine and minister to him in a way that is otherwise only socially acceptable in parent/child relationships or relationships between spouses. The patient's *right to privacy* relates to his right to expect that, in return for the trust he shows in surrendering himself into their care, the caring staff will respect his confidences and respect the dignity of his person. The right to privacy is not about the right to private treatment or the right to be nursed in a private ward, although it may include both. It is more fundamentally about respect for the fact that patients surrender some of their privacy on entering clinics or hospitals and that staff should be sensitive to the fact that different parties have different degrees of sensitivity to their loss of privacy, and that some patients will have special need for privacy in public institutions. Respect for the dignity of a patient's person and respect for the principle of confidentiality really go together as two sides of the same right to privacy.

The *right to treatment* is recognised in most societies as a moral right, but in Britain this right is recognised in law — in the 1948 legislation whereby the British National Health Service was established and medical treatment was made available to all as of right. Although individual doctors have a right to refuse to take on individual patients, they are ethically obliged to provide first-aid assistance, if no other medical practitioner is available. The right to treatment does not include the right to any specific treatment, for even if the doctor has agreed to take on a patient, he is not obliged to provide any treatment demanded by the patient. He retains the right to exercise his professional judgement about what the most appropriate treatment should be. Correspondingly, the patient has the right to ask for a second opinion without prejudice to his continuing contract with his doctor. The patient is dependent on the doctor as an expert in the diagnosis and treatment of physical and mental illness. In accepting the patient as his responsibility, the doctor undertakes a contract to care, to alleviate symptoms and, where possible, to offer therapy. In relation to the patient's right to treatment, the doctor has a corresponding duty to care and to do no harm to the patient. We have seen that the law recognises this right in a positive sense, but it also recognises a negative right. A patient has an absolute legal right to refuse treatment, and treatment given without the patient's consent is actionable in law and treated as criminal assault. (That is, unless the patient is incompetent to give consent — by reason of extreme youth, insanity or unconsciousness.)

The rights of the dying are these same ordinary rights of patients, which flow from the very nature of the doctor/patient contract, except that they may take on a greater importance and poignancy because the dying patient is so vulnerable and needs others to be sensitive to and to protect his rights.

The responsibilities of caring professionals are correlative to the rights of patients and also contingent upon the situation in which they operate, for example, as single-handed practitioner, part of a primary health-care team, part of a group practice or part of a hospital team with other institutional responsibilities. It is perhaps useful to distinguish between four different, but related senses of responsibility:

1. personal moral responsibility — responsibility *for* one's own actions;
2. professional or fiduciary responsibility — responsibility *for* the care of someone else;
3. professional accountability — responsibility *to* a higher authority;
4. civic duty — responsibility *to* wider society (Thompson, Melia and Boyd, 1983).

Although personal moral responsibility is perhaps the fundamental sense in which we understand responsibility, fiduciary responsibility is of particular importance and relevance to professional responsibility in caring relationships. Personal moral responsibility relates to the circumstances in which one is ordinarily held responsible for one's own actions, and praised or blamed for them; namely, when one knows what one is doing, has acted voluntarily and without duress, and when one can discriminate between what is right and wrong. Fiduciary responsibility (from the Latin *fiducia*, meaning trust) is acquired when someone is entrusted into your care (for example, a child or dependent patient) or when a patient voluntarily entrusts his life into your hands. Having responsibility for the care and treatment of patients and the right as a professional to make decisions on their behalf, concerning their best interests, is a matter of fiduciary responsibility, and the power or authority of health professionals to do these things derives from the trust which the patient and society place in them.

Professional accountability, or answerability to one's fellow professionals or superiors and to society through the courts, is a necessary consequence of being entrusted with responsibility for the care of others. Fiduciary responsibility can be abused (professionals can attempt to 'play God') and it is necessary that the rights of patients should be protected and that professionals should be answerable to society which gives them the power, status and authority to take life-and-death decisions on behalf of others. Civic duty is the other side of professional responsibility, namely, to exercise professional judgement to advise about the staff, facilities and resources required to provide an adequate standard of health care, and to use individual and collective professional influence to ensure that the well-being of patients is protected.

Because not much curing is done where patients are dying, the scope and nature of professional responsibilities change. There is a need for professionals to recognise when it is inappropriate 'to strive officiously to keep alive' and wiser and kinder 'to settle for comfort'. Because of the changed situation and changed expectations in the pre-death phase, professional and patient need to reassess their respective rights and responsibilities — both in the interests of truth and better terminal care.

The Autonomy of the Dying Patient

It is generally recognised that the doctor exercises fiduciary responsibility on behalf of and in the best interests of his patient, or at least pious medical rhetoric suggests that the prime purpose of medical treatment is to facilitate the full recovery of the patient, including the recovery of full independence. However, the way in which medical power is exercised often encourages dependence and frustrates the recovery of autonomy in the patient. In fact, some doctors find the suggestion that people should be encouraged to take responsibility for their own lives unacceptable because it would undermine their authority and control over 'their' patients. This is a particularly sensitive area with dying patients.

The Royal College of Nursing Code of Professional Conduct (1976) states equally firmly: 'Nursing care should be directed towards the promotion, or restoration, as far as possible, of a person's ability to function normally and independently within his own chosen environment.' Now although this may be the ideal and may, in practice, apply to ordinary patients, it is arguable that nurses are also reluctant to allow the dying the autonomy which they sometimes demand. This is all the more paradoxical because of the changed status of the dying patient, relative to the health-care team.

In many ways the public debate about euthanasia and the right to die is not about the rights and wrongs of suicide or assisted homicide, or the sacrosanctity of the doctor's clinical autonomy, and even less about hair-splitting distinctions between acts and omissions, active and passive euthanasia and the principle of double effect. It is fundamentally about the need to respect and enhance the dignity and autonomy of the dying.

It is a fact that there has been an enormous increase in public interest in euthanasia and voluntary euthanasia. However, these two things are often confused and it is perhaps necessary to explain that euthanasia (from the Greek *euthanatos*, meaning a good death) has two distinct meanings in current debate. In the technical sense, euthanasia relates to the possibility of doctors acting on their own judgement to hasten the death or terminate the lives of patients whose condition is hopeless. Voluntary euthanasia refers, on the other hand, to the possibility of patients authorising their doctors to terminate their lives under certain conditions specified in advance in a signed/sworn statement, completed when they are in full possession of their faculties. It is difficult to assess to what extent euthanasia is actually practised by doctors. Some would recoil in horror at the suggestion that they ever perform acts of 'assisted suicide' or 'homicide'; others would regard the 'easing of the passage of the dying' as part of good medical practice. It is difficult to draw the line, and what is involved is partly a matter of definition, but more fundamentally a matter of sensitive interaction between doctor and patient and co-operation in terminal care.

The campaign to legalise voluntary euthanasia has led to several attempts to put Bills before Parliament in Britain, but none has been successful because public opinion is not ready to accept that it is either legally practicable or morally defensible. However, there has been a vast growth in media interest in the topic, an enormous output of scholarly papers and books on the subject, and surveys commissioned by the Voluntary Euthanasia Society (1970 and 1976) have shown in one case that out of a sample of 2000 interviewed, 69 per cent were in favour of voluntary euthanasia, that even 52 per cent of Catholics interviewed were not opposed to is, and that an increasing number of elderly people were in favour of it. The public controversy concerning the EXIT 'Do-it-yourself suicide kit' and the number of subscribers who applied for it suggest that there is a widespread public concern about the rights of the dying.

This social phenomenon begs for some explanation. One plausible explanation might be derived from an observation of Pope John XXIII in his encyclical letter *Pacem in Terris*; when people start clamouring for their rights, it is usually a sign of deep-felt sense of outrage at injustice. It can be argued that the demand for the right to a good death,

or even the demand for the right to die, *is* based on real feelings of outrage on the part of the public at what they witness of the predicament
of those dying in our modern hospitals and the indignities and injustices
they suffer.

Analysis of the various surveys done by societies campaigning for
the legalisation of voluntary euthanasia show the following.

1. That people are anxious about the helplessness of patients in large
   impersonal institutions – where continuity of care is poor and where
   patients have little choice about their lives or circumstances.
2. People are anxious about the depersonalisation of care where machines take over, where the patient can be literally lost sight of in the
   maze of technological wizardry.
3. People are anxious about professionals striving officiously to keep
   patients alive, about unnecessary tests, investigations and surgery,
   about overweening paternalism and the risk of medicated survival
   or loss of control.
4. People are anxious about the poor standards of terminal care, not in
   the specialist units, but in general medical and surgical wards where
   the majority of people die, and about the general indignity of dying.

Although there is some evidence that general standards of terminal
care are improving, there is ample evidence that the injustices are real.
There are good grounds why people are clamouring for their rights,
clamouring for more dignity in death, clamouring for more autonomy
for the dying. There is a considerable irony in the lines from T.S. Eliot's
Four Quartets when applied to contemporary health care:

> The whole earth is our hospital
> Endowed by the ruined millionaire,
> Wherein, if we do well, we shall
> Die of the absolute paternal care
> That will not leave us, but prevents us everywhere

> (East Coker, part IV)

The image of divine providence is mimicked by the pretentions of
medical power, at least in the minds of the public. Doctors, as the
priests of our secular society, preside over and to some extent control
all the crucial *rites de passage* from birth to death. At one level, popular
concern with euthanasia represents a revolt against the medicalisation
of death. It is a kind of 'anti-clinical' backlash against the loss of

personal autonomy in areas affecting the most private and important events in our lives.

Because death has been privatised, medicalised and institutionalised, the ethics of terminal care have to be seen in an institutional setting. It has become a matter of *medical* ethics. However, it is arguable that the real issue is not one of medical ethics in the traditional sense – that is, about what moral direction to give doctors in caring for the dying – but rather, the issue is one of the autonomy of the patient, how to return some measure of choice and control to the dying, how to promote and facilitate their autonomy and respect their dignity. The issue is all the more poignant because dying patients, by and large, are elderly, institutionalised and relatively helpless – lacking in dignity and power.

This is what is disappointing about the response of professionals and the churches to the campaign to legalise voluntary euthanasia. They tend to have missed the point. The medical establishment failed to see that the challenge of EXIT was to face the question of the autonomy of the dying. The recent Vatican *Declaration on Euthanasia* similarly gets side-tracked into discussion of the validity of hair-splitting distinctions (Catholic Truth Society, 1980). It is relatively liberal in its interpretation of the traditional distinctions between acts and omissions, active and passive euthanasia and the principle of double effect. But it is a conservative document in so far as it sees the ethical issues as primarily ones of the scope and nature of medical responsibility and the medical definition of death, rather than a problem which needs to be viewed from the vantage point of the dying patient.

However, it is important to pause and ask how far patient autonomy goes. Not only will there be differences between the ideal and the practical circumstances of individuals in their different degrees of intelligence, capacity for independent thought and action, and actual physical condition. In many cases the issue may be academic, because patients are unconscious or have lost their grip. Nevertheless the problem remains for the lucid patient. How much autonomy should he be allowed? How can we protect the rights and dignity of the dying, whether or not they are capable of defending themselves? Still, given the will to promote patient autonomy, how far does it go? Does the right to a good death imply the right to die? How do we square the demand for patient autonomy, the demand for voluntary euthanasia, for example, with the fact that many dying patients are unconsultable, and that death itself is an involuntary process? Or how do we reconcile the rights of the dying with the rights of relatives and caring staff? The fact is that we cannot dismiss the euthanasia issue, or believe that the provision of better death technology will remove the question. The very nature of good terminal care presupposes in ideal circumstances the knowing participation of the patient in decisions relating to his care and management. Where do we draw the line between voluntary euthanasia and the patient's rights to some share in decisions about how, where and possibly when he dies?

Communication and the Rights of the Dying

Although the chapter devoted to communication emphasises that skilled and sensitive communication is crucial to good terminal care, there is hardly a chapter in this book which does not mention its importance. That is not only true of chapters where we might expect it to be mentioned, such as those on pastoral care, nursing and social work, but it is a key element in Chapter 11 on the psychological aspects of the treatment of chronic pain; and is also presupposed as part of the philosophy informing the chapters dealing with practical matters.

Communication and the Right to Know

We have argued that patients in general have the right to know, based on the actual or implied contract whereby the patient gives information about himself in return for information about his condition — his diagnosis, prognosis and treatment. Without relevant and appropriate information, the patient cannot give informed consent to treatment. Unless the patient is incompetent, it is illegal to give treatment without the informed and voluntary consent of the patient. However, it is questionable whether these legal and moral rights are always fully respected when the patient is dying. Although the caring professional has always to exercise discretion about when and how to share the truth with someone with a terminal illness, he does not have a moral or legal right to withhold information from the patient. In fact experience in specialist terminal-care units has shown not only the need for a policy of openness about death, but has indicated that it is both desirable and in some cases essential for the patient to be told the truth so that he may co-operate in decisions relating to his care and management.

A great deal has been said and written about truth-telling, and some professionals go through agonies of conscience about whether to tell the truth or lie to patients. It has often been pointed out that it is seldom, if ever, necessary to deceive patients and a policy of doing so can only lead to disillusionment and distrust when the truth is discovered. It is not even really a matter of choosing to tell or withholding the truth, but rather of how much to tell, when to tell and by whom and in what manner the painful truth should be shared with the patient.

It is a fact that most patients know the score and are relieved to be told. Such research as has been done with terminally ill patients confirms this claim. Several recent studies with dying patients in units where the policy is not to tell patients have shown that between 80 per cent and 90 per cent of these patients nevertheless do know that they are dying (Abrams, 1966; Benoliel, 1970; Hinton, 1972 and 1979; Parkes, 1966). This is not really surprising, because patients pick up this information from many different sources. The conspiracy of silence deceives no one except perhaps the conspirators. Patients compare their symptoms and treatment with other patients, pick up clues from conversation with hospital staff (including porters and domestic staff). They observe their own bodies and feel that they are not getting better, and they infer a great deal from the non-verbal communication of nurses and medical staff (hushed voices, telling looks, silent passing of the bed, over-solicitous care, etc.). The work of Hinton and others suggests that most patients are grateful to be told the truth,[1] even if only to put an end to the dreadful uncertainty — and although some patients may not want to discuss the matter, there is little evidence to support the fear of many professionals that patients will 'give up', 'turn their faces to the wall' or 'go to pieces' — provided they are given proper emotional support and time to work through the shock and grief reactions which may be the immediate consequence of being told. Some evidence tends to suggest that the condition of many patients improves on being told and that it makes them more determined than ever to live as long and as fully as possible.

The policy of many units to tell patients only if they ask is not a satisfactory response to the patients' right to know if the atmosphere of the unit is not conducive to intimate and confidential communication, if staff do not make themselves available and create time and opportunities to explore with patients how they are feeling and what their fears are. The fact is that the right kind of circumstances for open and trusting communication have to be created, and staff have to be specifically selected or trained for sensitivity and counselling skills. Good communication does not happen by accident, and even the best communicators have to learn their skills — whether by training or painful experience.

It is often said that if doctors and nurses were better communicators, a lot of difficulties would disappear. This is misleading because it does not identify the particular kinds of communication skills that are required. The fact is that most doctors and nurses are highly skilled communicators − at least they are masters of certain styles of managerial and manipulative communication. Both are used to using their knowledge and expertise and the highly selective disclosure of information as a technique for controlling patients, for securing their co-operation and compliance. Knowledge is power and the balance of power between professionals and patients is an unequal one. Not only is it necessary for professionals to learn to share their knowledge with patients in such a way that promotes their autonomy and self-respect, returning to them some measure of control over their lives; it is also necessary for caring professionals to learn a whole new style of communication. This may be difficult when both parties have been accustomed to the other style of communication − where doctors and nurses give the orders and patients meekly say: 'You know what is best.' However, a start has to be made somewhere, and in the context of caring for the dying, both staff and patient may be moved to discover new possibilities for sharing and mutual support (Fletcher, 1973).

Engaged, truthful, interpersonal communication is costly both in terms of time and emotional energy; this is why it is easier to fall back on either managerial communication or giving the bald facts. Sharing the truth with someone, particularly threatening or painful knowledge, is not just a matter of communicating information, but demands truthfulness. Truthfulness includes having a sense of responsibility for the truth you share and for the person with whom you share it. Only a cynic will 'tell the truth and be damned'. The crucial thing about sharing the truth with someone that they are dying is whether or not you are prepared to accept the responsibility that that entails − to provide continuing emotional support while they work through the stages of grief and shock which may follow. The most charitable construction that one can put on the fact that some doctors and nurses feel they cannot tell patients the painful truth is that they recognise that within the limits of a busy hospital ward, with all the demands of other patients, they simply cannot spare the time or make the commitment to provide the needed continuing support. The fact is that people's rights do not mean anything, unless we assist them to realise their rights. A patient's right to know depends critically on the goodwill and commitment of those who are prepared to make sacrifices which truth-sharing entails.

Communication and the Right to Privacy

We have said that the right to privacy includes respect for the patient's confidences and respect for the dignity of his person. Skill in communication is involved in both. Respecting a patient's confidence is not just a matter of not telling a patient's secrets, but is more fundamentally a sensitive exploration of the boundaries of trust and secrecy, and responsiveness both to the patient's needs and the demands of the objective situation. Although medical and nursing staff usually regard confidentiality as a primary duty in virtue of the trust placed in them, there is a risk that they will either interpret this duty too rigidly in a way that does not serve the patient's best interests or they may end up paying lip-service to confidentiality in a way that can undermine the trust and confidence of the patient.

In the context of team management in modern hospital care, and perhaps more particularly in a hospice, a system of extended confidentiality tends to apply. It is taken for granted that sensitive information may be shared within the caring team. This, it is argued, is necessary in order to provide continuity of care and is ultimately in the best interests of the patient. This is acceptable where the patient understands that the information which he shares will be passed on, where appropriate, to others involved in his care. It is certainly the case that many people recognise that they cannot expect the same degree of privacy in a public institution that they expect in a doctor's consulting room or their own home, and they understand that different standards of confidentiality apply. Some professionals, as a consequence of too strict a view of confidentiality, may become over-scrupulous about passing on sensitive information. However, nothing should be taken for granted and, where possible, the limits of confidentiality should be discussed with the patient. A kind of confidentiality contract should be negotiated, for that leaves both parties free and enhances confidence. This is necessary, because trust can be crucially important and the choice of a confidant by a patient with a burden to share may depend vitally on their confidence that their secrets will not be passed on without their consent.

Sharing of secrets is one of the first gestures of affection and trust between friends or lovers. The choice of a particular doctor or nurse as the person with whom to share a secret is a most important gesture of trust, as it may also be a cry for help. Secrecy is not the enemy of truth, but may be the guardian of truthfulness in sensitive relationships with vulnerable individuals, as it is with children. Ability to keep secrets is a test of fidelity, and involves the recognition by the confidant of a responsibility to protect the one who has shared his secret until he feels strong enough to face exposure to others. This is why we all intuitively recognise an obligation to keep people's secrets. Truthfulness is a matter both of fidelity to those with whom we share the truth, particularly about ourselves, and discrimination about when it is appropriate to encourage someone to allow you to share their secret with someone else who may be able to help them, or even to take it upon oneself, for their sake, to tell someone's secret if it is vital for their good. However, the latter course is a heavy responsibility.

A particular difficulty with dying patients arises when a spouse or caring relative is told the patient's prognosis and then forbids the doctor or nursing staff to tell the patient. Should doctors or nurses feel duty-bound not to tell the patient? On first principles, it may be argued that the spouse or relative has no right to prohibit the patient being told. To whom does the doctor or nurse have the primary responsibility? Whose life is at stake? Whose confidences are they anyway? Clearly the patient has a primary right to know, regardless of what relatives may say. The caring staff may have to risk the displeasure of relatives if they do tell, but they also have a responsibility to explore with the relatives why they are afraid of the patient being told. They may have to be asked whether they are protecting the patient or really trying to protect themselves from the grief involved and evading the responsibility to provide the dying patient with the support he needs. They may also need to see the mutual sharing of the truth as an opportunity for constructive grief work, which will make the ultimate separation easier to bear because the issues have been faced and some of the emotional burden shared. On the other hand, professionals should respect the judgement of relatives as to the likely vulnerability of the patient and may be helpfully guided by them when the patient is ready to be told. However, they cannot be bound by promises to relatives and have to be responsive to the needs and enquiries of the patient.

Respect for the dignity of the person of the dying patient does not only mean protecting him by screens from public gaze when he is being dressed or toileted, or providing him and his relatives with privacy to talk together without disturbance, or attentiveness to physical comfort in both important matters as well as lesser ones, like attention to pressure areas, dryness of mouth, odour and physical appearance. All these things are important expressions of respect for the patient's right to privacy. However, the more difficult and complex area relates to the whole question of the assessment of the patient's quality of life and the sensitive response to his needs in the attempt to improve and enhance his quality of life. Quality-of-life assessments can be notoriously subjective, but as the author of Chapter 1 points out, it is possible by the use of a variety of objective criteria to identify the needs of patients and to make more informed judgements about the direction of their management.

Talk of management in the same breath as quality-of-life assessments can smack of the worst type of professional paternalism. The variability of different patients' needs and responses to their circumstances demands that the caring team is sensitively and imaginatively responsive to the particular needs of each individual.

In practical terms, the right to privacy refers to the patient's right to some say in decisions regarding his management; for example, whether he is to be treated at home or in hospital or referred to a specialist terminal-care unit. Here, the interests and needs of others have to be taken into account and the patient's right to die at home may be contingent upon the skills and coping capacities of his family and the availability of supportive services and other resources. The right to privacy relates to the right of the patient to freedom from officious medical and nursing attention and unnecessary tests and investigations. Although decisions to carry out tests and investigations may fall within the compass of the doctor's clinical judgement, if he cannot hope to cure, but only palliate, the patient has an enhanced right to be counselled and to have some right to choose.

Who presides over the last rites – the doctor or the patient? In times past, when there was less that doctors could offer the dying, it was possible for the dying adult to be given a special dignity and the opportunity to command attendance of relatives at the death-bed. Death-bed scenes where the dying conducted the last rites themselves, with the doctor and the priest in the background, may have been scarce and may even exist only in fiction, but they symbolise an important alternative to the indignity of death where the patient is powerless in the hands of an institution, denied respect for his autonomy or right of choice, and isolated from meaningful contact with his loved ones. Once again, it is important to emphasise that good communcation is essential, if the patient's rights are to be properly respected and the patient allowed as much dignity and autonomy as possible.

Communication and the Right to Treatment

In the context of terminal care, the right to treatment does ultimately mean the right to a good death, to a death with dignity. The achievement of a good death is not just a function of skilled medical and nursing care and the right death technology, but more fundamentally a function of the creation of the right environment of support, co-operation between the whole caring team, and sensitive response to the needs of the whole person — physical, emotional and spiritual. At the most basic level, the right to treatment entails for the dying the right to adequate and competent terminal care, that is, proper pain control, alleviation of distressing symptoms such as breathlessness, nausea, depression and incontinence, as well as attention to lesser things such as dryness of mouth, pressure areas, odour and the physical appearance of the patient. However, it also entails a right to good emotional and spiritual support, and this cannot be imposed upon patients by staff whom they find unhelpful or uncongenial. Both sensitivity and humility are required by psychological and spiritual counsellors to recognise when they are not needed or wanted, or where it would be more appropriate to bring in someone else with other gifts and a different personality.

The issue of what constitutes treatment may be unclear, until a firm decision is made that therapeutic intervention is no longer appropriate. The patient's right to treatment does not entail upon the caring team the obligation to try every last and extreme remedy. 'Treatment' includes both therapy and tender loving care. Palliative care is none the less treatment for being confined to symptom control, and 'settling for comfort' is treatment, even if it is not therapy. However, where possible and where appropriate, patients have a right to know when the switch is made from therapy to terminal care.

As has been ably demonstrated in Chapter 12, the question of pain control is a complex one, and the proper management of the patient's needs may involve a variety of strategies, all of which presuppose good communication with patients — careful titration of pain-killing drugs to suit the individual needs of patients, treatment of anxiety/depression, which aggravates the pain and complicates management, by a combination of psychotherapy and drugs, or more radical surgical and other means to achieve nerve blocks. To some extent, the recent intensive study and research on pain control has changed the locus of discussion about the risk of shortening the patient's life, if the doctor accedes to the patient's demand for heavier and heavier doses of opiate drugs. The principle of double effect — namely, that the secondary effect of suppressing respiration and possibly putting the patient's life at risk was morally acceptable, provided the primary effect of relieving pain was the one intended by the doctor — was invoked to justify medical practice when pain-control methods were more crude. The patient's right to proper pain control can be met with a more skilled response, one that carries reduced risk and may even lead to prolongation of the patient's life through an improvement of his quality of life. Nevertheless the old dilemmas are not removed and may surface elsewhere.

It needs to be emphasised that, like all other rights, the right to treatment is not an absolute right. Just as the patient cannot legitimately demand that the doctor give him some treatment that will rapidly terminate his life, the patient's right to refuse treatment cannot be regarded as an absolute moral right either (whether they are in full possession of their faculties when they refuse treatment or not). It may be that the law recognises that a patient has an unconditional right to refuse treatment, but it can be argued that if there is a real chance that a treatment may cure one, one does not have an unconditional right to refuse such treatment. This is a sensitive area and one where great skill, wisdom and practical experience is needed when clinical decisions are made to give hazardous treatments which may shorten the life of the patient, or where doctors decide to try a treatment which the patient refuses. However, it must be emphasised with respect to dying patients, who know and accept that they are dying, that they have a right to refuse unnecessary tests and investigations, a right not be artificially resuscitated, that they have a right to refuse further treatment and go home to die. How seriously are the protests of patients taken? How often are they treated against their will? Clearly, the unhappy cases are likely to be cases where communication between patient and carers has been poor or has broken down.

Ideally, the death of a patient should be the conclusion of a process of good consultation, co-operation and supportive communication between the patient and his carers. Nevertheless questions remain. How far does the right to treatment or right to refuse treatment extend? When it is a matter of days/hours, should doctors stand in the way of patients who want out? Should doctors advise or assist patients to commit suicide? What reasons can a secular culture offer patients as a reason for continuing to live and to suffer? Christians insist that we do have a right to a good death, but not a right to die. The hospice movement is in many ways a Christian response to the pressure from the voluntary euthanasia lobby, to so improve the standard of terminal care that the demand for voluntary euthanasia becomes unnecessary. Paradoxically, however, the more hospice care is concerned to promote the autonomy, dignity and rights of the dying, the more their staff must face the challenge of co-operating with the patient in planning his terminal care, assisting him to a good death.

Good terminal care requires and presupposes the active and voluntary co-operation of the patient in the management of his own death. The open and frank recognition of a situation as terminal and the conscious decision to switch from therapeutic measures to palliative care raise in acute form the question of the patient's right to some say in where, how and when he dies, and his right, so far as he is able, to make of his death a meaningful personal act and significant event. The question is how far medical and nursing staff are prepared to facilitate these possibilities.

Institutional Models of Death and Dying, and the Limits of Professional Responsibility

Because death in modern society has become increasingly privatised, medicalised and institutionalised, there is a risk that caring professionals will acquire greater rather than lesser power over the lives of dying patients, that they will develop more and more efficient drugs and death technology, more skilful techniques for counselling, reorientating and managing patients, more total control over the ministration to their physical, emotional and psychological needs. There are risks inherent in the institutionalisation of death not only of a science-fiction processed, packaged and delivered thanatological service, but of overweening professional power which like Eliot's God 'will not leave us but prevents us everywhere'. The issue of patient autonomy and the protection of rights of patients is a real issue as we enter the era of institutionalised terminal care, just as it is a real issue how we shall educate caring professionals into a proper understanding of their role and the ultimate limits of their responsibility.

At present there is a real risk that cancer death will become a paradigm of death. Judging by stereotypes in literature, films and the media, this is already the case in the public mind. Cancer is associated in the public mind with the most horrible kind of death — death which is inevitably painful, protracted, distressing to the patient and relatives, and necessarily involves loss of dignity. Members of the hospice movement have attempted to explode these myths by showing that in most cases pain and other distressing symptoms can be controlled, patients can be enabled to live fulfilling lives almost to the very end, and with proper care dignity can be preserved until death. Nevertheless the hospice movement has tended to emphasise the stereotype. Hospices tend to have provided care for cancer sufferers and those suffering from other chronic degenerative diseases. Much of the early research on terminal care was concentrated on cancer patients because death can be anticipated and proper terminal care can be planned. Psychiatrists like Hinton, Kubler-Ross and Murray Parkes, who were some of the first to stimulate inquiry into the mental state of the dying and the bereaved, did so with cancer patients because they often remain lucid and able to communicate until the end.

However, there are several ways in which the interest of professional thanatologists can skew the perception of the nature of death and dying in modern society. The fact is that the cancers account directly for only 20 per cent of all deaths, and although they may account for the highest percentage of deaths in women between the ages of 35 and 60, nevertheless a majority of deaths are relatively sudden. Cancer deaths affect a younger age-group of patients who may excite more of our sympathy and attention, but the majority of people dying (between 60 per cent and 70 per cent) are more elderly, tend to die after relatively short episodes of acute illness and do not die in centres of excellence like teaching hospitals or hospices, but in acute medical and surgical wards, where the ethos of staff is geared to saving lives not terminal care (Cartwright *et al.*, 1973). The risk is that terminal care will become a speciality of a few highly motivated individuals, rather than part of the armamentarium of all doctors and nurses. Those concerned with terminal care have a responsibility to educate the public as well as other professionals to an acceptance of these facts of life, and death!

There is also a risk that by concentrating on cancer death and the hospice model, we shall be encouraged to idealise the peaceful, resigned, accepting death. Kubler-Ross's account of the five stages of dying (1970) tends to suggest that ideally the patient is assisted to move through the successive stages of shock and denial, anger, bargaining and depression until he wins through to acceptance and hope. (Some earnest thanatologists have actually attempted to process patients through these stages!) The hospice ideal of a 'good Christian death' consecrated by post-Victorian Christian piety has also emphasised the ideal of peaceful resignation to God's will and acceptance of death in a spirit of faith and hope — what Cecily Saunders describes as 'going out with all flags flying'. However, we must ask whether this is the most appropriate view of death, either on practical or on theological grounds.

Is there not here a danger that the Christian ideal of a good death fits all too conveniently with the demands of the medical and nursing staff for co-operative, acquiescent, passive and compliant patients? Difficult patients, patients who are not co-operative, who die pro-testing, angry, unreconciled, despairing, are an embarrassment and a nuisance. Is there not a possible risk of connivance between Christian piety and medical convenience to pressurise patients, albeit subtly, to conform to a stereotyped pattern of dying – convenient, happy, institutional death?

In actual fact the death of Christ is an ambiguous model – at least in the various Gospel accounts. Christian theology has at various times emphasised the humanness of Christ's angry protesting cry of dereliction from the Cross; alternatively, it has emphasised his death as a Voluntary Sacrifice, or act of Celebration or Affirmation. The model of his death as one of Obedient Resignation is only one of several possible interpretations, but it is the one which has most appealed to recent Christian piety. The humanistic tradition has encouraged respect for and tolerance of a wide variety of expressions of what it means to be human, in the various ways that men may affirm their dignity of dying. In the context of human suffering and faced with the mystery of death, we should perhaps learn to say with the Roman poet Terence: 'I am a man, and I reckon nothing human alien to me.'

Bertrand Russell (1957), contemplating his own death, said:

> I believe that when I die I shall rot, and nothing of my ego will survive. I am young and I love life. But I should scorn to shiver with terror at the thought of annihilation. Happiness is none the less true happiness because it must come to an end, nor do thought and love lose their value because they are not everlasting.

Dylan Thomas (1966), contemplating the death of his father, said:

> Do not go gentle into that good night
> Old age should burn and rave at the close of day
> Rage, rage against the dying of the light
> . . .
> And you, my father, there on that sad height
> Curse, bless me now with your fierce tears I pray
> Do not go gentle into that good night

Rage, rage against the dying of the light.

Nietzsche (1958), ruminating on his own death, said:

Many die too late and some die too soon
Strange as yet soundeth the doctrine: Die at the right time!
I show you the death that consummates
– a spur and solemn pledge to the living
My death I commend to you, free death
that cometh unto me, because I will it.
Free for death and free in death,
A holy nay – sayer when the time is past to say Yea.
Thus he is at home with death and with life.

Ladislaus Boros (1965), speaks of the moment of truth:

Death gives man the opportunity of posing his first completely personal act. Death is, therefore, the moment above all others for the awakening of consciousness, for freedom, for the encounter with God, for the final decision about his eternal destiny.

These existential statements of poets and philosophers may appear to be far removed from the actuality of death – where the majority of people die peacefully, gradually losing consciousness and without great drama or emotional crisis. However, the very variety of these envisaged modes of dying should open our eyes to the different hopes and aspirations of men, make us question our own assumptions and make us, like Terence, more tolerant of the infinite range and variety of forms in which the beauty and dignity of human life can be expressed.

Note

1. Compare Hinton (1979) and Parkes (1966). Also, in a recent unpublished study conducted by staff of St Columba's Hospice, Edinburgh, 85–90 per cent of patients interviewed before admission knew that they had a terminal illness and most found relief and comfort in being able to discuss the subject openly.

References

Abrams, R.D. (1966) 'The patient with cancer, his changing pattern of communication', *New England Journal of Medicine*, 274, 317–22

Aries, P. (1976) *Western Attitudes toward Death. From the Middle Ages to the Present*, tr. P.M. Ranussi, Johns Hopkins Press, Baltimore, Md

Benoliel, J.Q. (1970) 'Talking to patients about death', *Nursing Forum*, 9 (3)

Boros, Ladislaus (1965) *The Moment of Truth: Mysterium Mortis*, Burns and Oates, London

Boyd, K.M. (1977) 'Attitudes to death, some historical notes', *Journal of Medical Ethics*, 3 (3)

Cartwright, A., Hockey, L. and Anderson, J.L. (1973) *Life Before Death*, Routledge and Kegan Paul, London

Catholic Truth Society (1980) *Declaration on Euthanasia*, CTS, London

Choron, J. (1973) *Death and Western Thought*, Collier Books, New York

Fletcher, P.M. (1975) *Communication in Medicine*, The Rock Carling Fellowship, Nuffield Provincial Hospitals Trust, London

Hinton, J. (1972) *Dying*, Penguin Books, Harmondsworth, ch. 8

Hinton, J. (1979) 'Comparison of places and policies for terminal care', *The Lancet*, 6 January

Illich, I. (1975) *Medical Nemesis: The Expropriation of Health*, Trinity Press, London

Kubler-Ross, E. (1970) *On Death and Dying*, Tavistock Publications, London

May, W.F. (1975) 'Code, covenant, contract or philanthropy', *Hastings Center Report*, 5

Nietzsche, Friedrich (1958) 'Of Free Death', from *Thus Spake Zarathustra*, Pt 1, J.M. Dent, London

Parkes, C.M. (1966) 'The patient's right to know the truth', *Proceedings of the Royal Society of Medicine*, 66, 536

Royal College of Nursing (1976) *The Rcn Code of Professional Conduct*, RCN, London

Russell, Bertrand (1957) *Why I am not a Christian*, Allen and Unwin, London

Thomas, Dylan (1966) 'Go not gentle into that good night', in *Collected Poems*, J.M. Dent, London

Thompson, I.E. (1979) *Dilemmas of Dying – A Study in the Ethics of Terminal Care*, Edinburgh University Press, Edinburgh, ch. 5

Thompson, I.E., Melia, K. and Boyd, K.M. (1983) *Nursing Ethics*, Churchill Livingstone, Edinburgh, ch. 5

Tillich, Paul (1952) *The Courage to Be*, Yale University Press, New Haven

Voluntary Euthanasia Society (1970) *A Plea for Legislation to Permit Voluntary Euthanasia*, VES, London

Voluntary Euthanasia Society (1976) 'Report of an opinion poll', *Guardian*, 14 October 1976

23

SPECIALIST PALLIATIVE-CARE SERVICES

Ivan Lichter

The focus of palliative-care services was initially on the plight of the terminally ill, particularly those suffering from incurable cancer. Impetus for the establishment of services to assist these patients was aroused by the example of St Christopher's Hospice and others that began working in this field. The need to provide relief for the terminally ill and the ability of the hospice team to do so are now well established. The hospice philosophy, which includes palliative care, is already extending beyond the hospice to influence the care of other patients.

We are seeing a change in the pattern of disease and with it a change in the needs of our patients. Infection has been largely controlled and many other diseases are capable of accurate diagnosis and curative management. At some time in the future, medical care is likely to be involved almost exclusively with non-curable degenerative disease, when patient care will be largely palliative, aimed at giving relief and support.

For the present a description of palliative-care services must concentrate on those that have been established to provide for the terminally ill. This is justified on historic grounds and on the present availability of such services. The hospice movement has provided a model on which palliative care can be based, in whatever sphere it is applied.

The Need for Hospice Care

The care of the terminally ill is often limited, deficient or inappropriate. Minimal care and attention may be offered because 'nothing more can be done'; on the other hand, the patient's problems may be seen in terms of his disease, rather than his needs as a person, resulting in undue emphasis on investigation and the subjection of the patient to unwanted aggressive treatment, when recovery is no longer possible.

About 60 per cent of people in Great Britain die in hospitals and other institutions, rather than at home. In acute-care hospitals, the orientation of staff and facilities is towards cure so that the environment is not conducive to palliative care. The dying patient requires more personal care than can be given in an acute ward, where the demands of the work make it possible for his suffering to be overlooked, and he is likely to feel isolated and abandoned. There is much unrelieved physical distress, depression and anxiety among patients dying in general hospitals, and chronic-care institutions are no better suited to the needs of the dying. Parkes (1978) showed that although home care for terminal cancer patients can be successful, it too is often associated with unnecessary suffering. He came to the conclusion that there is a need for an in-patient unit which is willing to take over whenever family or patient become over-anxious, or symptoms emerge which cannot be adequately relieved at home.

Among the major impediments to good terminal care are lack of knowledge of the therapeutic possibilities and inability of staff to deal comfortably with the dying person. Selected and motivated staff with specialised training are required to achieve excellence in terminal care. It is also helpful if there is a special place which exists solely to meet the unique needs of the dying patient. There is concern also for family members who feel helpless in the face of the patient's distress and who, with the patient, face psychological, financial and spiritual difficulties.

The Hospice Concept

Today, the word hospice signifies a home or hospital designed for the care of those with incurable illness and a relatively short life expectancy. In the hospice, care is aimed at the alleviation of distressing symptoms, especially pain, and the improvement of the quality of life for the patients, together with practical and emotional support for the relatives.

The modern hospice dates back to 1905, when the Irish Sisters of Charity founded St Joseph's Hospice in Hackney in the East End of London. They continue to provide care for some 600 cancer patients each year. But the hospice movement as such can be said to have begun in Great Britain when Dame (then Dr) Cicily Saunders, working at St Joseph's Hospice, developed a comprehensive system of care for the terminally ill and their families. In 1967, she established St Christopher's Hospice in London, which became the model for hospice care. The manifest success of the principles of care for the terminally ill practised at St Christopher's Hospice and at some of the earlier hospices established shortly thereafter (like St Luke's Nursing Home in Sheffield and St Barnabas' Nursing Home in Worthing) aroused extraordinary interest in the subject of terminal care in health-care professionals and the public. The early hospices were developed and administered by people of great dedication, compassion and ability, and their example was responsible for a rapid expansion in the growth of hospices and a variety of other specialist services for terminal care in Britain, the United States and Canada, and to a lesser extent in other countries. In the United States there are now well over 200 hospice programmes; in Canada more than 25; and several in other countries. In the last five years, probably over 400 programmes, institutions or community efforts of one kind or another have been developed for the care of the dying in different parts of the world.

Britain

In Great Britain in the 1970s there was a proliferation of facilities and services specialising in the care of the dying, in particular for people with advanced cancer. There was enormous support from voluntary groups, who collected substantial sums to pay for the setting-up of hospice services. The earliest developments were independent charity nursing homes and hospices. Between 1975 and 1980 the number of terminal-care units more than doubled. The greatest growth was in 'continuing-care units', which appeared within the National Health Service; these were most often built by the National Society for Cancer Relief and situated in the grounds of NHS hospitals, but with the running costs subsequently met by the NHS. There are also a number of Marie Curie Homes and several Sue Ryder Homes which provide essentially nursing care. Even more rapid has been the growth of home-care services. Almost all have been established since 1975, many funded wholly or partly by the National Society for Cancer Relief. Most of these specialist domiciliary services are based on in-patient units, some on hospital support teams, though home-care teams also exist independently. The most recent development has been the hospital support or symptom-control team, based within existing general hospitals and providing specialist advice on symptom control and patient counselling.

A survey on 'Terminal cancer care: specialist services available in Great Britain in 1980' was undertaken by Barry Lunt (1981), under the auspices of the Wessex Regional Cancer Organisation and the University of Southampton. The study reported that in January 1980 there were 63 separate services in Great Britain providing 55 in-patient units, 23 home-care services, and five hospital support teams in various combinations. Two-thirds of the services consisted of an in-patient unit alone.

The remainder were various combinations of in-patient unit, home-care team and symptom-control team, the most common being a home-care team associated with an in-patient unit. Of the 23 home-care services. only five were independent of any other type of service. There were five symptom-control teams, all of which were associated with home-care teams and two with in-patient units also.

United States of America

Although several hospitals run by religious orders such as Calvary Hospital in New York City were already in existence, it was not until the work of Dame Cicily Saunders in Britain that widespread interest in the care of the dying developed in the United States. Dr Sylvia Lack, who had worked with Dr Saunders in London, was involved with the establishment of Hospice Inc., New Haven, Connecticut, which triggered off the American development of the hospice movement. Since then the number of hospice programmes has increased rapidly. They are largely of the home-care type; in-patient hospice services are generally hospital based.

About 80 per cent of the care of the terminally ill is undertaken in hospitals and nursing homes. The role of the hospice is yet to be determined by the federal government. There are indeed many physicians who are critical of the establishment of special terminal-care facilities. There is concern about continuity of patient care, which they feel might be better served by co-ordinating existing programmes and making better use of these. There is fear that hospices will lead to excessive fragmentation and over-specialisation, tending to relieve hospitals and physicians of their true responsibilities. There are also formidable problems concerning financial reimbursement for hospital services by third-party insurers, and considerable legislation and other difficulties in establishing hospice in-patient facilities.

Enthusiasm for hospice programmes in the United States may be waning. Whether hospice care remains viable will depend to an extent on the willingness of the medical bureaucracy to accommodate the hospice within its framework. There will also be a need to change some of the certification and reimbursement plans, and some aspects of Medicare and Medicaid to accommodate this new mode of care.

Canada

In Canada most of the development of hospice care has occurred in the university teaching hospital setting, adapting the hospice model of Britain to fit the structure of an active treatment hospital. In

Montreal, the Palliative Care Unit established by Dr Balfour Mount provided an innovative approach to hospice care, and remains a model of excellence.

Several other hospices are now in existence, as well as hospital-based palliative-care consultation services. The importance of this aspect of care has been recognised by the endowment of a Chair of Palliative Care at the Faculty of Medicine, University of Western Ontario, where a palliative-care unit will be established which will institute an education programme for students of medicine and other health-care disciplines.

Other Parts of the World

In Australia and New Zealand, several hospices and home-care services have been established; in South Africa, small beginnings have been made in several centres to provide specialised care for the terminally ill; and in the Netherlands and India, there are plans to provide hospice care. In Sweden, the aim will be to give better care to dying patients along the lines of existing social structures by training all groups of medical professionals, rather than by establishing hospices.

Providing Care

As our skills in investigation, diagnosis and treatment have improved, the scientific approach to medical management has tended to diminish concern with our role of giving care and comfort. This deficiency was recognised particularly in the treatment of the dying patient, and hospice care was designed to meet the special needs of terminally ill patients, providing appropriate care when cure is no longer possible. Comprehensive continuing care comprises in-patient facility, home care, day unit, out-patient clinic, domiciliary consultation, consultation service to hospital departments and bereavement visits.

Although many patients prefer to spend their last days at home and manage to do so until near the end, most patients die in hospital. The final admission for the majority lasts less than two weeks and is most commonly needed to give rest to an exhausted or anxious family. Others require admission because the family situation is unsuitable or because relatives are unable to cope with caring for the patient at home; frequently the patient welcomes admission so as not to be a burden on the family. Some in-patient beds are therefore necessary to care for the dying; earlier evidence suggested that their needs could best be met in a hospice environment.

The Free-standing Hospice

A hospice is an in-patient facility designed to bring relief to the patient and his family, and to establish an environment in which the individual can adjust emotionally and spiritually to his approaching death. The hospice is able to help those dying patients for whom the acute hospital is not appropriate and those for whom ordinary community services are no longer adequate. Although the main concern has been for patients with advanced or terminal malignant disease, some hospices – like St Christopher's Hospice – also accommodate long-term patients such as those with motor neuron disease.

Hospices give careful attention to the relief of pain and have a vigorous approach to the control of all symptoms that interfere with the patient's comfort, combining clinical expertise with a philosophy of personal care. The patient's needs are attended to by a collaboration of many disciplines working as an integrated team. Hospice staff can offer time, a relaxed informal atmosphere, care for the whole person and the skills developed in constantly dealing with similar problems. To do this they have a high nurse:patient ratio, with staff selected for their personal qualities and professional ability.

The hospice philosophy encourages open communication between patient, family and staff. Hospice staff have an insight into the ways in which patients perceive their illness and their symptoms, are sensitive to their suffering, and are concerned to help them and their families share their feelings of fear, sadness, anger and love. Staff who feel comfortable talking about these problems are able to assist them in coming to terms with their emotions, in coping with the approach of death and in finding peace. They help the patient maintain his individuality and dignity, and to live as fully as possible in the time that remains. And they assist the family in dealing with the stresses that the illness imposes during the illness and after death.

Patients are admitted to the unit for family relief and for treatment to achieve symptom control, followed either by discharge or by further care in the unit during the last days of the patient's life. The majority of units will also admit patients for basic nursing care. Weekends away or admission and discharge as required can be arranged. Patients are frequently returned home if home care or out-patient clinic support can be provided.

The family is welcomed to the hospice at all times. Family members are encouraged to help in the care of the patient, assisting in such tasks as feeding, bathing and taking the patient for walks, or helping in any of a number of ways that are open to them. Patients are encouraged to bring prized possessions from home, children are allowed to visit, and pets are permitted. Physiotherapy and occupational therapy, including diversional therapy, are usually available to improve mobility and independence and help to maintain morale.

Voluntary services provide an opportunity for involving the community in the work of the unit as well as giving support to hospital staff. Volunteers function as friends and companions to the patients and family members, assist with tasks such as providing transport for patients, help with gardening, flower arranging, social clubs and fund raising, act as beauticians, manicurists, hairdressers and chiropodists, or assist with other services.

In Britain, it has been found that of the units thought to be adequate for local needs, the median level of provision is 44 beds per million of population (Lunt, 1981). Although there is a wide range, the most common size of unit is 21–30 beds in wards or bays with four to five beds. The ideal hospice in-patient facility provides a home-like environment, preferably situated near good transport facilities so that patients can be readily visited. It may be custom-built, or a converted home or building, or it may be situated in an existing nursing home. The hospice setting is designed to provide attractive surroundings for living, emphasising light, colour and comfortable patient spaces. The décor, carpets, curtains, pictures and furniture are intended to produce a homely atmosphere. Ideally, there are areas for privacy and also for gatherings of patients' families and friends. There are often kitchen facilities to warm and serve family-prepared meals or snacks at any time of day or night, and an informal dining area where patients and family can eat and talk together. Rooms are available for family members to sleep overnight, and there is frequently a small chapel or 'quiet room'. The supportive physical environment encourages a sense of security for the patient, and of belonging and participation for the family. An attractive setting can do much to elevate the mood of the patient and to allay the anxieties of relatives who have been unable to care for the patient at home.

The hospice is a resource centre for teaching medical students, doctors, nurses, clergy, social workers and other health professionals who frequently visit for varying periods of time to gain an insight into the principles of hospice care. Several hospices provide training courses for qualified nurses and many conduct a variety of in-service training programmes. Hospices also carry out research programmes on aspects of caring for the dying.

A number of studies have shown that the hospice is effective in achieving its aims of care and support for patients and families. Parkes (1979) evaluated the in-patient services at St Christopher's Hospice and showed that patients were less often thought to have suffered severe pain and other distress than patients at other hospitals. Spouses of St Christopher's patients spent more time at the bedside than at other hospitals, and patients themselves valued their presence, which appeared to allay fear.

What the hospice has done is to set a standard of care rooted in an ethic of caring. In the hospice, something more than good symptom control and personal care for the patient can be provided. The environment created by appropriate architectural design and more especially by what St Christopher's staff call 'the corporate feel of the house' are special features of the hospice. Hinton (1972) noted that 'the importance of morale and sympathetic understanding in a unit devoted to the care of dying people cannot be over-estimated, and added to this major contribution to their physiological comfort may be an enhanced subjective effect of drugs'.

These benefits apply not only to the terminally ill cancer patient. A review of 100 cases of motor neuron disease treated at St Christopher's Hospice (Saunders, Walsh and Smith, 1981) reported that most patients and families showed an impressive ability to handle their deterioration in a hospice setting. A major difference was made to the patient's quality of life and to the support of the family by a determined programme of symptomatic treatment coupled with a positive attitude.

Finally, we should consider the question of cost. In Britain, it has been shown that the cost of maintaining a patient in a National Health Service hospice bed is about 50-60 per cent of the cost of a teaching hospital bed and 60-70 per cent of a general hospital bed. Moreover hospice patients spend more time at home — at any time the hospice is likely to have at least half its patients in their homes, where it offers specialised consultation and support to families, and liaison with the patient's own doctor, district nurses and other community services. The findings in the United States and elsewhere have been very similar.

Of the many fine hospices, only a few can be mentioned to illustrate specific aspects. St Christopher's Hospice (Figure 23.1) directed by Dame Cicily Saunders, is an independent charity hospice that has support from, and firm links in policy and practice with, the National Health Service. It now has 62 beds and accommodates 17 residential elderly. The hospice is staffed by two full-time consultants and one part-time senior consultant, three registrars and two research fellows, together with a physiotherapist, occupational therapist, speech

Figure 23.1: Improving the care of patients with advanced and terminal disease far beyond their walls — St Christopher's Hospice, London

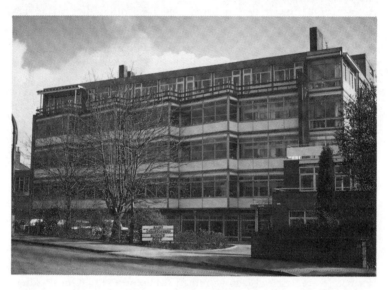

therapist, three full-time social workers and 160 volunteers. The consulting services of a pain clinic, an anaesthetist, psychiatrist, oncologist and radiotherapist are also available. The hospice provides a home-care service working closely with primary care teams, and out-patient and consultative services. A very active study centre provides a multi-disciplinary programme available to staff from other special centres and from the general fields of medicine, nursing and the allied professions. In the year 1980/1 there were about 3000 visitors of all disciplines from the United Kingdom and 400 from overseas for half-day and day visits. St Christopher's has a long-term programme of clinical research into the relief of pain and other terminal distress, and is involved in psycho-social studies into the support needed by dying patients and their families.

Sir Michael Sobell House (Figure 23.2) is a 20-bed National Health Service hospice unit situated in the grounds of The Churchill Hospital in Oxford. It was one of the earliest Macmillan units that were built under the aegis of the National Society for Cancer Relief with money raised by appeal, and on completion handed over to the National Health Service. The full-time Physician-in-Charge is Dr Robert Twycross,

Figure 23.2: Combining clinical expertise with a philosophy of personal care — Sir Michael Sobell House, Oxford

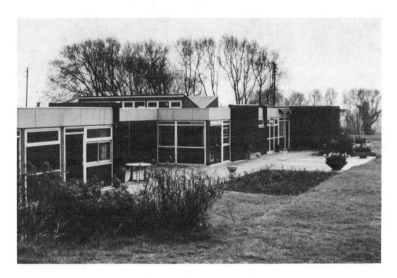

whose background includes research in pain control. While maintaining the principles of hospice care, there is an emphasis on a scientific approach to the evaluation and treatment of symptoms, with meticulous attention to assessment of mechanisms of pain and their relief. Situated as it is, the radiotherapy, medical and surgical services of the hospital are readily available, including access to the regional pain clinic. The unit runs a home-care service, a day unit, an out-patient clinic and a consultative service within the hospital as well as a domiciliary visiting service. The hospice has increasing involvement in research, and in teaching within the unit and in the medical and nursing schools at the John Radcliffe Hospital and at post-graduate centres in surrounding counties. All clinical and medical students and nurses in training receive lectures, and medical students spend two half-days at Sir Michael Sobell House. The post of Senior House Officer is part of a rotational training scheme for general practitioners. A six-week course for nurses approved by the Joint Board of Clinical and Nursing Studies is held twice yearly and two residential courses for doctors are held in the university biennially.

The Countess Mountbatten House in Southampton (Figure 23.3), directed by Dr Richard Hillier, is a Macmillan hospice unit (NHS) of

Figure 23.3: Friendly spaces for patient care — Countess Mountbatten House, Southampton

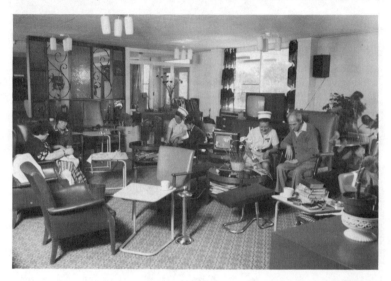

25 beds with a domiciliary care service for about 75 patients, providing symptom control, psycho-social support and rehabilitation. There is an out-patient clinic at the unit and an advisory service to local hospitals with regular ward rounds in the departments of radiotherapy and oncology. The unit has emphasised the provision of home care in collaboration with family doctors and a regional advisory function within the NHS system. An extension is planned for education and research.

Local conditions and facilities call for individual approaches. In Lower Hutt, New Zealand, the Community Domiciliary Nursing Trust, which had for many years been providing extended nursing care in the community, established the Te Omanga Hospice, a seven-bed in-patient facility housed in a converted dwelling (Figure 23.4). The hospice is associated with the home-care programme and together these provide a wide range of services, under the directorship of Dr Richard Turnbull.

In Wellington, New Zealand, the Mary Potter Hospice occupies a converted geriatric ward in the Calvary Nursing Home administered by the Little Company of Mary. A comprehensive hospice service is provided and medical students from the Wellington Clinical School visit the unit as part of their training.

Figure 23.4: Hospice — a place of care. The place is different, but the care is the same -- Te Omanga Hospice, Lower Hutt, New Zealand

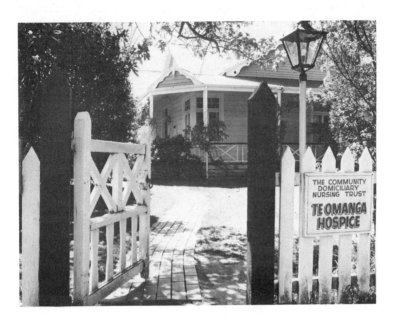

Day Units

Some hospices have day units to meet the needs of patients who may attend either for medical or social reasons. Patients may require continuing supervision and adjustment of medication, or may need to attend to provide some respite for the family or to give them time to carry out their other functions.

St Luke's Nursing Home in Sheffield has promoted this approach to care (Wilkes, Crowther and Greaves, 1978). The hospice, directed by Professor Eric Wilkes, has a day hospital for patients with advanced cancer and for the chronic sick (about 20 per cent of the total), aimed at improving comfort and prolonging independence and to enable both patients and their families to lead less restricted lives. The day hospital is an integral part of the terminal-care unit and was purpose-built, containing baths, showers and toilet facilities suited to the disabled. It also has a physiotherapy department and an occupational and recreational therapy room, an area for lunch and a hairdressing and beauty salon. In charge of the unit is a sister, assisted by three nurses who do a great deal of basic nursing. The unit has a social worker and trained volunteers working under qualified physiotherapists and occupational therapists. It is open five days a week and patients attend from 10.00 a.m. to 3.00 p.m., being transported to and from the unit by volunteer drivers.

Half the patients attending the day hospital with pre-terminal cancer have social and emotional needs, a quarter need general nursing care, and the remainder require more effective control of symptoms. The chronically sick patients attend mainly for social reasons, some having a special need for social stimulus and better support for the family. Patients attend the unit for as long as they need, 85 per cent coming once a week and some with special problems two or three times a week. It is convenient and reassuring to have the day hospital integrated with the in-patient unit where the patient is to be finally admitted. When the day unit has a rota of nurses that is common to the terminal-care unit, if admission is later needed, patients will be in the care of familiar and trusted staff.

Despite the difficulties of transporting sick patients to and from the unit, it is believed that the day hospital has resulted in a general improvement in care. Services of this type could be developed within existing hospitals to give support to home-care teams.

The Hospice within the Hospital

Many patients cannot be nursed at home in their last days and in-patient beds are required for their care. The difficulty and indeed the advisability of funding the establishment of free-standing hospices must be considered, especially if existing hospital beds are under-utilised, as is the case in some parts of the United States. Recent developments have shown that a variety of alternatives other than the free-standing hospice can successfully be applied to provide the skills learned from the hospice in caring for the terminally ill and their families.

The 'in-hospital' hospice unit is a segregated ward area in a hospital with a staff of physicians, nurses and social workers responsible for in-patient care and usually providing support for home care given by existing community services. The earliest 'in-hospital' hospice unit in a large teaching hospital was that established by Dr Balfour Mount in Montreal; it provides a comprehensive programme and remains a model for this type of hospice service (Mount, 1976). The Palliative Care Unit was instituted in a converted ward of the Royal Victoria Hospital in Montreal in 1975. The service comprises an in-patient ward, a hospital-based home-care programme, an out-patient clinic, a consultation service to the remainder of the hospital, and a bereavement follow-up service. There is a close link between the Palliative Care Unit and active oncology, ensuring constant interaction between the 'care system' and the 'cure system'.

In 1980, the Royal Victoria Palliative Care Service evolved into the McGill Palliative Care Service, with the potential for assisting in the development of similar programmes in other McGill teaching hospitals. At the Royal Victoria Hospital there are now 18 hospice beds and there is a 21-bed unit at the Montreal Convalescent Hospital. The service employs a large nursing team, which in the palliative-care wards provides six nursing hours per patient per day. It has a strong physician leadership of five full-time and two part-time medical staff, who can call upon the full range of psychiatric, medical and surgical specialty consultants available at the Royal Victoria Hospital. They are assisted by an occupational therapist, a music therapist, a co-ordinator of pastoral-care services and a co-ordinator of volunteers directing 180 volunteers. The consultative service is provided by two full-time nurses and two part-time physicians with a multidisciplinary support team. Home care is undertaken by a staff of four full-time nurses, who call in team members as required and mobilise other resources from the community. There is strong emphasis on education and research and the centre serves as a teaching resource for terminal care in Canada.

The hospice unit can be incorporated into different forms of medical practice. The Hayward Clinic in California has been integrated into the Kaiser-Permanente health-care system which is a large, pre-paid, group-practice, medical-care delivery system. The clinic has been developed within the hospital and the hospice team of nurses, volunteers and social workers work under the direction of the patient's own physician.

The 'in-hospital' hospice can appropriately be quite a small unit. At Weybridge Hospital in Surrey (a cottage-type general practitioner hospital of 41 beds), a six-bed continuing-care unit for terminally ill patients has been established in a ward of the hospital (Crail, 1980). The unit is maintained within the National Health Service and the patients' own general practitioners are expected to look after them. Patients are able to return home to be looked after by community nurses, who are encouraged to visit the patients while they are in the ward so as to familiarise themselves with pain and symptom control. In Wales there are eight two-bed NHS 'mini-units' attached to existing hospitals, providing hospice services.

When a hospice service is integrated into the functioning of a general hospital, the patient and family see the hospital as remaining concerned with the patient's needs. Hospice care can be viewed as an extension of treatment previously given with merely a shift to an alternative type of care.

In the hospital, the hospice unit has ready access to specialist consultant staff and hospital resources. Despite the fact that curative treatment is no longer envisaged, a significant number of patients receiving palliative care require further investigations to determine suitable treatment (Twycross, 1980). In the hospital, there is also easy availability of a radiotherapy unit, where appropriate treatment may often rapidly give excellent pain relief. Hospital staff are likely to request earlier consultation with the hospice team, making their services available to the patient at a time when they can derive most benefit. The hospice care service within a hospital has great potential for disseminating information and the skills of good palliative care. By example, it influences staff attitudes and care in the rest of the hospital to the benefit of the living as well as the dying. At the same time the hospice working within a hospital is likely to maintain clinical standards in keeping with high-quality scientific medicine.

In Montreal, it has been found that there is a requirement for ten hospice beds for 500 general hospital beds. It would be unrealistic to construct free-standing hospice facilities for all patients requiring terminal care in the present economic climate or probably at any time. A feasible alternative is this type of provision of hospital beds within an existing institution.

There are significant economies in the running of an integrated unit which does not require a separate administration, separate kitchens, laundries and other services. Moreover better symptom control enables patients to leave hospital sooner, particularly when there is the backing of a home-care service. An in-hospital hospice service can thus ease pressure on acute beds and save badly needed health-care resources.

The Hospital Support Team

When there is no designated in-hospital hospice unit, the needs of the dying patient are not generally well met, except where the health-care team in the acute-care ward has a special commitment to the care of their dying patients or where assistance is provided by a terminal-care support team. The symptom-control or hospital support team offers advice to medical and nursing staff in the care of individual patients with terminal cancer who are being cared for within an ordinary hospital setting. The symptom-control team may be associated with a home-care service or care may be provided by hospital-based physicians, nurses, social workers and chaplains.

A comprehensive service of this type based on an earlier programme pioneered at St Luke's Hospital in New York is that provided at St Thomas's Hospital London, where Dr Thelma Bates has established a multidisciplinary consultative symptom-control team (Bates *et al.*, 1981). It works within the hospital and in the community, using facilities that already exist in the National Health Service. The team offers advice and help for hospital patients and support for their families at the request of the patient's doctor, but does not assume their management; it has no beds of its own and patients remain in their own wards under the care of their own doctor and the ward nurses. In the community, on request from the general practitioner, the team works alongside the patient's own doctor and the existing community services, giving help without overlap of facilities. An out-patient clinic service is also provided. The unit now has four nursing sisters, a part-time social worker, a hospital chaplain and two doctors. In the future, a day-care centre is to be established and the use of volunteers is anticipated. Research is planned and medical-student teaching will be extended.

A support team can assist clinicians who prefer to be responsible for the continuing care of their patients. This type of service is inexpensive and has many of the advantages of an in-hospital hospice unit, but it does not have the special hospice atmosphere nor the advantages to be derived from the ability to assume total management of the patient in a hospice unit. For these and other reasons, hospice care may be more appropriate for some patients.

Support teams may meet difficulties in trying to establish a service. Hospital consultants may be reluctant to seek advice, especially regarding the care of a patient whose initial problem lay in their own sphere of expertise. Some may be anxious that the support team will wish to take over management, or there may be a fear that caring for terminally ill patients in their wards will block beds, although experience has shown that beds are more likely to be released by prompt and effective relief of symptoms. Some ward sisters may be reluctant to have on their wards staff belonging to another service.

Integrated In-hospital Support Services

Variants of the 'in-hospital' hospice or support team have evolved to meet local needs and resources. The Montefiore Hospital in New York has an integrated oncology service, where patients receiving palliative treatment (for example, chemotherapy) and those requiring only symptom control are treated in the same ward.

A programme to provide hospice-type care for terminally ill patients has been instituted at the Albert Einstein Hospital, a 422-bed general hospital serving a community of 1-2 million in North East Bronx (Dauber, Margolies and Spangenberg, 1980). Terminally ill patients are not segregated and care is given in general medical or surgical units. The service is provided by the hospital health-care staff without special funds and with little additional support.

At the North Tees General Hospital a nursing officer provides care for dying patients, with chaplains assisting in giving emotional support to relatives (Morris, 1981). Patients are referred by the consultant and the ward sister. After discharge from hospital, some patients continue to be seen with the approval of the general practitioner. Discussions are always held with the community nurse regarding treatment and care.

A basic form of in-patient service may be provided by a single hospice-trained nurse. Such a service was instituted at the Brompton Hospital in London and functioned very successfully.

On my own service (a thoracic surgical unit) in Dunedin, New Zealand we have adopted what is perhaps the most basic approach to palliative care and one which any hospital consultant can apply in his wards. Hospice-type care is provided by the existing ward staff, doctors, nurses, medical social worker, physiotherapist and occupational therapist, supplemented by a hospital chaplain and liaison psychiatrist. The team meets on the ward at least once a week, together with the hospital-based community nursing liaison sister and the local Cancer Society liaison officer. Family doctors, domiciliary nurses and ministers of religion in the community are invited when appropriate. Although the service was started seven years ago to care for terminally ill patients, before very long no distinction was being made between dying patients and others on the service. The clinician holds a ward round each week with the chaplain, medical social worker and psychiatrist seeing every patient, so that any needing their further services do not feel singled out or apprehensive. The needs of all are considered at the weekly meeting of the full team held at the same session. Home-care services are provided by the existing comprehensive hospital-based community nursing and domiciliary services. Needs are discussed with the community nurse liaison officer, who sees all patients before discharge, sometimes together with the nurses who will be looking after the patient at home. She also reports back regularly, and seeks advice in case of need, regarding all patients being cared for in the community. Extensive use is made of the medical social worker in the support of the family during the patient's period of care and in the period of bereavement. Consultation with other specialists is readily available and palliative radiotherapy is frequently used. The team is able to offer only limited assistance to patients in other wards.

Members of the team have from the outset been enthusiastic about the multidisciplinary hospice-type approach to patient care. Caring for the terminally ill in this setting has occasioned no stress; in fact, nurses are much more comfortable in an atmosphere of open communication and are keen to come onto the service. No extra staff have been employed and no additional expenditure incurred. Medical students attached to the unit are totally in sympathy and comfortable with the free communication and personal approach to patients that is practised on the ward.

The benefits of this type of care are extended to patients and family from the time of initial investigation and diagnosis, through curative or palliative treatment, to terminal care and bereavement, providing continuity of care by the same team in familiar surroundings. Giving this type of care and support in the earliest stages avoids many of the problems that may be encountered in terminal illness. Intractable terminal pain and distress due to physical and emotional demoralisation are seldom seen under these circumstances.

It may be that a system whereby each clinician, with his team, gives total care for his patients will prove to be the ultimate answer, with hospice units providing back-up and example. This will only become possible when a large body of doctors, nurses and other health-care workers have received training in palliative and supportive care.

Home Care

The desire of many patients to be cared for in their own homes is generally recognised. The patient is in familiar surroundings and can benefit from the emotional and psychological support of the family. The family are a vital part of the home-care team and they must know what is involved in caring for the patient at home. To be successful, home care must be accepted by both patient and relatives. Families who are able to manage the care of the terminally ill patient derive great satisfaction and benefit.

Wilkes (1965) found that about half the patients die without any period of difficult nursing and that one-quarter need only minimal medical care. About 20 per cent are difficult to nurse for less than two weeks and in only 15 per cent of cases does the period of difficulty last over six weeks. However, 14 per cent of patients dying of cancer at home are cared for by relatives themselves over 70 years of age.

When the decision is taken to care for the patient at home, care is usually supervised by the family doctor, assisted by district nursing and home-help services. The trusted family doctor who is acquainted with the family and their individual circumstances has much to offer. In Britain, general practitioners usually visit terminally ill patients on a regular basis. They may, however, be handicapped in having little experience in caring for the dying. When admission to a hospital or other institution is requested, it is usually as a result of social and nursing problems arising in connection with the family.

Hospice home-care services can assist the family doctor to care for the patient at home. These are specialist domiciliary medical or nursing services specially set up to offer advice and/or practical help in caring for patients with terminal cancer who are living at home. The nursing staff provide advice to general practitioners and district nurses, counselling of patients and relatives and bereavement follow-up. This they are able to do because of their experience in caring for the dying, and their appreciation of the role of the primary health-care team. To a varying degree doctors, social workers, occupational therapists and physiotherapists may provide back-up service, offering advice and visiting patients when requested. In Britain, medical input, where specifically allocated, is between one and two medical sessions per week for each home-care nurse. Otherwise medical advice is obtained by home-care nurses on an *ad hoc* basis.

Home-care services attempt to integrate the various existing community services such as nursing, home help, meals on wheels, linen and appliance services, and volunteer support of various kinds with a hospice or hospital service, providing continuity of care between these services and the general practitioner. Twenty-four hour cover is available to provide security and comfort for patients and their families, who may experience anxiety and a feeling of helplessness when frightening or upsetting symptoms occur. Effective supervision of this kind can only be given by a nurse who is familiar with the treatment and the drugs used for the control of symptoms. All the skills of the hospice-trained nurse are required to provide relief for the patient and family. Where possible, the hospice home-care nurse should be backed by a hospice consultant who can give advice and support. Better still are those home-care services that include a hospice doctor who is able to make home calls and provide the diagnostic and management skills of the hospice consultant.

It has been found that home-care services can best meet needs when associated with an in-patient unit. Nevertheless, improving community services to upgrade home care can reduce the need for in-patient beds by enabling patients to spend more time in their own homes. Such home-care services cost considerably less than in-patient care.

A very comprehensive home-care service is provided by Hospice Inc., New Haven, Connecticut. It was established in 1974, based on the successful home-care service introduced by St Christopher's Hospice in 1969. The service is directed by a full-time hospice physician and staffed by a multidisciplinary team consisting of an additional physician, nurses, a social worker, a clinical pharmacist, clergy, other professionals as needed, and volunteers.

The Macmillan Home Care Service operating out of St Joseph's Hospice, directed by Dr Robin Pugsley, provides a remarkable service for a population of 800,000 in a London area of 30 square miles. The service, caring for about 100 patients at any one time, is staffed by three doctors, eight or nine nurses, two social workers and a physiotherapist, who are all on-call 24 hours a day, sharing patient care with the general practitioner team. X-rays, laboratory tests and specialist consultations can be obtained in the patient's home, and the care provided enables two-thirds or more to die at home. Patients are seen only with the general practitioner's consent, after which prescribing is done mainly by the hospice doctor. Hospice domiciliary staff liaise regularly with the community nursing officer, and hospice liaison notes are kept in the patient's home when both hospice and district nurses share care. The service looks forward to employing a specialist nurse for the care of dying children and co-operation in a symptom-control team in the local teaching hospital.

In Edinburgh, the St Columba's Hospice home-care team successfully co-operates with existing services and now consists of three doctors and four nurses (Doyle, 1980). It provides an advisory service, supporting nearly 300 family doctors and community nurses within the City of Edinburgh (population 0.5 million), as well as an extensive community medical consultation service for 1.25 million people and a 'symptom-relief' consultation service in the local hospitals. There is a sitter service for home patients and a 24-hour telephone advice service. Referrals are made to the home-care service by general practitioners and consultants. When seen at the invitation of the consultant, prior to discharge home from hospital, the formal consent of the patient's family doctor is first obtained. The general practitioner retains clinical responsibility and continues to visit, advise, issue prescriptions and, when necessary, decides on admission on consultation with the

Medical Director of the home-care service. The service is part of a hospice programme based on a 30-bed in-patient unit which has a rapidly developing educational role. The hospice is directed by Dr Derek Doyle who is also on the teaching staff of the University of Edinburgh Department of Medicine.

The general experience has been that when home-care services are available, families are willing to try to care for the patient at home, if they are assured of ready access to an in-patient bed in case of emergency or extreme stress. The patient spends longer at home, though most require hospital admission in the last days. Admission, when it becomes necessary, is almost always because of stress on the relatives or the impossibility of providing further support. In less than 10 per cent of cases is the admission because of difficulty in controlling physical symptoms.

The introduction of hospice home care always requires tact and diplomacy. District nursing services may see the introduction of a hospice team into the community as an intrusion into an area of care traditionally their own. General practitioners may feel that they are in the best position to know about the background of their patients and to care for their needs, and may consider the new service an interference in their field that would tend to diminish their status. Generally, however, after initial suspicion, home services have been well accepted.

The Choice

It might be advantageous to incorporate care of the dying patient and family into existing medical practice and community health-care systems. The hospital may be the best and most cost-effective setting for organising in-patient terminal care and for integrating with existing community health-care agencies in order to co-ordinate home and hospital care functions. Such a system also ensures an easy transition between active treatment and palliative care.

Each community must determine what is best for its own particular needs and what is feasible in terms of staff, resources and finance. If only a home-care service can be supported, this can indeed provide effective help, particularly if specialist medical consultation is available. Where an elaborate home-care service cannot be provided, a single, trained nurse can give valuable assistance.

In-patient facilities must be provided and this may be in the form of an in-hospital unit of one type or another or in some areas by a free-standing hospice. The latter has many advantages, but it will not be feasible to provide this type of service wherever in-patient care for the dying is needed.

Geriatric Care

With an increasingly elderly population, chronic illness assumes even greater importance. Although no appropriate measures for diagnosis and treatment are withheld on the grounds of age, management may need to be modified in the older person by reason of overall prognosis, of disturbance to the person which is in excess of the expected benefit, or for a number of other reasons (Chalmers, 1980). The aim is to improve functional capacity by curative measures or by palliation, and by helping the patient to cope with disability.

When ground is steadily being lost over a protracted period, the time comes when a decision must be made to settle for patient comfort, rather than further attempts at cure. Providing relief and assistance with the perceived problems is not 'giving up', but 'active pursuit of positive relief'. For the elderly, care is often long-term and must be total care that ensures an appropriate balance between social and health services.

Home Care

Chronic disease intrudes compellingly into the lives of the elderly, who require a wide variety of ancillary services if they are to be properly cared for. To meet this need, there has been an increase in the range of domiciliary services provided in recent years to augment those of the primary care team of general practitioner, community nurse, health visitor and social worker. Services available to the elderly living in their own homes may include district nursing, home aid, medical social work, equipment loan, laundry, meals on wheels, occupational therapy, physiotherapy, day care and a variety of community-based volunteer services.

Day Hospital and Day Centres

The day hospital is part of the hospital service, but closely linked to the community services. The day hospital can provide facilities for clinical examination, investigation and treatment of patients who are able to be cared for at home. It can help with the rehabilitation of patients, provide social contacts and give support for patients in order to maintain them in the community. Relief can be given to relatives for a regular period during the week.

Day-care services can share in-patient rehabilitation facilities such as physiotherapy and occupational therapy; hospital patients are then able to mix with patients who have similar problems and have achieved discharge. Day centres may be run by local authorities or in sheltered-housing complexes for the maintenance of the moderately disabled. They undertake the social and recreational function of the day-care unit and give relief to relatives, but do not undertake medical or rehabilitative functions.

In-patient Care

Half of the people who die in the United Kingdom each year are over the age of 75 years. More than half die in hospital, and of those who die at home, some 20 per cent have a period of hospital care during the year before they die. Patients need to be admitted to an institution if adequate nursing care cannot be given at home, or when it is necessary to give respite to a relative who has borne the burden of nursing, or less frequently for medical reasons.

Patients should be nursed in a bright, sympathetic atmosphere that provides technical expertise, comfort and mental stimulation. Continuing-care wards for the elderly should provide rehabilitative activity and nursing which emphasises caring and support. Relatives and friends must have access to patients and to staff and be allowed to help with care. A significant number of those admitted to geriatric wards will have their terminal illness there. The best units provide a high standard of care for continuing-care patients and for those who are expected to die.

Pain Clinics

Special clinics for the relief of pain are usually staffed by a number of consultants and generally include a physician, surgeon, neurologist, neurosurgeon, psychiatrist, anaesthetist and other disciplines as appropriate. The pain clinic has at its disposal a wide variety of interventions to relieve pain, usually treating chronic pain that has lasted several months, and intractable cancer pain.

Chronic pain is frequently a multifactorial problem which may best be managed through a multidisciplinary approach. Initially, the patient is seen by a member of the staff who is most likely to be able to help. If the problem requires it, further consultation is arranged, sometimes seeking the joint opinion of a group.

Staffing and Training

The hospice or palliative-care team encompasses many disciplines and includes nurses, medical social workers, physiotherapists, occupational therapists, chaplains, other paramedical staff and frequently volunteers. Many nurses and other health professionals learn their skills by working in an established hospice, most of which provide in-service training programmes. This is the best training for palliative care. Courses that focus on technique alone are likely to lose sight of the essential spirit of the hospice, which is a special quality of commitment to the patient.

Medical Staff

Experience has shown that good palliative care is best provided by a team that includes a doctor. He should be skilled in the evaluation of symptoms and their relief, especially in the control of pain. In the hospital setting, the team doctor may undertake palliative care in addition to his normal duties, when the work does not warrant a full-time appointment. A more extensive hospital-based service might well include a general practitioner as well as a hospital consultant.

There is now a small number of medical specialists skilled in palliative care by virtue of considerable hospital experience. They have come from a wide range of backgrounds including family doctors and consultants in oncology and a number of medical and surgical specialties. The requirement is more for an attitude to patient care than a particular medical experience.

Palliative care requires good clinical judgement and skilled medical management. Changing symptoms necessitate immediate additions and revisions of therapy. Rapid control must be achieved before a pattern is established that is more difficult to alter; relief is urgent when the patient has little time left. The patient must maintain his confidence that comfort can be provided and distress eased.

For doctors, working in a hospice remains the only way of learning about the care of the terminally ill. A number of hospices in regions that have a medical school provide basic instruction for medical students which will ensure that, in future, doctors are better equipped to provide hospice-type care. For the present, few trained medical personnel are available, although more young doctors are now involved in terminal care.

In the hospices in Britain, Lunt (1981) found that broadly there were two arrangements for providing routine medical staff cover. Doctors worked in the unit either full-time or for certain specific sessions, or were available 'as needed'. 'As needed' cover was usually provided by a local general practitioner or by the medical staff of the ward in the hospital where the unit is situated. The majority of units relied on outside doctors to provide cover, with only eleven units (mostly NHS) entirely staffed by doctors working full-time or part-time in a unit. Only ten units had a full-time consultant or medical director, although 17 more had part-time consultants.

When it comes to the establishment of a hospice unit, more formidable problems are to be anticipated. Most hospices have encountered difficulties in the earlier stages, and the successful development of a hospice service requires drive and dedication of an extraordinary degree. One has only to spend a short time in the outstanding hospices to appreciate that what is remarkable about these units is the considerable charisma of those who have created them and the energy and zeal with which they have pursued their objectives. Despite wide public support, there has been professional caution and suspicion and there is a continuing need for sensitivity and diplomacy in dealing with colleagues who may see the service as a threat, and criticism of the care already provided by them. To maintain hospice development, there will be a continuing need for leadership by people with the unique attributes of those who established the earlier hospices.

Nursing Staff

Nurses provide much of the patient contact and are carefully selected, usually by intensive interview. It is important to determine the nurse's motivation for working in a hospice service and whether she has a realistic perception of hospice work. It is unwise to employ those who have been bereaved within the past year; an attempt should be made to assess how previous bereavement and stress have been coped with. It is also well to be aware that those who have a driving need to give and be needed are at risk from burn-out. Emotional stability is a vital asset. Nurses who work in a hospice must have the appropriate nursing training and experience. For those who will be giving home care, experience in community nursing and a knowledge of community resources are an advantage. Ultimately, staff are employed for their personal qualities as much as for their skills, and are usually engaged for a three-month probationary period to determine whether they are suited to the work.

The Joint Board of Clinical Nursing Studies provides two courses in the care of the dying patient and his family, most of the clinical experience being given in a specialist centre for the care of the dying, usually a hospice. In the United States, the Connecticut Hospice also provides a six-week training programme for the continuing-care team.

A recent study (Lunt, 1981) showed that independent charity hospices employed 1.17 full-time equivalent nurses per bed, whereas in the National Health Service the figure was 0.87 nurses per bed. However, the ratio of trained to untrained nurses was higher in NHS units. Almost all units had a Nursing Officer or Matron. For home-care services, the workload varied widely, with a median of 15 patients per full-time nurse, and an annual median of 64 new patients/year/full-time nurse in the NHS services and 45 in the charity services.

The Specialist Hospice Nurse

There is already a body of highly trained specialist nurses, who have gained their skills and expertise in the hospice service. It has been recommended that training should include hospice philosophy and goals; theoretical and clinical aspects of hospice care; physical assessment, symptom control, and the assessment and management of pain; identifying needs of patient and family; an understanding of loss, grief, crisis, death and dying, bereavement, and the impact of cancer on the patient and family unit; exploration of attitudes and feelings towards the terminally ill; the multidisciplinary approach and community resources; and ethical issues in cancer treatment in the terminal stages of disease.

The specialist hospice nurse is, however, just as likely to be a good nurse of pleasing and friendly disposition, with innate sensitivity and understanding who has gained her special skills working in a hospice and who has received a variable amount of in-service education.

The specialist hospice nurse must be able both to work independently and as a member of a team, and should have skills in observing and evaluating physical symptoms and emotional problems. The specialist nurse participates actively in symptom control, adjusting dosage as required and giving support and advice where necessary.

Paramedical Staff

The arrangements for social work, occupational therapy, physiotherapy and other health-care staff vary. Some units employ full or part-time staff as part of the unit team, some units share staff with other hospital departments, whereas some have trained people working on a voluntary basis.

Volunteers

Volunteers constitute a unique component of the hospice team. Their work is greatly valued and hospices of any size generally have an organiser of volunteer services and provide training for their volunteers.

Stress

Stress on staff may result in so-called burn-out, when the care-giver is not able to cope with stress in an adaptive manner. Burn-out has been defined by Pines and Maslach (1978) as 'a syndrome of physical and emotional exhaustion, involving the development of negative self concept, negative job attitudes and loss of concern and feeling for clients'. Hospice nursing may entail considerable stress, yet there is little published evidence about rates of staff turnover to support the commonly held opinion that there is a high-rate of burn-out among hospice nurses.

Burn-out is usually due to a number of factors, rather than one particular stress, and does not occur suddenly. When it develops there are physical, emotional and behavioural manifestations that can readily be recognised. The burn-out subject may describe fatigue, inablity to relax, headaches, gastrointestinal disturbances, loss of appetite, weight change, sleeplessness, respiratory problems and frequent colds. There may be an increase in the use of alcohol and cigarettes or drugs, and irritability, depression and paranoia. Powerlessness and lessening of job satisfaction may be felt. Behavioural changes may be manifested in increasing isolation from fellow workers, absenteeism and decreased effectiveness, and serious changes in interpersonal relationships involving family and friends. Friel and Tehan (1980) reviewed burn-out in a hospice home-care service. They related stress to work environment and to endogenous factors.

The hospice nurse has an important role in decision-making and the home-care nurse, who visits alone, may carry the additional stress of a heavy caseload. Hospice nurses spend a great deal of time with anxious and apprehensive patients and families who require support and assurance. In addition, they have to bear the burden of frequent death and will inevitably become emotionally involved with some of their patients, suffering feelings of loss when the patient dies. Working with dying patients is also a constant reminder of one's own mortality.

An important source of stress is inadequate training, so that the nurse feels incompetent to deal with the problems she meets in the care of the dying patient and family.

In the earlier stages of the establishment of a hospice service, additional tension and stresses are engendered by the need to integrate the service into the existing health-care system, especially if there is resistance or a feeling of competition. The hospice facility is an idealistic one which promotes a sense of mission and a deep personal commitment to the care of the dying patient. Staff therefore have high expectations of themselves. There may be a sense of urgency to relieve physical symptoms and a feeling of responsibility to be available at any time and to respond to patients or relatives who wish to discuss their problems. Nurses will feel disappointed, if they are unable to meet these goals consistently.

Prevention

Burn-out may be prevented or alleviated by appropriate measures. Administrators must recognise the problem and take measures to ease stress by creating suitable work environments and conditions, and by providing appropriate support. A private, attractive place for the hospice home-care team to work in while at the central office is helpful. Nurses should have their own common room, where they can meet and talk freely and should have adequate breaks for relaxation. Days off should be arranged to suit their preference; and frequent short vacations should be encouraged. Opportunity should be given for rotation to other types of work such as volunteer training and other hospice projects. Care must be taken not to overburden home-care nurses, whose stress can be alleviated by having other team members occasionally accompany them on home visits.

In hospices like St Christopher's, stress is diminished by the mutually supportive, self-contained, close-knit community of staff who tend to remain for a period of time, and who appreciate one another as individuals. In such an environment stress may be recognised by understanding colleagues who can provide opportunities for ventilation of problems. A variety of patient and staff programmes gives additional relief from the cares of hospice work. Importantly, strong leadership and a sense of mission are a source of emotional support.

An important means of avoiding undue stress is to ensure that health-care personnel are properly trained, so that they are able to deal confidently with the problems of patients and their families. Such training should include development of interpersonal skills to enhance communication and abilities in counselling.

Combined ward meetings provide an opportunity for reviewing and discussing difficult problems related to patient care. Support and guidance is given by the consultant, so that the responsibility of decision-making is shared. It is helpful also to hold regular meetings where frustrations and concerns can be expressed.

Nurses are subjected to the reactions of patients and family and may be required to deal with feelings of anger, frustration, depression and anxiety. They will also have to manage their own feelings associated with caring for the dying patient and his family, and should have access to a mental health specialist who can help them deal with stresses and personal problems. At other times they may prefer to seek advice and help from the matron, the social worker, the chaplain, or their nursing colleagues. Not all problems are about work, but may include home and family difficulties.

Team members must have a realistic perception of the stresses involved in the work and take a personal responsibility for their emotional needs. A stable personal life and a supportive family and friends reduce stress and increase feelings of self-esteem.

It is preferable for staff to live away from their place of work so that they can spend their free time in a different environment, mix with people unconnected with their work, and pursue a variety of interests. In this way, they can bring something of the outside world into the restricted lives of their patients. Part-time staff, many of whom are married and have families, can make a special contribution in this way. They are also liable to suffer less stress.

The Way Ahead

Experience has already shown that hospice-type care can be applied in any setting by the organisation of currently available services. There should therefore be no serious obstacle to its wider incorporation into the pattern of traditional medical practice. This will require improved communication with all those providing care.

To date, most of the effort has been limited to patients dying with cancer, especially in the last three months of life. Less has been done for those whose illness takes a more protracted course. Yet much distress can be avoided by early palliation and support, which may also make the terminal stages less painful. A stated objective of hospice care is to assist the patient to live the life that remains as fully as possible. This can best be done before serious disability limits achievable goals. Care at this stage is no doubt outside the scope of the hospice; yet it is a sphere where much useful palliation can be provided.

In a report by the Wellington Health Services Advisory Committee, New Zealand (1981), it is noted that in their area the interval between recognition of terminal illness and death was 44-7 weeks (50 per cent due to cancer and 28 per cent to cardiac disease). There is thus a need for palliative care to be offered before it becomes terminal care.

Little support has been provided for those with chronic conditions other than cancer that may lead to death over a longer period of time. There is need for extension of the hospice philosophy to encompass not only the dying, but all those in distress, whether their illness be terminal, chronic incurable disease or even short-lived acute illness. A greater awareness of the therapeutic possibilities for providing relief of disturbing symptoms and appreciation of the emotional distress which is so often a component, coupled with a reorientation of attitude towards giving 'total' care, will affect the general approach and practice of professional staff in whatever sphere they work.

For the provision of palliative-care services in the future, there will probably be greater concentration on symptom-control teams or support nurses in hospitals, and of home-care teams that work closely with the primary care team of the family doctor, the community nurses and the home-care services (Lunt and Hillier, 1981). Even where minimal resources preclude a sophisticated home-support team, care can be improved by making available trained nurses to work within the community. These services, supported by day-care facilities, can reduce the requirement for in-patient beds.

When beds are required, integrated care within hospitals or hospice-type care delivered within general hospital ward services provide workable alternatives that can be established in any hospital. For those who would be better cared for in a hospice unit, the 'hospice within the hospital', providing care within the framework of existing institutions, may prove the most realistic solution.

It is unlikely that there will be any great expansion in free-standing hospices. There will, however, continue to be a need for special units that serve as models of expertise, disseminating their skills and, above all, their attitudes and continuing to carry out their function of teaching and research. Hospices associated with schools of medicine and nursing will provide for doctors and nurses in training, as well as for other health service personnel.

A recent survey by Dr Colin Murray Parkes (1983) has revealed a heartening improvement in the care of the terminally ill in general hospitals. Medical and nursing professions which had come to concentrate on curative treatment and on technical skills are learning to place appropriate emphasis on palliation, on caring, and on seeing the patient and his family more clearly as persons needing relief in their distress.

References

Bates, T., Hoy, A.M., Clarke, O.G. and Laird, P.P. (1981) 'The St Thomas' Hospital terminal care support team', *Lancet*, i (8231), 1201-3

Chalmers, G.L. (1980) *Caring for the Elderly Sick*, Pitman Medical, Tunbridge Wells

Crail, R.B. (1980) 'A pilot scheme in continuing care', *Practitioner*, 224, 126-7

Dauber, L.G., Margolies, E. and Spangenberg, S.E. (1980) 'Hospice in hospital', *New York State Journal of Medicine,* 80 (11), 1721-3

Doyle, D. (1980) 'Domiciliary terminal care', *Practitioner*, 224, 575-82

Friel, M. and Tehan, C.B. (1980) 'Counteracting burn-out for the hospice caregiver', *Cancer Nursing*, 3, 285-93

Hinton, J. (1972) *Dying*, Penguin Books, Harmondsworth

Lunt, B. (1981) *Terminal Cancer Care: Specialist services available in Great Britain in 1980*, Wessex Regional Cancer Organisation and University of Southampton, Southampton

Lunt, B. and Hillier, R. (1981) 'Terminal care: present services and future priorities', *British Medical Journal*, 283 (6291), 595-8

Morris, W.A. (1981) 'Care of the terminally ill in a district general hospital', *British Medical Journal*, 282 (6260), 287

Mount, B.E.M. (1976) 'The problem of caring for the dying in a general hospital: the palliative care unit as a possible solution', *Canadian Medical Association Journal*, 115 (2), 119-21

Parkes, C.M. (1978) 'Home or hospital? Terminal care as seen by surviving spouses', *Journal of the Royal College of General Practitioners*, 28, 19-30

Parkes, C.M. (1979) 'Terminal care: evaluation of in-patient service at St Christopher's Hospice', *Postgraduate Medical Journal*, 55, 517-27

Parkes, C.M. (unpublished) ' "Hospice" versus "hospital" care: re-evaluation after 10 years as seen by surviving spouse'

Pines, A. and Maslach, C., (1978) 'Characteristics of staff burn-out in medical health setting', *Hospital and Community Psychiatry*, 29, 233-7

Saunders, C.M., Walsh, T.D. and Smith, M. (1981) 'A review of 100 cases of motor neuron disease in a hospice', in C.M. Saunders, D.H. Summers and N. Teller (eds), *Hospice: The Living Idea*, Edward Arnold, London

Wellington Report of the working group of the Wellington Health Services Advisory Committee (1981) *The Care of the Terminally Ill*, Wellington Health Services Advisory Committee, Wellington

Twycross, R.G. (1980) 'Hospice care – redressing the balance in medicine', *Journal of the Royal Society of Medicine*, 73, 475-81

Wilkes, E. (1965) 'Terminal care at home', *Lancet*, i, 799-801

Wilkes, E., Crowther, A.G.O. and Greaves, C.W.K.H. (1978) 'A different kind of day hospital – for patients with preterminal cancer and chronic disease', *British Medical Journal*, 2, 1053-6

Recommended Reading

Ajemian, I. and Mount, B.M. (1980) *The Royal Victoria Hospital Manual on Palliative Hospice Care*, Arnon Press, New York

Doyle, D. (1979) *Terminal Care*, Churchill Livingstone, Edinburgh

Lack, S.A. and Buckingham, R.W. (1978) *The American Hospice,* Hospice Inc., Hospice Institute for Education and Training and Research Inc., Newhaven, Conn.

Lamerton, R. (1980) *Care of the Dying*, Penguin Books, Harmondsworth

Saunders, C.M. (1978) *The Management of Terminal Disease*, Edward Arnold, London

Saunders, C.M., Summers, D.H. and Teller, N. (1981) *Hospice: The Living Idea*, Edward Arnold, London

Twycross, R.G. and Ventafridda, V. (1980) *The Continuing Care of Terminal Cancer Patients*, Pergamon Press, Oxford

Wilkes, E. (1982) *The Dying Patient*, MTP Press, Lancaster

24 AIDS AND ADAPTATIONS

Peter J. Swarbrick

Whether one is considering providing a specific aid to assist in the management of severe disability or considering adapting existing domestic appliances – furniture or the house itself – it is perhaps obvious, but probably in need of emphasising, that the aid or adaptation should improve the quality of life of the patient for whom it is provided. It is obviously important that the individual sees it as fulfilling such a function and will in fact therefore make use of it, whether it is a cheap and simple modification of a commonplace article or a lavish, complex and specially designed piece of apparatus. The fact that a significantly high proportion of aids are not used regularly indicates some lack of thought – either as regards the initial suitability of an aid, or inadequate instruction in its use, or monitoring of its continued effectiveness.

However, what is possibly more common, and less to be condoned, is the failure to provide aids – either through ignorance of their existence or of the means of obtaining them, or because it is considered that the expectation of life is so short that it is 'not worth it'. Apart from the fact that prognosis in terms of time in many so-called 'end-state' conditions is extremely difficult to predict accurately, there is a moral responsibility to make this time as worthwhile as possible. It is easy to allow the feeling that medical treatment has 'failed' to influence excessively one's attitude in the further care of the individual.

Purposes of Aids and Adaptations

To the patient:

> to relieve pain and discomfort;
> if possible, to give greater independence, especially in such personal activities as dressing and toileting, and thereby maintaining or improving self-respect;
> to relieve what may be at times considerable guilt at the help required from the carer.

518

To the carer:

to relieve physical stress whether short or long-term;
to relieve emotional stress to enable him or her to continue to cope
with caring;
if possible, to enable that carer to have more free time.

Although consideration is given here mainly to the home situation,
many general points apply within a hospital or similar institutions.

Pertinent Points in Aid Provision

Plan Ahead

It is important to try and anticipate what the next stage in an individual's requirement for aids and adaptations will be for a variety of reasons.

1. One may be able to prevent an unwanted condition; for example, it is better to prevent a pressure sore, rather than to give the carer extra work and the patient increased pain from treatment of an established sore.
2. An earlier provision of an aid may give someone a greater degree of independence; for example, the provision of a wheelchair while the patient is still able to self-propel is a much more positive approach than waiting until one is needed purely to enable a carer to move the individual to and from the toilet.
3. Some aids for adaptations may take a considerable time to be provided or to carry out, because of financial or bureaucratic constraints.

Look for Simplicity

The simpler the aid, the easier it is to use and the less chance it has of going wrong. For example, an air-cell pressure-relieving mattress is often more comfortable for the patient and certainly has less problems than many electrically-operated mattresses which not only frequently break down, but often produce a persistent wearying noise.

The other highly relevant point about simplicity in an aid is that it *should* be much cheaper, whether commercially produced or home made. The help that it gives may be totally out of all proportion to its costs. For example, a spoon or fork can have its handle thickened by foam rubber, enabling someone with stiff, weak or unsteady fingers to feed him or herself; a simple sliding board may enable someone to transfer from bed to chair.

Predict Problems Likely to be Caused by the Use of an Aid or Adaptation and Get Expert Help in Provision of Aids

These points are complementary to each other. It is important that the professional providing the aid is familiar with its use and also able to explain to and train the patient and the carer in the correct, efficient and *safe* use of the aid. It is also important to be able to predict the effect that the use of the aid will have on other aspects of the local environment. An obvious example of this is the provision of a mobile hoist. Pain and distress may be caused to a patient because of the methods used to lift him or her, both by professional as well as non-professional carers. A considerable amount of physical strain is also imparted to the lifter. In a number of instances these problems can be overcome by the correct use of a mobile hoist. However, for safe use of a hoist, experience and training in the correct choice of sling and manipulation of the hoist is required. Use of the hoist is also much more time-consuming in most instances and also, particularly within limited areas within the home, there may be problems in moving it from one room to another, or within a room. Unless the professional concerned gives a considerable amount of training and support to both the carer and the patient, a potentially highly useful item of equipment will not be used, and continuing distress will be caused to them both.

Who Has the Expertise? There is still a tendency on the part of doctors to undervalue the knowledge and expertise of other professions in the assessment of needs of severely disabled patients. This is unfortunately combined with a lack in medical training of providing an understanding of the possibilities that aids provide. One should therefore perhaps consider the roles of other professionals.

The Nurse. In fact probably of all professionals, the nurse has the most involved contact with the patient and is possibly the person that should be able to assess most clearly an individual's needs. However, once again his or her training has been geared to the nurse being the active giver and the patient the passive receiver of care. As most training is received in acute units, where the stress is on carrying out a task as efficiently and as quickly as possible, it is very difficult to adjust to a situation where it is better for the patient to be allowed more independence, but which may be more time-consuming, at least in the short term, for the nurse. Training has also been geared to the idea that there will always be another more or less skilled assistant available to help, for example, in lifting and transferring a patient. However, back strain amongst hospital nurses sharing a lifting task is highly prevalent — the problem is obviously even greater in home surroundings, where there may be only one person to attempt to lift.

The Occupational Therapist. Of all professional staff, whether in hospital or community, who are involved in the care of a disabled patient, the occupational therapist has in fact received the most training in assessing those problems associated with disability and in using aids to overcome these difficulties. Many hospitals still do not have an occupational therapy department, and many departments which do exist are not adequately used by the physicians. The patient can be taught to transfer to and from bed, bath and toilet, and also the appropriate handling of a wheelchair. Liaison of the hospital therapist with the community therapist, who can assess needs within the patient's own home enables adaptations to be carried out as appropriately and as expeditiously as possible, with subsequent training in and monitoring of the effectiveness of the facilities supplied.

The Physiotherapist. The physiotherapist is probably involved to a much lesser extent at such an advanced stage and is most likely to be asked to advise on perhaps the most suitable walking aids. On the other hand, one must not consider that maintenance of walking for as long as possible is most suited to any individual's need — half an hour's painful limited walking can be more exhausting and achieve a fraction of that achieved by a whole day in a wheelchair.

The Speech Therapist. The speech therapist should be thought of in a wider sense of dealing with communication problems. This becomes particularly relevant in, for example, degenerative neurological disorders such as motor neuron disease, where the intellect may be painfully alert to the inability to communicate. The speech therapist is able to assess whether as much can be achieved by a simple inexpensive speech board as by going to the expense of providing one of the increasing range of electronic communicator devices.

The Clinical Psychologist. The clinical psychologist does not provide any actual physical aids, but may be the person best able to establish the true needs of the individual as opposed to the needs perceived by the professional.

The important thing obviously is that no matter whose expertise and advice is sought, communication between professionals should be good and there should be a willingness to accept different ways of looking at the problem than perhaps one is used to.

Monitoring the Use of Aids

It is not sufficient simply to provide an aid and instructions in its use. Regular monitoring of its effectiveness must be carried out. If an aid is not being used one might ask the reasons why. Is it because it is inappropriate; wrong size; incorrectly adjusted; or, having once been useful, is it no longer suitable following the progression of the condition? Apart from monitoring being of immediate help to the patient, it also enables recycling of sometimes expensive equipment for the earlier use of others.

Avoid Overprotectiveness

Because of the severity of the condition and a high degree of dependency of the patient, there often is fear on the part of the carer that the greater independence provided by an aid or adaptation will expose the patient to increased risks of injury, etc. Although this is possibly so, the degree of risk has often been exaggerated. In any case, within reason and as long as the risk is explained to and understood by the individual and family, and accepted by them, its dangers are far outweighed by the benefits – both physical and psychological – that this extra independence provides.

It is impossible and would be totally impracticable to attempt to provide a list of aids and adaptations available. The most important thing for any person thinking about their use is to be able to gain access to the appropriate provider of equipment or advice.

APPENDIX

Examples of Simple Aids

These are commercially available and relatively cheap or able to be home-made.

Toileting	— Toilet seat raise — surrounding rails
Bathing	— Bath seat and board
Grooming	— Long-handled comb or brush
Dressing	— Fastenings made of Velcro, long-handled shoe-horn
Feeding	— Modified or special cutlery
Sitting	— High chair or chair raised on blocks
Writing	— Adapted pen or pencil
Reading	— Book-rest, rubber thimble to turn over pages
Transferring	— Sliding board, blocks under bed or chair
Pressure Areas	— Sheepskin
Aids to Mobility	— Walking frames, crutches, tripod walker

More Complex Aids

Bathing	— Fixed bath hoist
Transferring	— Hoist, either fixed gantry or electrical — which may be patient operated — or mobile, attendant operated
Pressure Areas	— Pressure-relieving mattress or wheelchair cushion, air suspension beds, cast body shell
Mobility	— Wheelchair, self or attendant propelled, standard or purpose built or adapted electric
Environmental control	— Remote control or electronic systems of varying degrees of complexity and cost, e.g. Possum

Adaptations to Home

These may involve greater or smaller structural alterations. Most are

523

relatively expensive. Examples are:

Ramping at outside door for wheelchair.
Provision of lift whether on stair or directly vertically between rooms.
Building on of additional purpose-built room, e.g. bathroom.
Widening of doorways to accommodate other equipment, e.g. mobile hoists or wheelchairs.

Responsibilities for Providing Aids and Adaptations Within the United Kingdom

The provision of those aids and adaptations undertaken by statutory bodies are fairly well defined. What is variable is the ability and desire of statutory bodies in different parts of the Country to provide these services. A useful guide is the NHS Memorandum, 1976 (GEN) 90 quoted subsequently, but basically the provision of aids and equipment is the responsibility of:

1. The Health Authority where (a) they are directly related to the management of an illness, especially to facilitate the patients domiciliary nursing care or to the rehabilitation of the patient from hospital; or (b) skills in a particular discipline within the nursing service are more appropriate to the prescription and use of aids required on medical and nursing grounds, e.g. the provision of walking aids by physiotherapists.
2. The Local Authority Social Work or Social Services Department where the aids or equipment are required to help the disabled person achieve a greater independence within his or her own home and are predominantly of a domestic character, e.g. aids to daily living.

Where structural adaptations to houses are required to make them suitable for handicapped people the local Housing Authority may:
(a) carry out such adaptations to their own houses with the aid of a Housing subsidy or
(b) contribute to the cost of such adaptations to privately owned houses where the work is unsuited to other grant aided improvement work.

Provision of wheelchairs is made through Artificial Limb and Appliances or Vehicle Centres which are situated in the main centres of population throughout the United Kingdom and are administered jointly by the National Health Service and the Department of Health and Social Security or Scottish Home and Health Department.

Provision of Mobile Hoists comes into a grey area — the responsibility for this varies in some parts of the country and it would be advisable to contact the local Social Services or Social Work Departments or the local Health Authority to establish if there is a local policy.

Mobile Aid Centres

These are travelling exhibitions which tour the country. Contact the organisers for details of places to be visited.

Mobile Aids Centre, Scottish Information Service for the Disabled, 18-19 Claremont Cres., Edinburgh, EH7 4QD

Travelling Exhibition of Aids, Royal Association for Disability and Rehabilitation, 25 Mortimer St, London, W1N 8AB

Visiting Aids Centre, Spastics Society, 12 Park Cres., London, W1N 4EQ

Rehabilitation Engineering Movement Advisory Panels (Remap) Thames House, North Millbank, London SW1P 4QG

A voluntary organisation of engineers with 40 different regional panels which offers technical expertise to help solve specific problems.

Publications

(a) *Equipment for the Disabled,* 2 Foredown Drive, Portslade, Sussex, BW4 2BB. Compiler E.R. Wiltshire, published by: Oxford Regional Health Authority. A series of booklets, regularly reviewed, listing and illustrating equipment, both manufactured and self-made. Advice is offered on selection, and solutions to various problems suggested. Titles in Series:

Wheelchairs	Hoists and Walking Aids	Housing & Furniture
Personal Care	Disabled Mother	Outdoor Transport
Communications	Home Management	Clothing & Dressing
Leisure & Gardening	Disabled Child	for Adults

(b) *Provision by Health Boards and Local Authorities of Aids and Equipment for Disabled People and Adaptations to their home,* NHS Memorandum (1976 (Gen) 90. This defines the areas of responsibility in Scotland for providing aids and adaptations and also acts as a useful *aide-mémoire* of the range of aids available.

(c) Peggy Jay – *Coping with Disablement,* Consumers Association, 1976. A practical manual which covers the common areas of difficulty and offers some of the more usual solutions – including simple 'Do it yourself' aids. It gives general advice on selection of the more appropriate type of aid, and on the avenues of approach for obtaining the aids.

(d) Christine Tarling – *Hoists and their Use,* Heinemann, 1980. This book has gathered together information on the different types of hoists with the object that those caring for severely disabled people can choose the correct equipment. It examines training in the use of hoists and slings.

(e) *Home Made Aids for the Disabled,* British Red Cross Society, London, 1969.

(f) *Rehabilitation Today,* Update Publications, London, 1977, Stephen Mattingly, Ltd. Particular chapters:

Ch. 12 – Aids and Appliances
Ch. 13 – Wheelchairs and Powered Vehicles
Ch. 18 – The Severely Disabled

(g) Nichols – *Rehabilitation of the Severely Disabled Vol. II – Management,* Butterworth, London, 1971. The main part of this book provides a particularly lucid guide to general problems of highly dependent patients with detailed suggestions for aids and adaptations and also deals with particular problems caused by specific disabilities. Several appendices provide specific solutions to individual functional problems.

(h) Sidney Thwart – *Handicapped at Home,* a Design Centre Book in association with the Disabled Living Foundation, it provides practical advice on ways to plan and equip homes for maximum independence.

(i) Gloria Hale (ed.) *Resource Book for the Disabled,* Imprint Books, Ltd, London, 1979 (also available in USA, Canada, South Africa and Australasia). A general book aimed particularly at the individual and his or her family in giving specific advice on, among other things, aids and adaptations and the way to obtain them.

(j) Darnborough and Kinride — *The Directory for the Disabled*, 1st edn 1977, especially sections:

(2) Aids — their provision and availability

(3) House and Home

Information about Aids — USA

1. *Accent on Information,* PO Box 700, Bloomington, Illinois 61701. A computerised retrieval system, which provides information on a variety of subjects. A search request form may be sent for which lists different categories including aids and adaptations.

   Accent on Living's Buyer's Guide is a 70-page booklet which lists the names and addresses of manufacturers of products for the disabled and related publications. Companies in the list will all send catalogues on request.

2. *Institute of Rehabilitation Medicine,* 400 East 34th Street, New York, 10016. Publishes many books and leaflets and periodicals dealing with aids to daily living. Write for publication list — includes list of commercial sources for adapative equipment.

3. *National Rehabilitation Association,* 1522 K Street, NW Washington DC 20005. Membership open to everyone concerned with problems common to all disabled people — various publications and pamphlets.

4. *Federal Information Centers,* in 77 major cities will direct individuals to the correct federal, state or local agency needed. The telephone number appears in the telephone directory under 'US Government, Federal Information Centre'; or write to General Services Administration, Washington DC 20405 for a leaflet 'Federal Information Centers'.

5. *Publications*

   (a) Lowan and Klinger — *Aids to Independent Living — Self-help for the Handicapped*. A classic compilation of aids, and advice covering almost every area of daily living.

   (b) *Sources of Information on Self-help Devices for Handicapped*. An annotated bibliography free from the National Easter Seal Society for Crippled Children and Adults, 2023 West Ogden Ave., Chicago, Illinois, 60612.

Information on Aids — Canada

Canadian Rehabilitation Council for the Disabled (CRCD), Suite 2110, One Tonge St, Toronto, MSE 1ES. A national federation of voluntary organisations who are concerned with and committed to helping the physically disabled. Provides among other services the following:

1. *Technical Aids and Systems for the Handicapped, Inc.* This is a technical aids supply centre under the auspices of CRCD, with the responsibility to market, distribute and service technical aids for the handicapped which are unavailable through other means.
2. *Resource Manual of Canadian Information Service for the Physically Disabled.* A Directory of Services available in Canada, listed by province. Updated regularly. Available on subscription.
3. Regular Publications — *Rehabilitation Digest* — has regular Bulletins on Technical Aids.

Information on Aids — Australia

1. Australian Council for Rehabilitation of Disabled (ACROD), Bedford and Buckingham Streets, Surryhills, New South Wales, 2010 — National Federation of Voluntary bodies conducting programmes to disabled people. Provides information service and publishes 'Directory of Services for Disabled People'.

Information on Aids — New Zealand

1. *Provision of Aids and Adaptations* in New Zealand is either through the Hospital or Domiciliary Occupational Therapists, all of whom are employed by the local Hospital Boards, in other words by the National Health Service. The Occupational Therapists advise on requirements and supply these from the Hospital Boards' stores.
2. *New Zealand Resource and Disability Centre,* Palmerston North Hospital, Private Bag, Palmerston North. The Centre has an associated aids display centre and is able to provide advice on aids and adaptations.

INDEX

529